SUPERVISION OF LEARNING AND ASSESSMENT IN HEALTHCARE

Sara Miller McCune founded SAGE Publishing in 1965 to support the dissemination of usable knowledge and educate a global community. SAGE publishes more than 1000 journals and over 800 new books each year, spanning a wide range of subject areas. Our growing selection of library products includes archives, data, case studies and video. SAGE remains majority owned by our founder and after her lifetime will become owned by a charitable trust that secures the company's continued independence.

Los Angeles | London | New Delhi | Singapore | Washington DC | Melbourne

5TH EDITION

SUPERVISION OF LEARNING AND ASSESSMENT IN HEALTHCARE

NEIL GOPEE

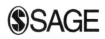

Los Angeles | London | New Delhi
Singapore | Washington DC | Melbourne

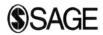

Los Angeles | London | New Delhi
Singapore | Washington DC | Melbourne

SAGE Publications Ltd
1 Oliver's Yard
55 City Road
London EC1Y 1SP

SAGE Publications Inc.
2455 Teller Road
Thousand Oaks, California 91320

SAGE Publications India Pvt Ltd
B 1/I 1 Mohan Cooperative Industrial Area
Mathura Road
New Delhi 110 044

SAGE Publications Asia-Pacific Pte Ltd
3 Church Street
#10-04 Samsung Hub
Singapore 049483

Editor: Laura Walmsley
Editorial assistant: Sahar Jamfar
Production editor: Sarah Sewell
Copyeditor: Sharon Cawood
Proofreader: Bryan Campbell
Marketing manager: Ruslana Khatagova
Cover design: Sheila Tong
Typeset by: C&M Digitals (P) Ltd, Chennai, India
Printed in the UK

Library of Congress Control Number: 2022942516

British Library Cataloguing in Publication data

A catalogue record for this book is available from
the British Library

ISBN 978-1-5297-7593-8
ISBN 978-1-5297-7594-5 (pbk)

At SAGE we take sustainability seriously. Most of our products are printed in the UK using responsibly sourced
papers and boards. When we print overseas we ensure sustainable papers are used as measured by the PREPS
grading system. We undertake an annual audit to monitor our sustainability.

CONTENTS

LIST OF BOXES, TEMPLATES, FIGURES AND TABLES

Boxes

Tables

ABOUT THE AUTHOR

I am currently employed as Lecturer at the Faculty of Health and Life Sciences at Coventry University, and have previously also been Associate Lecturer at the Open University for mentorship and Post-Graduate Certificate in Education courses. My role as external examiner at various higher education institutions in my subject areas has further broadened my insights into the two subject areas that I teach and research: first, teaching, learning and assessment in relation to undergraduate and postgraduate students; and second, leadership and management in healthcare settings.

I first qualified as a nurse a few decades ago and worked in general surgical nursing before moving on to complete the registered mental health nurse course. Through my nursing career, a combination of clinical experience in primary care and general intensive care nursing has also been complemented by attendance at numerous professional development short and long courses, including various workshops on writing for publication, and also completing my doctorate in continuing professional education at the University of Warwick.

My first peer-reviewed article was related to the evaluation of a novel mode of delivery of the Enrolled Nurse Conversion Course, based on my then nurse tutor role. By the turn of the millennium, as nurse education programmes became more established in UK universities, this opened up further authoring opportunities, and I negotiated with Alison Poyner, Commissioning Editor at SAGE Publications, to write the *Mentoring and Supervision in Healthcare* book, the first edition of which was published in 2007; this is the fifth edition, with the title and content adjusted. Along the way, I also worked with SAGE to write the *Leadership and Management in Healthcare* book (up to its third edition), and *Practice Teaching in Healthcare* and *Leading and Managing Healthcare* textbooks (published in 2022). I have also written chapters in edited books and had a range of peer-reviewed articles published.

ACKNOWLEDGEMENTS

I would like to acknowledge the constructive guidance provided by the editors at SAGE Publications, especially Alex Clabburn.

I would like to acknowledge and say thank you to:

- Natasha Taylor, Curriculum Lead/Associate Professor (Simulation), Coventry University, for writing Chapter 4 – Application of Simulation to Healthcare Students' Learning; and for components related to paramedic practice in other chapters.
- Dalvir Kandola, Lecturer in Midwifery, University of Leicester, for providing insights into the supervision of midwifery students' learning and assessment in **practice settings**, and for contributing to the midwifery components in Chapter 6.
- David Hopkins, Senior Lecturer for Operating Department Practitioners (ODP) programmes, Coventry University, for a case study related to an underachieving ODP student, presented in Chapter 8.

LIST OF ABBREVIATIONS

AHP	Allied health professions
BACP	British Association for Counselling and Psychotherapy
CAIPE	Centre for Advancement of Inter-Professional Education
CCG	Clinical commissioning group
CHEF	Care Home Education Facilitator
CINAHL	Cumulative Index to Nursing and Allied Health Literature
CIPD	Chartered Institute of Personnel and Development
CLE	Clinical Learning Environment
CLEI	Clinical Learning Environment Inventory
CLES+T	Clinical Learning Environment, Supervision and Nurse Teacher
CLiP	Collaborative Learning in Practice
CNO	Chief Nursing Officer
CPD	Continuing professional development
CQC	Care Quality Commission
CSP	Chartered Society of Physiotherapy
DHSC	Department of Health and Social Care
EBHC	Evidence-based healthcare
EBM	Evidence-based medicine
EBP	Evidence-based practice
GMC	General Medical Council
GP	General Practitioner
GROW	Goal, Reality, Options, Will/Wrap up (model)
HCPC	Health and Care Professions Council
HEE	Health Education England
HEI	Higher education institute
IATE	Institute for Apprenticeships & Technical Education
IPE	Inter-professional education
IPL	Inter-professional learning
MORA	Midwifery Ongoing Record of Achievement

NCIHE	National Committee of Inquiry into Higher Education
NEWS	National Early Warning Score
NHS KSF	NHS Knowledge and Skills Framework
NICE	National Institute for Health and Care Excellence
NMC	Nursing and Midwifery Council
NQB	National Quality Board (NHS)
NVQ	National Vocational Qualification
ODP	Operating department practitioner
OSCE	Objective Structured/Simulated Clinical Examination (at times referred to as OSCA, with the substituted letter A signifying Assessment)
PAD	Practice Assessment Document
PARE	Practice Assessment Record and Evaluation
PCA	Patient-controlled analgesia
PDP	Personal development plan
PEF	Practice education facilitator
QAA	Quality Assurance Agency for Higher Education
RAPSIES	Recognition, Analysis, Preparation, Strategies, Implementation, Evaluation, Sustaining (framework)
RCN	Royal College of Nursing
RCT	Randomised controlled trial
RM	Registered midwife
RN	Registered nurse
SBE	Simulation-based education
SCPHN	Specialist community public health nurse
SDL	Self-directed learning
SMART	Specific, measurable, achievable, realistic and time-limited
SOLER	Sit squarely, open posture, lean towards the other, eye contact, relax
SOP	Standards of proficiency
SSSA	Standards for Student Supervision and Assessment
STEP	Social, technological, economic and political
SURETY	Sit at an angle, uncross legs and arms, relax, eye contact, touch, your intuition
SWOT	Strengths, weaknesses, opportunities and threats
VARK	Visual, aural, read–write and kinaesthetic
WBL	Work-based learning

INTRODUCTION

The Rationale and Scope of this Book

The aim of this book is to provide well-founded knowledge of the principles of teaching, learning and assessment that healthcare professionals as **practice learning** supervisors and assessors in practice settings can apply to their day-to-day duties towards learners and healthcare profession students based on proven principles and research. Only a handful of university-based preparation courses on how to teach and assess health profession students and other learners replaced the previous, widely available mentoring (and similar previous teaching, learning and assessment) short course in nursing and midwifery. However, parallel well-designed guidance is available and mandatory in some instances for health and social care professionals involved in teaching and assessing students (e.g. practice educators for allied health profession students), at **pre-registration** level and post-qualifying.

Supervision of practice-based learning and practice assessment are significant dimensions of the professional duties of nurses, midwives and allied healthcare professionals, in particular in relation to supporting the educational preparation of pre-registration students. The practice learning supervisor role is also known by other titles, such as clinical educator, practice educator and clinical instructor in different healthcare professions, and in non-UK countries, and appropriate educational preparation for such roles is required in nursing and midwifery (be they university based or healthcare trust based) so as to enable supervisors of learning to perform these roles competently (see Glossary at the back of this book for a brief explanation of different roles).

Different versions of these roles have evolved over the years and various research findings on facilitation of practice learning and student assessment have been published. The roles, responsibilities and educational preparation of supervisors of practice-based learning and assessors of practice competencies for nursing and midwifery students are delineated in *Standards for Student Supervision and Assessment* (SSSA) (Nursing and Midwifery Council [NMC], 2018a). The mentor role has thereby been replaced by '**practice supervisor**' and '**practice assessor**' roles, and also the new '**academic assessor**' role, with the requirement for all to work in collaboration.

Although the standards for practice supervisors and assessors in the NMC's SSSA publication are mainly for nursing and midwifery students, they were based on general principles of **facilitation of learning** and student assessment in healthcare settings so that they are mostly also applicable to the other health and care professions, such as allied health professions (AHP), social work and medicine. In the current scene of inter-professional learning, reciprocal supervision of learning and student assessment between health professions has been happening quite effectively for at least a decade, where permitted.

This book explores in detail the necessary standards, competence areas and outcomes for effective supervision of practice-based learning and assessment. To do so, the book draws on the wider contemporary and previous knowledge of the dynamics of practice learning supervision and similar roles across different professions, as well as research and current policies, and aims to support **registrants** to acquire the knowledge and skills that are necessary to fulfil the necessary standards for practice learning supervision and assessment. It thus brings together and builds on the existing knowledge of principles and practices of enabling and supporting learning and student assessment in various current health and care arenas. Thereby, it also constitutes a firm backdrop for healthcare professionals to further develop and enhance their expertise in teaching and assessment.

All health and social care registrants should be able to fulfil the role of practice supervisor for nursing and midwifery students, as indicated by the NMC, as long as it is within their areas of competence, and they have had appropriate educational preparation. Both recently qualified registrants and those who are more experienced, as well as previously qualified mentors, should find this book useful, as should those who were prepared for these roles through the older 'teaching and assessing' courses.

This book is a direct result of my numerous years of experience of teaching and examining on mentoring and 'teaching, learning and assessing' courses, as well as my experience as a registered nurse in adult nursing and mental health nursing, along with the need for a textbook that reflects current policies and research findings on practice learning supervision comprehensively. In addition to current knowledge in the field, this textbook also recognises the challenges encountered by both newly qualified and more experienced practice learning supervisors, often doing so within resource constraints, role changes and changing healthcare workforce profiles. It examines the day-to-day and longer-term issues and challenges in the supervision of practice learning, and explores potential solutions, where possible supporting them with relevant theories, frameworks and contemporary research findings. The ensuing implications with regard to responsibility and accountability are also necessarily explored.

The Structure of this Book

As just indicated, this book is firmly based on current knowledge in the field and is structured to ensure that it also addresses all NMC's (2018a, 2018d) standards and frameworks for student supervision and assessment. These standards, which can be easily applied to other healthcare professions as well, are based on the recognition that all registrants' roles include teaching and supporting learning, along with being role models of the highest standards of care for health and care service users.

Standards for practice-based teaching and learning have been available for almost two decades, and they have been revised a few times, leading up to the current NMC's (2018a) SSSA directive, and those in the Health and Care Professions Council's (HCPC) (2017) *Standards of Education and Training*. This textbook draws on the wider principles and practice of effective supervision of practice learning and student assessment in health and social care, and also addresses the NMC's (2018a, 2018d) and HCPC's (2017) standards for doing so, examining and analysing these functions, and supporting them with relevant research related to these roles.

Chapter 1 begins by examining practice learning supervision as an entity in its own right. It starts by unravelling the exact nature of the duties of practice learning supervisors, and of the term supervision, and differentiates them from other similar or overlapping roles, such as clinical instructors, practice educators, practice education facilitators (PEF) and preceptors. The common aim of all these roles is to facilitate healthcare profession students and learners' acquisition of **clinical intervention** skills, knowledge and appropriate values as they develop into proficient healthcare professionals.

A range of rationales for these roles is then identified, which is followed by the various factors that enable practice learning supervisors to fulfil their role effectively, including ways in which they build effective working relationships with their learners. Subsequently, the necessary personal and professional attributes of effective practice supervisors are explored. The nature and likely detrimental effects of poor or adverse forms of supervision are also discussed, followed by an examination of different models and approaches to practice learning supervision.

Then, Chapter 2 takes a detailed look at how learning occurs. It examines why and what learners learn, significant different perspectives on learning, teaching and education, and learning theories, styles and approaches to learning, including use of learning contracts and learning agreements.

Chapter 3 builds on how learners learn and explores the principles of teaching and facilitation of learning. The chapter starts by ascertaining the range of people whom healthcare professionals teach, followed by the reasons for teaching and learning. It then focuses on various ways in which practice learning supervisors enable healthcare students to learn healthcare delivery skills, utilising both formal and informal teaching and learning opportunities.

An analysis of facilitation of learning, as distinct from teaching, is presented, which is followed by key perceptions and research-informed major views and approaches in teaching. The levels and stages of skill acquisition (taxonomy levels) are explored, and the types of knowledge associated with skills are considered, along with levels of knowledge acquisition. Steps in lesson planning for structured short teaching sessions for teaching skills and knowledge are then ascertained, followed by an examination of different teaching methods and the use of different teaching aids, including those for students with disabilities.

Entitled 'Application of Simulation to Healthcare Students' Learning', the content of Chapter 4 complements those in preceding chapters on how learners learn and on facilitation of learning. To do so, the chapter examines the fundamental reasons for simulation-based learning, the different types of simulation, and the increasing range of mechanisms or tools for simulation-based education (SBE) that are available to health profession educators to choose from. Ways of ensuring effective application of SBE, governance of teaching by simulation, and supporting students through SBE, are also addressed.

Then, Chapter 5 focuses on the attributes that are important to make healthcare settings effective learning environments, and on ways in which practice supervisors can maintain and enhance the learning culture in practice settings. Research related to **clinical learning environments**, which underpins the development of the tool for regular **educational audits** of practice placement areas, is then discussed. The audits aim to ascertain the psychosocial factors and learning resources (human and material) for facilitation of the acquisition of practice competencies by healthcare profession students.

Students' perspectives on practice placements such as their expectations and their practice objectives are considered, and then an examination of the part played by national guidelines and local policies on practice placements follows. Issues related to practice placements are also examined. The utilisation of **learning pathways** (based on patients' journeys through healthcare systems), which can be incorporated into learning contracts and can play an important role in ensuring the success of practice placements, is also explored to a good extent.

Underpinning effective practice-based learning supervision is the practice supervisor's leadership, which is the focus of Chapter 6. A practice supervisor's leadership essentially constitutes being a role model of the highest standards of evidence-based, person-centred practice, as well as in proactive tentative planning of students' learning during practice placements and assessment of their practice competencies. Changing practice based on new evidence is integral to practice supervisors' leadership, which is explored in some detail in this chapter, and includes instances of leadership in the supervision of midwifery and AHP students' practice-based learning.

One of the principal purposes of practice assessors' education programmes is to equip assessors with the ability to assess students' clinical competence based on well-informed principles of assessment. Chapter 7 therefore focuses on the assessment of healthcare students' competence as the fundamental component of all educational programmes for skill-based healthcare professions, and includes practice supervisors' contributory role in the continuous assessment of students.

To explore the principles and processes of assessment, the chapter focuses on what assessments are, the various purposes of assessment of competence, who assesses and when, and differing ways in which they are conducted – and also provides a good understanding of the student's pre-registration programme and how to utilise the different methods of student assessment in care settings.

Under how to assess, in addition to different methods of assessment, the chapter explores key principles, such as levels of assessment and fairness of assessments, as well as student self-assessment and peer assessment. Validity and reliability as crucial attributes of assessments are then explored in some detail, the aim being to ascertain the student's fitness to practise.

Then, Chapter 8 addresses the management of assessments, which includes the planning of episodes of assessment, along with techniques for giving effective feedback to learners and the documentation of assessments. Pass or fail criteria are examined, followed by the academic assessor's role in ascertaining the achievement of proficiencies during the student's pre-registration programme and then at the point of registration.

Research findings over the years have highlighted various day-to-day problems encountered by both assessors and students in relation to assessment of competence during practice placements. Therefore, practice supervisors and assessors' leadership includes proactively and carefully planning students' assessment of competence, and also averting possible problems that could occur during student assessment. The assessor's responsibility and accountability come into play together with the use of 'professional judgement'. The use of action plans, and the reassessment of the student, are necessary components, and how intra- and inter-assessor reliability are achieved and monitored are also explored.

Chapter 9 concentrates on the evaluation of facilitation of learning by practice supervisors, and of student assessment. The nature and purpose of evaluation amount to practice supervisors self-monitoring the quality of their work with students. The chapter therefore considers what evaluation is, who is involved in the evaluation of learning facilitation and assessment, and how it is performed, including the use of models of evaluation. Consideration of the results of evaluations might trigger the need for further learning for learning supervisors, and consequently this chapter also examines continuing learning for practice supervisors and assessors, incorporating details of regular updates for practice supervisors and assessors, along with revalidation requirements and lifelong learning.

Each chapter in this book begins with an introduction to key concepts in the chapter and the chapter objectives, which is followed by the main text, a chapter summary and suggestions for further reading. A logical combination of text, illustrations, activities, reflection points and case studies is incorporated to engage the reader fully with the material in the book.

How to Use this Book

To examine the knowledge base, skills and attitudes required for effective practice learning supervision and assessment, and the achievement of care professions' standards for supervision and assessment, this textbook adopts an analytical and interactive style throughout, with a clear focus on the means of application of principles and theories of supervision of learning in various practice settings, and the assessment of students' practice competencies. Therefore, through action points and reflection points, the reader is encouraged to explore and apply concepts to their own practice and to their teaching and student assessment roles.

The action points usually ask the reader to consider a particular point or component and make some notes, while reflection points ask the reader to reflect on their own experience and knowledge prior to moving on to the subsequent concepts in the text. They thus allow practice supervisors and assessors to exercise the freedom and scope to be creative in enabling students' learning and assessment of their competence.

A number of case studies have been incorporated in the text as examples of situations that practice supervisors and assessors might encounter, so that the reader can explore ways in which they can manage the situation satisfactorily. Furthermore, the information in some of the boxes, for example a box in Chapter 1 titled 'Characteristics of Effective Practice Learning Supervisors', is derived from a number of workshops on the previous mentor preparation courses and current teaching and assessing modules. As events evolve, and because different practice settings have their own specific requirements and strengths, feel free to make further notes of your own on other components in addition to those in the boxes.

To summarise:

Chapter objectives

These identify briefly the key theories, concepts and principles covered in the chapter.

Action points

These ask you to consider a particular point and make some notes. They are obviously optional for the reader, but they endeavour to enable you to apply or explore the theories or concepts inherent within student supervision and assessment in your own practice setting.

Reflection points

These ask you to reflect on your own personal experience and potential actions, but can also be discussed with a peer or in a small group.

Text boxes

These highlight multiple aspects of a key theme.

Templates

These are examples of tools that you can use with your own students in your role as a practice learning supervisor or practice assessor.

Case studies

These are examples of situations that you may encounter when you become a practice supervisor or practice assessor, as they are based on previous actual supervision of learning and student assessment situations.

Chapter summaries

These remind you of the key points addressed in the chapter that you have just read and worked through.

Further optional reading

This is carefully selected learning material that will enable you to expand your knowledge further with regard to some of the main themes in the chapter.

Terminology

The term healthcare professional is used in this textbook to signify all health or social care employees, that is medical and non-medical, including nurses and all allied health professionals who hold a qualification that is recognised by either their national **regulatory body** (that is, the NMC, HCPC, etc.) or professional body. The term healthcare incorporates social care where appropriate.

The term learner is used to refer to everyone who wants or needs to learn healthcare skills, while students are those learners who are actually following professional education programmes leading to university qualifications. The terms practice competencies and practice objectives are also used interchangeably.

The term practice learning supervisor is used interchangeably with the NMC's practice supervisor role; and the terms 'learning supervision' and 'student supervision' are also applied interchangeably. Finally, the terms healthcare service user, care service user and service user, client and patient are all used in this book to incorporate anyone who avails themselves of health or social care provision in the UK.

The term 'registrants' refers to registered nurses (RN), registered midwives (RM) and all other healthcare professionals whose names appear on the NMC, the HCPC and other healthcare regulatory bodies' professional registers.

The Glossary just before the Index defines a range of other terminologies that are integral components of this book.

NMC and HCPC Guidance

The UK reader is strongly advised to have a good look through the NMC's (2018a) directive document *Standards for Student Supervision and Assessment* and the NMC's (2018d) *Standards Framework for Nursing and Midwifery Education,* or the HCPC's (2017) *Standards of Education and Training,* which essentially provide sound guidance on effective practice learning and student assessment.

1

EFFECTIVE SUPERVISION OF PRACTICE LEARNING

Introduction

As in many professions, nursing, midwifery and other health and care students on pre-registration (also referred to as pre-licensure, or pre-qualifying) courses acquire their clinical intervention skills predominantly in the clinical setting, where their learning is facilitated under the supervision of appropriately qualified registrants. Practice learning supervision is of course not a new activity, and the title 'practice supervisor' replaced the title mentor in nursing and midwifery practice education relatively recently (NMC, 2018a). Other health professions retained their alternative titles for practice-based learning supervision, for example 'practice educator' and 'clinical instructor', and even workplace supervisor.

The term supervision itself, in the context of learning, however, is not well researched and, therefore, the intelligence in this chapter is based partly on the research that is currently available, and on policy literature on supervisory activities in various professions. It is also partly based on similar previous and current roles, such as mentoring and practice education, as well as on the author's and colleagues' professional experience in nursing and healthcare.

The Health and Care Professions Council (HCPC) (e.g. 2021), the General Medical Council (GMC) (e.g. HEE, 2022a) and other healthcare regulators also specify particular requirements for supervising students' acquisition of clinical intervention skills and knowledge in healthcare settings. These are specifically explored in relevant sections of this book.

This first chapter on the supervision of students' learning in care settings starts by clarifying the meaning of the terms supervision and practice supervision, and differentiates them from similar and overlapping roles and titles. It then explores the various reasons for practice supervision for enabling practice-based learning, and the range of healthcare professionals who can perform the duties of practice learning supervisors.

Ways of performing the role effectively are then examined, followed by discussion on some potential problematic aspects of these roles, and the steps that can be taken to avert or resolve them. Thereafter, the chapter explores structured models and frameworks for effective practice education for health and care students, and culminates in proposing an informed framework for effective practice learning supervision.

Chapter objectives

1. Distinguish between practice supervision and similar roles that support learning for health and care students and learners.
2. Explain a range of reasons for requiring practice supervisor-type roles, in addition to facilitating students' acquisition of their profession's competencies.
3. Identify and evaluate a range of factors that can enable effective supervision of learning, including the personal attributes and responsibilities of effective supervisors, and establishing supervisory relationships with students.
4. Analyse the likelihood and effects of poor or faulty supervision and the actions that can be taken where it is likely to occur.
5. Analyse a number of approaches, frameworks and models of informed and systematic supervision of practice learning, that enable students' acquisition of clinical skills for safe, effective and sensitive practice.

Practice Supervision for Practice-Based Learning

For nursing and midwifery students' practice-based learning in healthcare settings, the publication *Standards for Student Supervision and Assessment* by the Nursing and Midwifery Council (NMC, 2018a) sets out details around how practice supervisors and practice assessors can perform their duties in the course of their daily activities, and do so effectively. The mentor role had been firmly established for facilitating learning in clinical workplaces during practice placement since the 1980s, and successful mentoring mechanisms gradually pervaded numerous other areas of learning (e.g. research mentoring, mentoring in medicine, youth rehabilitation mentoring, business mentoring). Coaching is another popular line of activity for facilitating skill-based learning.

For practice supervision, the NMC (2018a: 6) indicates firmly that it 'enables students to learn and safely achieve proficiency and autonomy in their professional role'. It indicates that all nurses and midwives are capable of supervising students, and recognises that student learning is also supervised by other health and social care registrants. The NMC consequently explains its 'expectations' of practice supervision, along with:

- practice supervisors' roles and responsibilities
- practice supervisors' contribution to student assessment and progression
- preparation of practice supervisors and subsequent ongoing support
- the organisation of practice learning.

As can be expected, the HCPC (2021) acknowledges practice learning supervision for allied health profession (AHP) students, and for AHPs continuing professional development (CPD), as well as for those returning to practice after a career break. The practice supervisor role, as well as impactful supervision activities, are examined in substantial detail in the course of this chapter.

The practice assessor role, which is separate from the practice supervisor's, is examined in full detail, particularly in Chapters 7 and 8. The aim of separating practice-based learning and summative assessment (see the Glossary at the back of this book for a brief explanation of key terms) roles in this way is partly to make the student assessment of competence more objective, fair and consistent (see Chapter 7 for an explanation of these terms), particularly in the light of several years of research that have identified possible problems with student assessment (e.g. Gainsbury, 2010; Christiansen et al., 2021). Furthermore, Professor of Nursing Macleod-Clark, who recommended this change, indicates that separating the opposite roles of support and supervision from assessment will mean that all registrants can be practice supervisors (Agnew, 2018: 14) and thereby 'vastly expand the pool of nurses involved in the training of students'.

On the other hand, dividing the role can add a further level of bureaucracy, according to Morley et al. (2017: 170), although research has repeatedly found that student supervision and student assessment are conflicting roles if both are undertaken by the same individual (e.g. Tweed et al., 2010; Hutchison and Cochrane, 2014).

Distinguishing Between Practice Supervisor and Similar Roles

The practice supervisor role is just one of several that support learning in practice settings and therefore there is some overlap in certain aspects of the supervision of learning roles in practice settings, such as in the personal qualities of registrants who willingly support learning, but there are distinct boundaries as well.

━━━━━━━━━━━ ACTION **POINT** 1.1 ━━━━━━━━━━━

Different education support roles and functions

To begin with, think of all post-holders in health and care settings who have a teaching role toward students of different care professions, and note them down. What are the differences between their roles?

You are likely to have identified a variety of post-holders who enable or support learning for students and other learners in practice settings, which might have also included practice facilitator, field instructor, buddy, clinical educator, peer learning, and so on. Although there are some common elements in the definitions, scope and remit of practice supervisor and similar roles, there are also differences. The most popular learning support roles are explained briefly next.

Practice supervisor

As a role that replaced the mentor role in nursing and midwifery in 2018, the practice supervisor role in supporting learning and continuous practice assessment of students is examined in detail later in this chapter.

Generally, the defining attributes of practice supervisors (also referred to as practice learning supervisors in this book) include being a role model, being a facilitator of learning, having good communication skills, being knowledgeable about the field of practice and aware of the principles of adult education, and so forth. Additionally, in various countries, the term clinical instructor is the equivalent of the practice supervisor role; and also in some UK professions, for instance in clinical psychology, where, the term 'protégé' is used when referring to the student receiving learning supervision (e.g. Barnett, 2008).

Practice assessor

The practice assessor is a relatively novel role for appropriately qualified, competent and experienced registrants, whose remit includes the assessment of students' achievement of practice competencies during practice placements, and thereby the NMC's (2018c) standards for pre-registration education, and uses student information provided by practice supervisors and others. Practice assessors also liaise directly with academic assessors to determine each student's fitness to progress from one part of their education programme to the next (e.g. year 1 to year 2), and eventually register with the NMC. Practice assessors for nursing students are not required to be from the same field of practice as the student they are assessing if they have suitable equivalent experience.

Academic assessor

This is another relatively novel role, usually a university-based lecturer with detailed knowledge of the proficiencies that students have to achieve during practice placements and whose progress they are nominated to oversee. The academic assessor works closely with practice assessors to determine each student's achievement of SOP identified for their year of study and, in the final year, their fitness to register with the NMC. Academic assessors must have appropriate preparation for the role, and more analysis of their duties is presented in Chapters 7 and 8 of this book.

Assessor

The term 'assessor' is often used as a generic title given to individuals who are appropriately qualified and experienced health or social care professionals whose educational preparation entailed developing skills in assessing students' level of attainment related to the stated practice competencies or outcomes (e.g. National Vocational Qualifications [NVQ] assessor).

Preceptor

A preceptor is 'a registered practitioner who has been given formal responsibility to support a newly registered practitioner through **preceptorship**', according to the Department of Health (2010: 6), and in the UK, the 'preceptor' is a first-level registrant who has had at least 12 months' experience within the same area of practice as the practitioner requiring support. Preceptorship comprises a period of structured transition for the newly registered practitioner during which they are supported by a preceptor, to develop their confidence as an autonomous professional, and to further develop their clinical intervention skills, values and behaviours (DH, 2010: 11).

The preceptor role emerged from the realisation that, for newly qualified nurses, the transition from being a student to being employed as a registered healthcare professional is a major leap in responsibility and accountability, which can also cause substantial stress, disillusionment and dropping out of the profession (e.g. Kramer, 1974; NHS Education for Scotland, 2017). However, although the preceptor role has been advocated for decades, and implemented successfully by several **healthcare organisations**, it remains problematic in some areas, particularly due to a shortage of registrants to staff those areas. Nonetheless, Moore (2018), the Department of Health (2010) and others describe well-received preceptorship frameworks for supporting newly qualified nurses, which includes a minimum of two weeks' **supernumerary status**, and protected time for both preceptor and preceptee.

Practice educator

While being largely similar to the practice supervisor role, the practice educator role refers to guiding and supporting allied health profession (AHP) students during their practice placement. The British Association of Social Workers (BASW) (2019: 3) defines a practice educator as a person who 'takes overall responsibility for the student's learning and assessment, utilising information from a range of evidence sources', which suggests that the practice educator role in social work is largely similar to the previous mentor role in nursing and midwifery.

The HCPC identifies the 'practice educator' as 'a person who is responsible for a learner's education during their practice-based learning and has received appropriate training for this role' (HCPC, 2017: 52). To fulfil the role of practice educator, the HCPC (2017: 44) requires that practice educators 'are trained and that this is followed up with regular refresher training and support'. The HCPC adds that if 'practice educators are involved in assessing learners, they should be prepared to do so through training in a way that is consistent across all practice-based learning on the programme'.

Fundamentally, the practice educator is required (1) to perform patient care duties safely and effectively, that is, in accordance with the procedures and clinical guidelines approved by the healthcare employer; (2) to facilitate learning for specific AHP students; and (3) maybe to assess students' competence, unless a designated assessor does this. Additionally, in radiography and other AHPs, practice educators can opt to undertake a short programme to become 'accredited' practice educators. However, there is some inconsistency in the title and the role internationally, with practice educator, mentor and preceptor titles being used interchangeably at the moment.

Practice education facilitator

The practice education facilitator (PEF) role in nursing and midwifery emerged largely from research by Phillips et al. (2000) that identified several problems with the then mentoring role. The purpose of the PEF role is to ensure that student experience during practice placements is successful by ensuring provision of support and guidance to practice learning supervisors and others who contribute to the student's learning in practice settings. A similar title and role applies to PEFs who are based in non-NHS nursing homes, which is known as care home education facilitator (CHEF) (NHS Education for Scotland, 2021).

This is a very important role as PEFs are also called upon to advise practice learning supervisors when students are struggling or failing to make progress in the achievement of their practice placement competencies. For students on practice placements, PEFs also organise dedicated group discussion sessions away from the practice setting for particular categories of students, for reflection and peer support purposes.

Research by Carlisle et al. (2009: 715) on the impact of the PEF role revealed that the PEF role is 'accepted widely across Scotland and is seen as valuable to the development of quality clinical learning environments, providing support and guidance for practice-based learning supervisors when dealing with "failing" students, and encouraging the identification of innovative learning opportunities'. Later, a study by Mathisen et al. (2022) found that PEFs have a key role in strengthening the clinical learning environment, particularly by their visibility and accessibility in the clinical area and their clinical credibility.

However, when Scott et al. (2017) examined the PEF role in healthcare trusts in London and the surrounding area, they concluded that there is a lack of consistency in the job definition of the role across healthcare trusts, and that PEFs feel undervalued and vulnerable to budget cuts. Nonetheless, in the context of the **Collaborative Learning in Practice** (CLiP) (e.g. RCN, 2022a) coaching model of learning supervision, PEFs are seen as key players in supporting placement learning, along with the 'clinical educator' who is appointed specifically for overseeing this mode of facilitation of learning.

Clinical instructor and clinical educator

These are general titles utilised in different countries to signify registrants with a substantial teaching role in clinical settings.

Lecturer-practitioner

Lecturer-practitioners are normally advanced or specialist practitioners who are contractually employed partly by the **healthcare provider**, and partly by the partner higher education institute (HEI). A study conducted to explore the likely differences in the roles of mentors, lecturer-practitioners and link lecturers, indicates that the then mentors tended to focus principally on individual students, lecturer-practitioners on the 'learning environment', and link lecturers on knowledge acquisition by students and the fulfilment of course requirements (Carnwell et al., 2007)

Personal tutor

Each pre-registration student is allocated to a nurse lecturer who acts as a personal tutor to the student, mostly for pastoral care-type duties. This role normally lasts for the duration of the three-year pre-registration course, and is also known by other terms such as 'academic adviser'.

Clinical supervisor

The terms clinical supervisor and educational supervisor signify practice-based teaching roles in medical education, for example, which entails doctors facilitating learning for medical students' learning during practice placement; and both clinical and educational supervisors are appropriately trained, prepared and supported in their educational roles, according to HEE (2019, 2022b) and the NMC (2018a). However, the term clinical supervisor also applies in the context of clinical supervision, which signifies the provision of peer support to clinical supervisee colleagues, which is provided in a structured way by applying a systematic approach to this activity, such as Waskett's (2010) 4S model of clinical supervision, comprising of structure, skills, support and sustainability; or Proctor's (2011) model of clinical supervision (explored shortly in this chapter).

Mentor

The mentor role prevailed for around two decades in nursing and midwifery until it was replaced recently by the practice supervisor, practice assessor and academic assessor roles (NMC, 2018a). The role was built on existing knowledge of the subject area, such as research on teacher training by Kerry and Mayes (1995), who indicated that effective mentorship includes:

- nurturing
- role modelling
- functioning (as teacher, sponsor, encourager, counsellor and friend)
- focusing on the professional development of the student
- sustaining a caring relationship over time.

Coach

Some of the learning supervision roles are still developing, including practice facilitator, buddy, coach and clinical educator. The more developed terms 'coach' and 'coaching' tend to surface repeatedly in nursing and other professions, and involve instructing and supporting the coachee to perform a skilled task, step by step. The Chartered Institute of Personnel and Development (CIPD) (2021a) indicates that coaching techniques are based on the use of one-to-one conversations to enhance an individual's skills, knowledge or work performance, and:

> Coaching aims to produce optimal performance and improvement at work. It focuses on specific skills and goals, although it may also have an impact on an individual's personal attributes such as social interaction or confidence. The process typically lasts for a defined period of time. (2021a: 1)

'Performance', 'specific skills' and 'goals' are key common words used in determining a common understanding of the term coaching, which in turn usually incorporates a more directive and prescriptive approach. This term, title and performance enhancement function of the coach, however, is more closely linked to sports, which involves training coachees using individually tailored programmes aimed at enhancing their physical performance, usually so that they are able to take part in competitions in specific sports.

Other prominent areas include life coaching (enabling the coachee to live a healthier and more fulfilled life); health coaching (enabling individuals with long-term conditions such as diabetes or Parkinson's disease to self-care); and business coaching (guiding someone who is starting their own business for the first time and helping them to succeed). These arguments see coaching very much from a management speak that includes productivity and efficiency, rather than the safety, effectiveness and compassion that are widely advocated in healthcare. As noted earlier in this chapter, coaching also features in the CLiP method of facilitating learning during practice placements, and is discussed later in this chapter and in Chapter 6.

In reporting on the findings of an audit of a new role termed 'clinical coach', whereby an appointed academic coaches underachieving (also referred to as 'marginal' or 'at risk') student nurses during practice placements, Kelton (2014) indicates that a systematic approach to clinical coaching can significantly enhance students' successful completion of the placement. Clinical coaching entails the appointed clinical coach, that is a new resource, providing additional support and guidance to the identified student. Another application of coaching in healthcare is management coaching, as discussed under 'Supervising students to learn management skills', later in this chapter.

Other, similar roles include **academic link lecturer** and practice teacher. Academic link lecturer refers to named lecturers, as a contact point between each practice setting, that have students on practice placements and the partner HEI. They are involved mostly when there is a student-related problem during placement that requires urgent action. Many of the previous functions of personal tutors and link lecturers have increasingly become part of the PEF's remit.

As for the practice teacher role, this was initially specifically adopted in recognition of the additional educational preparation required for the supervision of learning for students on specialist community public health nurse (SCPHN) courses. It used to refer to a registrant who had gained knowledge, skills and competencies as well as qualifications in both their specialist area of practice and in their teaching role, and utilised for the assessment of students on specialist or advanced practice courses. Practice teachers supervise learning and assess students who are on courses in the same specialism as the practice teacher (in health visiting, school nursing, occupational health nursing, etc.), but the title has only been sporadically used since 2019.

In summarising this section on practice learning supervisor and similar roles, it is clear that there are areas within these roles that overlap, and there are distinctions between them when prevailing national policy and professional bodies' definitions are considered. However, as these roles evolve, and different models of implementation are applied in different settings, endeavouring to disentangle the educational philosophy underlying these roles – such as differentiating between coaching and mentoring – is seen by Megginson et al. (2006: 5) as a 'sterile debate'. Nonetheless, for several of these roles, formal educational preparation is a requirement and national standards have to be achieved (e.g. BASW, 2019).

Unravelling Supervision and Supervisors of Learning

The meaning of the terms supervisor and supervision varies according to the context in which each applies. The dictionary (Brookes and O'Neill, 2017: 808) indicates that to supervise means: (1) to direct or oversee the performance, action or work of another; and (2) to watch over (people) to ensure appropriate behaviour.

In general, the term 'supervisor' thus tends to be used in the context of the management of workers to ensure designated tasks are completed to the specified standard, and on time. It also refers to individuals in management positions in organisations who have the authority by the employer to recruit staff for specified posts, assign duties, oversee the quality of their work, provide relevant training or professional development, and take disciplinary action when appropriate.

So, what is supervision in the context of pre-registration students' learning? With regards to the relatively recently implemented 'nursing associate' role, HEE (2017: 10) indicates that a supervisor is a 'suitably prepared professional trained to support students in practice', which is somewhat similar to the NMC's (2018a) practice supervisor role, but, in the context of nursing associate training, the supervisor can also be an appropriate manager.

Being 'suitably prepared' implies educational preparation for teaching and assessing duties, which, in addition to being a NMC (2018a) and HCPC (2017) requirement, is also because although a number of universities include a module on how to teach in their pre-registration programmes, which enables students to gain insights into how to teach other students (e.g. in the CLiP model of coaching discussed elsewhere in this chapter), service users and carers, they do not adequately educate them on how to assess students on their practice learning outcomes.

Supervision, on the other hand, is defined by Kilminster et al. (2007: 2) as: 'The provision of guidance and feedback on matters of personal, professional and educational development in the context of a trainee's experience of providing safe and appropriate patient care.' Moreover, Johnson (2017) suggests that supervision is relationship-based facilitation of learning, that also heeds ethical and legal parameters. All explanations of supervision, explicitly or by implication, indicate that its focus is on learning professional intervention skills that are person-centred, and that it is founded on the development of a trusting relationship that should be initiated by the supervisor, although, in healthcare, students are explicitly advised to proactively initiate interaction with their supervisor-to-be.

Alternatively, in the context of the application of supervision to health and social care professions, Hawkins and McMahon (2020: 3) refer to supervision as 'a joint endeavour in which a practitioner, with the help of a supervisor, attends to their clients, ... transforms their client relationships, [and] continuously develop[s] themselves, their practice and the wider profession'. The term supervision has thus long been widely applied to client-practitioner relationship-based professions such as social work supervision.

The term also has very specific meaning in the field of counselling, whereupon one or more highly experienced counsellors help less experienced or trainee counsellors to develop their practice in counselling interventions. The British Association for Counselling and Psychotherapy (BACP) (2018: 22) indicates that 'supervision provides practitioners with regular and ongoing opportunities to reflect in depth about all aspects of their practice in order to work as effectively, safely and ethically as possible'.

The BACP (2018) recommends supervision to anyone providing therapy-based services, working in roles that require regularly giving or receiving emotionally challenging communications, or engaging in relationally complex and challenging roles. Accordingly, the BACP (2018: 23) notes that 'supervisors and supervisees will periodically review how responsibility for work with clients is implemented in practice and how any difficulties or concerns are being addressed'. An effective interpersonal relationship is essential in both the above-mentioned aspects of supervision.

In the context of the supervision of practice-based learning, Johnson (2017) asserts that supervision is the formal provision of a relationship-based, work-focused education and training by approved supervisors. Johnson adds that 'supervisors bear clinical, ethical, and legal responsibility for their supervisees' work' (p. 8). Additionally, the term 'educational supervision', or academic supervision, tends to apply specifically to academics supervising students with their course project, research or dissertation.

Many elements of the above explanations of supervise, supervisor and supervision apply to practice supervisors enabling students' practice-based learning in nursing and healthcare pre-registration education. Implicit in the meanings of the word supervision is the implication that the supervisee (e.g. student nurse) is likely to have training needs, and is presumably motivated to learn to perform healthcare interventions to the expected high standard.

On examining the multiple approaches to learner supervision within healthcare professions, Nancarrow et al. (2014) perused several definitions of the term supervision in relation to placement learning, and noted that they all tend to include effective working relationships and an intentional support for learning that enables the sharing and enhancing of knowledge and skills. They note that definitions of supervision also apply to support mechanisms for practising professionals within which they can share clinical, organisational and developmental experiences with others in order to enhance knowledge and skills (p. 240).

An effective 'supervisory relationship' between supervisor and student is the most influential factor in student learning during practice placements and student satisfaction with practice settings as effective learning environments, according to research by Papastavrou et al. (2016), Suliman and Warshawski (2022) and others, who also indicate that the teaching and learning atmosphere is 'pivotal' for learning. Effective supervision is thus dependent on a strong relationship between student and supervisor, and also on the amount and content of feedback given to students, according to research on students' expectations and perceptions by Gratrix and Barrett (2017).

However, research on student social workers' 'field supervision', conducted by Cleak and Smith (2012), conclude that when the field supervisor is based on-site, this results in superior quality student supervision, while off-site, or external, supervision (also known as distant supervision or long-arm mentoring) was found to be the least effective. Nonetheless, Maynard et al.'s (2015) research suggests that off-site supervision can be very effective, by:

- careful planning and preparation for the placement
- selection of an appropriately motivated 'task supervisor' on-site
- communication among all involved
- knowledge of roles and expectations.

A popular framework for effective clinical supervision by Proctor (2011) provides another perspective as a more holistic model of effective learning supervision, as also advocated by Johnson (2017) and HEE (2019). Proctor's model comprises addressing the formative, normative and restorative aspects of supervision. *Formative* refers to the educational aspect of the supervisor–student relationship; *normative* addresses the clinical guidelines and procedures that must be adhered to; and the *restorative* component enables practitioners to develop resilience when they encounter challenging circumstances, by engaging in reflective conversation, for instance. In addition to all three aspects needing to be addressed for effective, appropriate supervision, Proctor indicates that their supportive function underpins the model, which incorporates the attitude, skill and intentions in the relationship (more on this later in this chapter).

The mechanism for effective practice supervision in nursing and midwifery is detailed by the NMC (2018a), which includes components such as:

2.4 practice supervision ensures safe and effective learning experiences that uphold public protection and the safety of people

3.1 serve as role models for safe and effective practice in line with their code of conduct

3.2 support learning in line with their scope of practice to enable the student to meet their proficiencies and programme outcomes

4.2 contribute to student assessments to inform decisions for progression.

These aspects of the practice supervisor role clearly indicate that it is a collaborative one, which is focused on students' learning healthcare intervention competencies that are set jointly between healthcare providers and the partner HEI, based on the NMC's standards for nursing and midwifery education. The NMC also indicates that all NMC-registered nurses and midwives are capable of supervising students, serving as role models for safe and effective practice; and that students may be supervised by other registered health and social care professionals as well, within an ethos of inter-professional learning (IPL), as long as the registrant from the other profession is fully proficient in their area of practice prior to teaching students.

A potential weakness of IPL in practice settings is that different care professionals can be protective of their cognate areas, and therefore might teach students only selective and superficial aspects of interventions. Such 'piecemeal' facilitation of students' learning risks being fractional and incomplete, which is why the supervisor of learning 'requires specific training and competence', according to Falender (2014: 6).

Having analysed the nature of the concept supervision and the practice supervisor role, we now explore which professionals can work as practice supervisors, and then give further reasons for the role, in addition to that of facilitation of students' learning in practice settings.

Who can be a Practice Supervisor?

As noted earlier, from 2019 practice education for nurses and midwives has been facilitated by practice supervisors, a role previously fulfilled by mentors. This change resulted in the availability of more registrants to support students on placement than was happening with the mentor role. There was a need for the wider availability of competent, clinically based supervisors of learning to enable students to learn clinical skills 'in the real world' of nursing so that they are 'fit for practice' (as noted by the National Committee of Inquiry into Higher Education [NCIHE], 1997). Nursing and midwifery students can be supervised in practice by NMC-registered nurses, midwives, nursing associates or other registered health and social care professionals.

However, despite all the reasons for the practice supervisor role discussed so far, it should not be presumed that all qualified healthcare professionals wish to undertake practice supervision work, for all or even some of the time. Some healthcare professionals feel that continual allocation of students to them all year round can be detrimental to their own effectiveness in carrying out their own workload, and they would like some space for reflection and to focus on their own professional development. Furthermore, concerns have been expressed by students and practice learning supervisors across healthcare that the quality and provision of educational and clinical supervision (has been) inconsistent and that this could negatively impact on patient safety, as well as on clinical placement experience that in turn can lead to burnout and retention issues, according to HEE (2019).

In the selection of practice supervisors, it is important to ensure that healthcare professionals have the motivation and the necessary skills and expertise for the facilitation of students' learning in practice settings, which include establishing an effective working relationship, coaching, giving feedback, maintaining standards and carrying out continuous assessment. Other writers and researchers identify similar lists of skills. Such lists initially appear simplistic but a whole range of micro-skills are required to undertake practice supervisor duties, and this can usually be developed through the appropriate educational preparation followed by experience.

The NMC (2018a) indicates that practice supervisors have to undergo preparation for the role, whereby HEIs, together with practice learning partners, must ensure that practice supervisors have an understanding of the proficiencies and programme outcomes they are supporting students to achieve, and that they should receive ongoing appropriate support for the effective supervision of and contribution to student learning and assessment. Furthermore, as all registrants who meet the NMC's criteria may be required to supervise learning, preparation for learning supervision is feasible on a mass scale, and it can also be streamlined by limiting the number of practice supervisors identified for each student, according to Highe (2020).

Rationales for the Practice Learning Supervisor Role

Practice-based learning and practice supervision are necessary requirements for supporting the learning of health profession students, including those who are following novel career pathways, such as student nursing associates, apprenticeship students in nursing and allied health professions (Council of Deans of Health, 2017; Institute for Apprenticeships & Technical Education [IATE], 2022a), and those on well-established programmes such as medical education. A more detailed examination of why we need practice supervisors for learners, however, reveals a number of reasons for this.

━━━━━━━━━━━ ACTION POINT 1.2 ━━━━━━━━━━━

Why practice learning supervisors?

To explore in more detail the wider reasons for practice supervisors being needed in healthcare students' practice education, consider and make notes of all the reasons you can think of for practice learning supervisor roles within healthcare.

When students on the previous mentoring courses were asked to cite as many reasons as they could think of for requiring mentors, they tended to be able to identify several, almost all of which apply to today's practice supervisor role. The reasons given include the need to ensure safe practice by learners, to enable students to achieve their course practice competencies, and to listen and act as a sounding board for any worries or fears that students might have around care interventions. Further reasons cited for practice learning supervision in nursing, midwifery and AHPs are listed in the box below.

Why we Need Practice Learning Supervisors in Nursing and other Health Professions

- For guidance and support
- To structure the working environment for learning
- For constructive and honest feedback

- For debriefing related to good/bad experience during placement
- As a link person with other areas
- As a role model
- To monitor the achievement of competencies
- As a friend and counsellor
- For encouragement
- To provide the appropriate knowledge base for nursing interventions
- For questioning
- For protection from poor practice
- To build confidence
- For sharing learning, i.e. learning from each other
- It is an NMC requirement
- To keep your own skills and knowledge up to date
- For integration of theory to practice
- For developing one's work skills in teaching and explaining
- To provide students with structured learning during practice placements.

One of the advantages of practice supervision is that students who have been on placement in the particular practice setting might be attracted to apply for a post in that setting after qualifying, and therefore it can have recruitment benefits. Furthermore, in healthcare and non-healthcare professions, practice learning facilitation roles have been implemented successfully in the form of management mentoring. In initial teacher training, mentoring has worked successfully for some time (e.g. Kerry and Mayes, 1995; Gov.uk – Ofsted, 2020).

Furthermore, mentoring new teachers results in benefits for both the student teacher and the mentor, whereupon the latter experiences professional stimulation and collaboration, personal fulfilment, friendship and support, motivation to remain current in one's field and networking opportunities; while benefits to the institution include more satisfied staff and greater scholarly productivity, according to Barnett (2008: 3), for example. The term mentoring continues to be applied in various arenas, including medical mentoring, which consists of a teaching-learning relationship that is confidential between two qualified doctors (Viney and McKimm, 2010), and is more akin to clinical supervision in nursing, midwifery and AHPs, which was explained earlier in this chapter.

Another reason for practice learning supervision is stated in the codes of professional practice for nurses, doctors, social workers and AHPs, which usually indicate that qualified practitioners have a duty to teach and facilitate students' learning during practice placements so that students develop their competence under supervision (NMC, 2018a: clause 9.4, for example), and therefore all registrants should fulfil the duties of practice supervisors. Similar requirements feature in healthcare professionals' job descriptions, which are also guided by the NHS Knowledge and Skills Framework (KSF) (CIPD, 2021b).

Practice supervision of course also provides registrants with the opportunity to plan and develop their teaching skills, which in itself is a feature of their own professional development and can constitute a stepping stone in their own career trajectory.

Yet another basis for practice supervision is the prevalence of work-based learning, which constitutes the practice-based development of skills and (practical) knowledge. Its main features are reflected in the social learning theory that was advocated by Bandura (1996) and which centres on learning skills by observing skilled professionals perform them first. Social learning theory therefore also involves practice supervisors being role models, and comprises a four-step process of learning (see Figure 1.1).

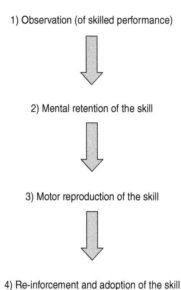

1) Observation (of skilled performance)

2) Mental retention of the skill

3) Motor reproduction of the skill

4) Re-inforcement and adoption of the skill

Figure 1.1   The four-step process of learning a skill

In more detail, the four processes of learning that the learner goes through are as follows:

1.   Observation of skilled performance:

- The individual observes a skilled performance (a 'modelling stimulus').
- The observed behaviour is seen as being useful and distinctive.
- The observer's level of arousal pertaining to the skill is raised.
- The observer is keen to learn the skill.
- The observer has previously felt positive reinforcement for learning skills.

2.   Mental retention of the skill:

- Step-by-step performance of the skill is mentally assimilated.
- There is mental rehearsal of modelled behaviour.

3.   Motor reproduction of the skill:

- The observer carries out observed behaviour of the skill and self-evaluates it in terms of performance under guidance of the expert.

4. Reinforcement and adoption of the skill:
   - The behaviour is reinforced by external reward such as praise or through self-reinforcement, and is likely to be adopted.

According to Bandura (1996), we do not possess any inherent behaviour patterns at birth except reflexes, and therefore learning occurs by observing other people, which is the essence of social learning theory and which therefore includes learning from social situations. In healthcare, learners (e.g. students and preceptees) learn and acquire practical skills by observing practice supervisors, and then following through the four processes identified in Figure 1.1.

Bandura's (1996) social learning theory had previously been termed 'observational learning' or 'modelling' and was built on behaviourist learning theory (see Chapter 2). It is a component of work-based learning, a concept that is examined in some detail in Chapter 5 in the context of learning in practice settings, and also resonates with Peyton's (1998) model of teaching healthcare intervention skill (discussed in Chapter 3).

Supervising students' learning management and leadership

In addition to clinical skills, healthcare students also develop management and leadership skills and knowledge from the very first year of their pre-registration programme, but in more focused ways during their final practice placement near the end of their course. Thereupon, in addition to consolidating their care intervention skills, they also learn the practicalities of organising, managing and leading care interventions for service users (e.g. NMC, 2018c).

More broadly, there have also been several endeavours to implement management coaching in various organisations, whereby trainee managers' learning is supervised by named highly experienced managers to enable those less experienced to develop their management skills. A small number of healthcare professionals have had experience of management coaching, whereupon the management coach function initially involves advising the trainee manager to explore the utilisation of particular management techniques, and takes a more directive approach. Then, when the trainee has developed substantial management skills, the role can become less directive; and, much later, coach–learner activities become more akin to those of 'buddies', i.e. equals.

As noted earlier in this chapter, clinical coaching has its benefits, and management coaching in healthcare entails guiding more junior registrants to develop their management and leadership skills, through one-to-one guidance and support that can enhance their organisational skills, as also noted by Coleman and Glover (2010). This also applies to more senior managers, such as the executive nurse, receiving coaching from independent appropriate personnel.

For finalist healthcare students, learning care organisation skills entail taking charge of a small group of service users' care, for example those in a bay in a hospital ward, and managing all their care during one shift of work. Managing care involves dealing with changes in the service user's condition, delegating tasks to other members of staff, risk assessment, and so on, but under the supervision of their practice learning supervisor. Management activities identified by Gopee (2022) that third-year students can learn, include:

- ensuring that everyone in the care setting follows health and safety rules for staff, patients and visitors
- managing resources – human and material
- co-ordinating care and motivating inter-disciplinary team members
- participation in management initiatives
- supervising learning, preceptoring, training and education
- managing the duty roster and identifying annual leave
- ensuring that all abide by the code of practice, e.g. confidentiality
- checking that individual monitors, handheld devices, computers, etc. are functioning correctly
- involvement in clinical governance activities, e.g. audits, collecting statistics.

For coaching, the GROW model (also referred to as: GROWing – which stands for Goal, Reality, Options, Will/Wrap up) is advocated (e.g. Connor and Pokora, 2017) as a framework for effective coaching. There are several other books on coaching, and short courses and modules are available from various organisations.

As should be obvious from the above reasons for the practice learning supervisor role, there are also several coincidental benefits in undertaking this teaching role, in addition to it often being a job role requirement for healthcare professionals.

Effective Supervision of Learning in Practice Settings

A number of factors need to be considered to ensure a comprehensive and systematic approach to the effective supervision of practice-based learning. In a systematic review of the supervision of practice learning, Jokelainen et al. (2011) concluded that the activity comprises two main themes, which are, first, facilitating student learning and, second, strengthening students' professionalism (professional attributes and identities). Four sub-themes were identified as well as a number of categories under each sub-theme.

To address effective supervision of learning, the following section explores student supervision from the following three perspectives to ensure it is implemented systematically and is effective: (1) the personal attributes of effective practice learning supervisors; (2) an effective supervisory relationship; and (3) the responsibilities and actions of practice learning supervisors that enable learning.

Attributes of effective practice supervisors

The personal characteristics of practice learning supervisors play a crucial part in enabling effective learning by students during their practice placements.

═══ ACTION POINT 1.3 ═══

Characteristics of effective practice learning supervisors

Make a list of what you consider to be the characteristics or personal attributes of a registrant who is effective in their practice supervision role, towards either undergraduate or postgraduate students. Consider their characteristics from such perspectives as personal qualities, approach/actions and skills.

Responding to Action Point 1.3 must have been straightforward, as all healthcare professionals have undertaken pre-registration programmes that included practice placements, and will have encountered practice-based learning supervisors (e.g. practice educators) who support learning. Some supervisors may have been excellent, while there may have been reservations held about others. Most of the characteristics of learning supervisors identified by groups of post-registration students are listed in the box below.

Characteristics of the Person Who is an Effective Practice Supervisor

- Is patient
- Is open-minded
- Is approachable
- Has a good knowledge base
- Has up-to-date knowledge and competence
- Has good communication skills, including listening skills
- Provides encouragement
- Is self-motivated
- Shows concern, compassion and empathy
- Has teaching skills
- Provides psychological support
- Acts as a counsellor
- Is diplomatic, fun and fair
- Is willing to supervise students' learning and to conduct continuous assessment
- Is versatile, adaptable, flexible
- Allows time and commits self to it
- Is confident
- Is enthusiastic
- Acts as an advisor
- Is honest and trustworthy
- Is trusting
- Is a role model
- Is non-judgemental
- Is a resource facilitator
- Is able to build impactful supervisory relationships.

The characteristics of practice learning supervisors noted in the box above can be grouped under three themes, which are (1) clinical **competency**, (2) ability to develop interpersonal relationships, and (3) personality traits such as being approachable, according to an integrative review by Collier (2018).

Effective supervisory relationships

Practice supervision activities, therefore, incorporate a number of factors that enable effective student learning, which include establishing effective supervisory relationships, creating an environment for learning, carrying out an evaluation of learning during the practice placements, and so on. Of primary significance is the need to establish an effective supervisor–student relationship, which encompasses the multiple concerted ways by which such relationships are developed and maintained, including continuing effective supervisor–student communication, the personal attributes of practice supervisors and the range of actions that they take to enable and support learning.

Research conducted to measure the quality of teaching and learning in practice settings reveals that the supervisory relationship between practice learning supervisor and learner is the most important factor contributing to effective clinical learning experiences (e.g. Bennett et al., 2012). A study conducted by Eller et al. (2014) found that there are eight components in effective supervisor–student relationships, including open communication and accessibility, mutual respect and trust, and role modelling.

'Establishing effective working relationships' is one of the areas in which practice supervisors have to be competent in order to enable students to integrate into practice settings and to support practice-based learning. However, for two individuals who are usually initially unknown to each other, adopting supervisor–learner roles presupposes that they are able to communicate with each other, develop a rapport and cultivate a 'working' relationship at the very least. The word *rapport* means 'a sympathetic relationship or understanding' or 'a close and harmonious relationship in which the people or groups concerned understand each other's feelings or ideas and communicate well' (Brookes and O'Neill, 2017: 778); and *relationship* refers to 'the dealings or feelings that exist between people or groups' and 'an emotional association between two people' (2017: 790).

So how are relationships formed between the two designated parties? According to Rogers and Freiberg (1994), counsellors and helpers build a trusting and working relationship by ensuring that certain 'core' conditions always prevail. These conditions are:

- acceptance (or unconditional positive regard) – of the individual for who they are (e.g. for their individual strengths and weaknesses) and through mutual respect
- genuineness – as a person, honesty
- empathic understanding – being able and willing to view situations from the other person's perspective.

These key conditions are explored in some detail in the context of student-centred learning in Chapter 3. Rogers and Freiberg (1994) emphasise that 'trust' underpins these key conditions, which they suggest, in reality, permeates all mutually beneficial relationships. It is akin to a 'psychological contract' between practice supervisor and learner, or between unwell person and carer, or between colleagues and friends. The two parties also have to be willing to spend time together to maintain this relationship and to work towards the achievement of practice objectives, for instance. Although the learner has to actively seek out relevant learning opportunities, the practice supervisor also needs to take actions that support the learner's learning, by, for example, familiarising themselves adequately with the student's educational programme.

Specific details on proficient 'Communication and relationship management skills' are provided by the NMC (2018c: 27–30) under Annexe A. Additionally, for research on how practice supervisors and learners develop trust in each other, see Hauer et al. (2015), noted under the Further Optional Reading section of this chapter; and for well-informed suggestions on ways of making students feel welcome and integrating then into the practice team, see Tremayne and Hunt's (2019) article in the same section.

Responsibilities and actions of practice supervisors that enable learning

In addition to the personal attributes of practice learning supervisors, other researchers have explored the 'roles' of mentors, which refer to the actions that they take to enable or facilitate learners' learning. Deducing from an earlier substantial study on various aspects of mentoring, Darling (1984) identified 14 roles that enable learning, which also apply to the practice supervisor role. These roles are being a/an:

- role model
- energiser
- envisioner
- investor
- supporter
- standard prodder
- teacher-coach
- feedback giver
- eye-opener
- door-opener
- ideas bouncer
- problem solver
- career counsellor
- challenger.

Ways in which practice supervisors feature as role models for learners and colleagues is briefly explored in Chapter 6 of this book in the context of the practice supervisor's leadership. Taking a broader perspective, however, Hall et al. (2008) explored teacher mentors' perceptions of their role in teacher training and found that it comprises nine roles and responsibilities for supporting the learning of individuals engaged in teacher training, which includes being a coach, a counsellor and a source of advice.

Research on the qualities of an effective supervisor in the context of practice learning seems non-existent, although the qualities of supervisors of doctorate students and of those in line management positions do exist. Alternatively, the HCPC's (2022) research identifies ten characteristics of effective learning supervision, which are presented in the box below:

Key Characteristics of Effective Supervision

1. Supervision is based on mutual trust and respect.
2. Supervisees are offered a choice of supervisor to secure a good match on a personal level, an expertise match and to meet cultural needs.
3. Both supervisors and supervisees have a shared understanding of the purpose of supervisory sessions.
4. Supervision focuses on sharing and enhancing knowledge and skills to support professional development and on improving service delivery.
5. Supervision is regular and based on the needs of the individual, and ad hoc supervision is provided in cases of need.
6. Supervisory models include one-to-one, group, internal or external or distance supervision.
7. The employer creates protected time, supervisor training and private space to facilitate supervisory sessions.
8. Training and feedback are provided for supervisors.
9. Supervision is delivered using a flexible timetable, to ensure all staff have access to sessions, regardless of working patterns.
10. Different types of supervision, including practice, professional and managerial supervision, are delivered by different supervisors, or by those who are trained to manage the overlapping responsibility as both line manager and supervisor.

Source: HCPC (2022)

ACTION POINT 1.4

Self-rating of practice supervisor's attributes

Based on either Darling's (1984) roles of the mentor or the HCPC's (2022) characteristics of effective supervision, consider and identify situations where you are in a practice supervisor-type role, or likely to be in the near future. Then:

- For each role or characteristic, do a self-rating of yourself using the numbers 1 to 4, with 1 indicating development or learning need, and 4 indicating proficient.
- Next, focus on one or two of the roles or characteristics on which you rate yourself as low, and consider why this is (e.g. lack of opportunity), and how you can develop your competence in that role.

The roles and responsibilities of the effective practice supervisor are regularly researched to ascertain the more contemporary nature and perceptions of this function. On exploring NHS and HEI managers' perceptions of learning support roles, Carnwell et al. (2007) found that the primary requirement of practice learning supervision comprises of clinical expertise, teaching skills and student support. However, they also identified the potential for role conflict, particularly if the supervisor has qualified only relatively recently and therefore is still enhancing their own repertoire of clinical skills.

No doubt a range of components that support learning can be identified. One of the key functions of the practice supervisor is to help the student integrate into the practice setting, which entails managing the practice placement, receiving the student and conducting initial, mid-placement and final interviews, which are supported by the use of learning contracts or learning agreements. 'Acceptance' of the student (Rogers and Freiberg, 1994) signifies that the practice supervisor accepts the student for their current levels of knowledge and competence, which will be either substantial or minimal.

ACTION POINT 1.5

Practice supervisor actions that support learning

In addition to having the characteristics of an effective practice supervisor, think of and make a list of a number of actions that practice supervisors can take to support learning.

As for managing the placement, designated practice supervisors may have been nominated before the student starts on the placement and would need self-preparation time beforehand to ensure they understand what the role requires of them. Time would also have been set aside for receiving the student and introducing them to the care team.

Seeing the practice placement from a student's viewpoint suggests that they might be experiencing different feelings in anticipation of the placement. They are likely to appreciate any prior information sent to them, which might include any preparatory reading that the student can undertake. On the first day, they tend to appreciate an introduction to the practice setting, making them feel comfortable about learning, a professional but friendly environment, student involvement and continuity of practice supervisors. These perspectives are consistent with 'empathic understanding', which is a key condition of effective supervisory relationships as already noted earlier in this chapter.

Furthermore, the NMC (2018d) and the National Nursing Research Unit (King's College London, 2020) have identified the need for protected time (referred to as 'supported learning time' by the NMC, 2018d: 9), but this has, at times, proved difficult to access, according to the RCN (2016: 11).

The HCPC's characteristics naturally reflect more contemporary learning supervision, and the roles identified in Action Point 1.4 are also referred to as 'Measuring Mentorship Potential'. Each of these roles can be explored in detail as a concept in its own right and, to illustrate this, consider, for example, the 'challenger' and 'supporter' roles.

During their practice placements, students are likely to encounter service-user care situations that they find challenging, and other situations that are less so, especially in the latter part of their pre-registration programme when they will already have acquired a range of clinical skills. How much support should the practice supervisor provide the student with when the latter encounters challenging situations?

▬Reflection point 1.1▬

Learning supervision support and challenge

Consider the practice supervisor's roles as challenger and supporter and think of patient care situations (or clinical interventions) in your workplace that, say, a second-year student will find highly challenging, and others that will be much less challenging. Often, practice supervisors have to comment on the level of initiative that their students have shown. So, think for yourself (or discuss with a peer) what level of support you would provide to your student if that student encounters highly challenging service-user care situations.

What is the result if the student consistently encounters situations that are of 'low challenge' to them?

Of course, students have to be supervised all the time, either directly or from a distance. There are various examples of situations that present high or low challenges for learners in practice settings, and the level of support required. Asking a third-year student nurse consistently to perform clinical skills for which they have already been signed off as competent would provide a lesser challenge to them, and lesser support might be required. But if the same student has not yet learnt how to provide care in epidural pain control, for instance, or catheterisation, then this would present a higher challenge and the student is likely to need a fair level of support.

Daloz (1989) explored the effects of different levels of challenge and of support, and concluded that high challenge and high support can lead to growth and the achievement of aspirations (or vision), while low support and low challenge can result in stasis and apathy. However, high challenge and low support, according to Daloz's findings, can lead to 'retreat and burnout' (see Figure 1.2).

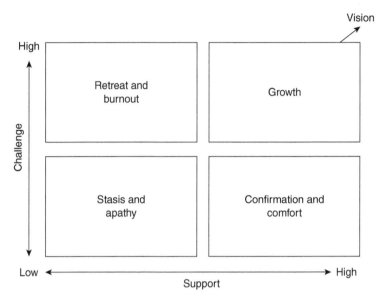

Figure 1.2   Effects of support and challenge on the learner's development

Source: Daloz, 1989

Issues Related To the Supervision of Learning in Care Settings

A common experience in nursing in the twenty-first century has been that nurses working in many practice settings feel that they are managing their workload with ongoing staffing constraints. Indeed, Phillips et al.'s (2000) research acknowledged that the then mentors were fulfilling this role as one of several other roles they had during any normal span of duty. Furthermore, despite 'protected time' for facilitating students' practice-based learning having been advocated for decades, the implementation of this mechanism has remained difficult to implement, mainly due to multiple demands on learning supervisors' time (e.g. King's College London, 2020).

Consequently, there is a risk that the student's learning experience can become fragmented and superficial, and the student is left with several service-user-related queries. The supervisor–student relationship can thereby also be affected negatively. When working within these constraints, knowingly or unknowingly, practice supervisors' actions (or inactions) could result in reduced attention to learning.

━━━━━━━━━━━━━ ACTION **POINT 1.6** ━━━━━━━━━━━━

How practice supervisors might hinder learning

Think of, and make notes on, a range of actions (or inaction) on the part of practice supervisors that coincidentally may be seen as discouraging or hindering learning in addition to those already noted above.

_____

Case Study 1.1 presents an example of recent poor supervision of practice-based learning.

━━━━━━ **Case study 1.1** ━━━━━━━━━━━━━━━━━━━━━━━━━━━━━━

Poor supervision of practice-based learning

Mel Alexis is a second-year student nurse on a rehabilitation ward. One day, she finished her shift early, having told the staff nurse in charge that she had a terrible headache, while in fact she was extremely upset regarding her placement.

That morning she had felt that the staff nurse had spoken to her in a very unprofessional manner, as she does to patients as well. This is what bothered Mel the most. She also challenged the staff nurse over her drug administration that morning. A patient was left her morning medication in a pot on the table but was unable to swallow it as she needed assistance due to her having a weak side and problems with her other hand. As Mel walked past the patient's room, the patient called her and indicated that she had not taken her tablets yet. As Mel was not the nurse who administered the drugs, she called the nurse to the room for her to administer the medication. The nurse said that she did not have time to do this but that the tablets were correct for the patient.

Mel agreed to assist in giving the medication but noticed three tablets lying on the table beside the pot. Mel asked the nurse what these tablets were and she was advised that they were morning medications as well. Mel doubted this as they were not in the medicine pot and asked the nurse why they were not in the pot, but the latter did not give an answer and instead picked them up and put them into the pot. The nurse then told Mel to assist with the medications and Mel made it clear that she did not feel that the medications were correct, as there seemed to be more tablets than the patient usually took in the morning. The nurse told Mel not to question her drug administration, so Mel felt that she had no choice but to assist the patient in taking the drugs.

This event highlighted Mel's unhappiness with this ward. She had started feeling like this on day one, when she was not introduced to any staff members or shown around. She had had to find things out for herself during her time on this ward and if she asked where something was, the staff said it would be quicker for them to get the item themselves rather than show Mel. As a second-year nurse, she was expecting to do many nursing activities but instead she felt that she was being treated like a support worker. Although Mel loves providing basic nursing care to patients, she expected a lot more from this placement than she was actually getting. Mel appreciates that on a rehabilitation ward nursing entails a unique set of activities, but she feels that she has yet to see what these activities are.

Mel says she has always wanted to be a nurse and really loves the job, but this ward has now made her question this and it makes her very sad to feel this way.

In response to Action Point 1.6, you may have felt that one of the problems that students have experienced in the past is the lack of opportunity to work with their practice learning supervisor. Actions on the part of practice supervisors that can discourage learning which you might have thought of are:

- lack of interest in students and in their learning needs
- lack of knowledge about the student's course
- lack of **evidence-based practice** or research utilisation
- having a hierarchical mindset and a lack of team approach
- not acknowledging the student's previous experience
- negative attitudes
- a reluctance to change practice.

There is a possibility that you have yourself witnessed poor supervision of learning, either directly or indirectly. Earlier research has identified the personality characteristics of practice-based learning supervisors that discourage learning. For instance, Darling's (1985) qualitative study revealed what she termed the characteristics of the 'galaxy of toxic mentors' (see Table 1.1).

Table 1.1   The 'galaxy of toxic mentors' (or practice supervisors)

Types	Features
Avoiders	Practice supervisors who are not available or accessible, also referred to as 'ignorers' or 'non-responders'
Dumpers	Throw people into new roles or situations and let them flounder, or let them 'sink or swim', often deliberately
Blockers	Actively avoid meeting the learner's needs by refusing requests, by controlling through withholding information, or by blocking the learner's development by over-supervising
Destroyers/Criticisers	Set out to destroy the learner by subtle attacks to undermine confidence, and open and public verbal attacks and arguments, questioning the learner's abilities and deliberately destroying confidence

The types of activities and demeanour identified by Darling in Table 1.1 are referred to by Proctor (2011: 26) as 'oppressive supervisor behaviour'. Based on extensive experience in management and decision-making, Heirs and Farrell (1986) explored the mindsets of individual employees who enable an organisation to progress with its aims, and those of people who block such development. While the focus is on looking for, and developing, 'talents' in junior employees, in reality the mindset of some employees can stifle the development of juniors and learners. The researchers grouped the problematic or disabling traits of those who block development as 'three mental poisons', in terms of the functioning of rigid minds, ego minds and Machiavellian minds (see box). Such ways of thinking are not always obvious, nor easily detected, but do affect learning adversely.

Rigid Minds, Ego Minds and Machiavellian Minds

The rigid mind:

- Has personal values that are set or stereotyped
- Is unable to see the positives in others' thoughts if they conflict with their own thinking
- Continually blocks the openness of more creative thinking
- Is loyal to traditional thinking and rejects novelty
- Appears to lack imagination or creativity
- Stifles the use of originality and encourages complacency.

The ego mind:

- Sees elements of a problem only in terms of self-interest and self-importance
- Is fairly ambitious and has a high opinion of their own abilities
- Looks after number one to the exclusion of other considerations
- Pays little attention to what others think and say
- Is unsociable and does not contribute to collective thinking
- Will betray colleagues and even the organisation if it serves their ends.

The Machiavellian mind:

- Quickly sees the range of likely outcomes of any decision
- Manipulates the feelings and ambitions of others to deceive
- Is devious and calculating
- Intimidates and engages in politicking
- Perpetuates worry in the organisation and is perpetually currying favour with superiors
- Is scheming, cunning and suspicious of subordinates.

Source: Heirs and Farrell (1986)

Then, in their study to explore students' experiences of practice placements, Gray and Smith (2000) found that while effective and good supervision of learning did prevail, the majority of students also experienced learning-inhibiting activities of some healthcare professionals in supervisory roles, including supervisors' lack of knowledge and expertise, having poor teaching skills, delegating unwanted jobs to students, breaking promises and intimidating students.

Although neither Heirs and Farrell's nor Gray and Smith's research are recent, it is useful to be aware of the risk of such behaviours occurring, and to prevent them from happening. More recent studies include Cant et al.'s (2021: 1) review of qualitative research on clinical placement learning, which identified 'Unsupportive instructors, a lack of supervision and not being included' in the team as factors that inhibit learning. Another systematic review and meta-synthesis by Panda et al. (2021) found that the attitude of clinical staff, instructors and significant others, which had a major influence on students' clinical learning, as well as the lack of a sense of belongingness and self-motivation to learn, and a perceived fear of making mistakes, were some of the demotivating factors. A lack of resources to facilitate need-based training, staff shortages, workload and inconsistencies between theory and practice, were also found to be key challenges in the CLE.

Darling (1985) makes a number of suggestions on how to manage 'toxic' supervisors of learning. For instance, the student can try to keep the relationship with the practice supervisor balanced by building a support network with other students or registrants within the team and drawing on their own personal strengths (for instance, problem-solving skills). However, line managers are often aware of practice supervisors who under-perform, and conversely Heirs and Farrell (1986) suggest that it is the responsibility of the organisation's managers to identify those employees who block development and learning. 'Poisonous' thinking endures but can be changed gradually through formal and informal meetings. Decisions about the delegation of responsibilities and roles need to be applied selectively and be overseen with the appropriate intensity or freedom.

At times, practice supervisors may be ineffective because of a lack of detailed knowledge of their student's educational programme (their course), regarding which the PEF should be able to advise. Other action that can be taken when ineffective supervision is detected is to implement co-supervision, which involves two or more practice supervisors jointly supervising the student's learning. Temporary non-allocation of a student to the ineffective practice supervisor is another alternative that might work. Managers can formally or informally ask the practice supervisor how well they feel they are fulfilling their practice supervision duties. The line manager may be able to confront the ineffective practice supervisor if poor learning supervision has been observed, or a complaint received. There are alternative strategies, but they will be dependent on local circumstances. The ethical aspects of poor supervision of practice learning are discussed in Chapter 8.

Approaches, Models and Frameworks for Effective Practice Supervision

Despite some likely practice supervisor behaviours interfering with students' learning, the practice supervision role comprises a necessary mechanism for supporting the learning of healthcare students. Due to the humane, personal and suffering-prevention nature of healthcare provision, professional education programmes have to be appropriately structured and their impact carefully monitored. The practice supervision of students therefore also has to be adequately structured, with an appropriate combination of directive and facilitative approaches that are adopted, depending on the existing knowledge and competence of each student.

The underlying principles on which practice supervisors base their role vary to some extent according to their personal beliefs and approaches to the supervisor role, and about student learning, and therefore determine their blueprint of how they fulfil the role, as well as the model of supervision that they apply.

The differences between the terms approach, model and framework are as follows. 'Approach' to practice supervision is personal to the individual and is based on their own life and professional experiences, and personal views and beliefs. It would therefore depend on the practice supervisor's beliefs about nursing, about undergraduate course design, and about student and learner populations and their styles of learning.

A 'model', however, can be defined as a research-deduced, and therefore informed, set of interrelated essential components that enable the activity to be executed comprehensively. A 'framework' takes this further, whereby the components of the model are utilised as key areas or sections for planning and implementing the activity, and may even have been empirically tested.

All three perspectives indicate a well thought-out and systematic approach to the student's placement experience to make it optimally effective. Very few frameworks for the supervision of learning and mentoring in healthcare have been available. Darling's (1984) roles of the mentor constitute such a model, while the NMC's (2008) eight domain standards for mentoring have been another. For supervision of learning, it should prove useful to examine other approaches and models of practice supervision that could be applied, such as those identified in Table 1.2. When using the CLiP model, for example, a clinical educator supports and coaches students, acts as a source of expert advice in such circumstances as under-achieving students, and contributes to enabling and maintaining the care setting as a learning environment (e.g. RCN, 2022a).

Table 1.2   Approaches and models of practice learning supervision

Collaborative Learning in Practice (CLiP) model	Entails appointing a 'clinical educator' to coach students' practice-based learning
Apprenticeship or coaching model	The practice supervisor is a skilled crafts person, and the learner learns by following instructions provided by the supervisor

Reflective practitioner model	Based on learning theories, e.g. **andragogy**, styles of learning and student-centred approaches, the practice supervisor is a critical friend and co-enquirer
Competence-based model	The practice supervisor enables students to learn specific practice objectives, and monitors and records their progress
Team practice supervision	A team of designated practice supervisors oversee one or more students' learning, which is also applied to team supervision for doctorate students, for example
Contract supervision	Formal supervision of learning that is time- or objectives-restricted for both supervisee and supervisor, e.g. when on practice placement at another institution
Dissertation supervision	Solely for one-to-one student guidance with their dissertation by a named academic supervisor
Personal coaching	A natural, mutual and self-chosen relationship for one-to-one coaching related to a specific task, and is usually terminated by mutual agreement

The approaches and models of supervision of learning identified in Table 1.2 can all be adopted or adapted for practice supervision, as deemed most appropriate locally. Furthermore, the RCN (2016) recently identified three non-UK models of learning supervision, which notably are also insufficiently researched, which are:

- Real Life Learning Wards (Amsterdam model): involves team-based mentoring and students are given responsibility for patient care early on in the placement.
- Dedicated Education Units (USA and Australia): also involves team-mentoring, but with an extra focus on creating a positive learning environment.
- Clinical Facilitation Model (Australia): the facilitator assesses the student, but their learning is facilitated by other registered nurses and by student 'buddying'.

In these models, there is more than one student per practice supervisor. In their systematic review of practice education, Jayasekara et al. (2018) found that dedicated education units and 'collaborative clinical placement' models result in enhanced engagement by students and constitute more effective learning environments. In the former model, the supervisor receives additional payment for the role, and the latter incorporates joint university–healthcare organisation appointments.

There are also other forms of supervision of practice-based learning, which include shadowing, inter-professional supervision, and e-supervision, which are concepts and activities that are transferable, and suggest flexibility as alternative forms of practice supervision. Electronic or e-supervision can be implemented successfully, whereupon the supervisor and the student communicate entirely via their computer or a similar device. Of course, internet-based mentoring (e-mentoring) is not a new concept as its feasibility has been demonstrated for some time.

With e-supervision, Bear and Jones (2017) researched factors that influence satisfaction with an internet-based practitioner–student learning relationship in which the business studies student participates in choosing their supervisor, and found that satisfaction with the supervisory relationship correlates with trust in the practice supervisor. Consequently, students view their practice supervisor as a role model, and have an agreed understanding of the objectives of the supervision during practice placement (also known as internship).

Long-arm or distant supervision is yet another form of learning supervision that tends to prevail primarily in certain areas of primary and social care where the practice supervisor would not generally be based at the same healthcare site as the student, and yet all criteria and activities constituting effective practice supervision are fulfilled.

━━━━━━━━━ **ACTION POINT 1.7** ━━━━━━━━━

Application of approaches and models of practice supervision

In your own experience of practice learning supervision activities, which of the approaches, models or frameworks referred to in the above sections apply to learning professional skills in your own practice setting, and why? Which one(s) are the most suitable? Make some notes.

The apprenticeship model, which is akin to coaching, has previously been applied mostly to the training of support workers, in that an apprentice often learns skills and crafts at the level of task performance, along with the necessary associated practical knowledge, unlike the holistic psycho-bio-social approach taken by nurses, for example. Johnson (2017) endeavoured to constitute an apprenticeship model of learning supervision based on Bandura's (1996) model of development of self-efficacy, but concluded that the latter covers an insufficient range of concepts for the effective supervision of learning for healthcare students.

The reflective practitioner approach is one that is frequently favoured within health profession circles, whereby practice supervisors take a less directive approach to practice-based learning. The competence model might also apply, but the reader needs to be aware of varying definitions of the term 'competence'. Some definitions see competence as the ability to perform a skill in accordance with agreed procedures and to incorporate practical knowledge, while others see it as incorporating **theoretical knowledge**.

Most of the under-researched models and approaches presented in Table 1.2 are not frameworks for practice supervision, although they can constitute systematic, comprehensive and often self-styled ways of supporting practice learning. Furthermore, there are also instances where students and practice supervisors can mutually select each other for their respective roles for facilitation, guidance, assistance and support with student learning. The notion that students can select their practice supervisor also has currency in some situations, such as if one of the members of the learning supervision team's job changes at short notice, or when the student is asked to select a supervisor from the practice supervision team.

Peer supervision (or peer teaching) is another emerging model of learning supervision, and Gilmour et al. (2007), for example, report on a highly successful peer-teaching programme in which second-year student nurses oversee first-year students' learning on their pre-registration university courses. Increasingly, the value of peer-learning supervision is being recognised and widely implemented (e.g. RCN, 2016: 11, 18).

However, we need to be aware of the previously noted shortcomings of peer teaching and peer learning in professional practice (peer teaching also being a component of the CLiP model of practice learning) whence we were advised to guard against the likelihood of senior students passing on poor practice to junior students, and possibly an incorrect knowledge base. Furthermore, one of the risks of peer teaching is that past mistakes are likely to be repeated even after qualifying, when the individual is no longer closely supervised and consequently the quality of care is compromised.

Furthermore, the evaluation of peer teaching during practice placement tends to indicate that some students feel that time spent teaching junior students is time sacrificed that could have been used for further developing their own clinical practice while working with their supervisor. Clearly, peer teaching by senior students needs to be encouraged, but it needs to be carefully structured so that the students who are on the verge of becoming RNs do not lose out from lack of access to their practice supervisor, nor from incidental learning. Additionally, any innovation or change in practice needs to be considered in the context of 'management of change', for the implementation to be effective (see Chapter 6 of this book for a discussion on management of change).

'Communities of practice' (also discussed in Chapters 2 and 5 of this book) is yet another form of peer supervision. Moreover, increasingly, as inter-professional working and inter-professional learning are being systematically operationalised, the concept of inter-professional learning supervision has also gained in popularity and credibility. For example, an evaluative research study on inter-professional supervision of learning conducted by Lait et al. (2011), found that:

- students also learned about the roles of other professions, as well as how to work together to provide patient-centred care
- inter-professional learning can be 'threaded' through all clinical placements, rather than being offered periodically on the three-year pre-registration programme.

The researchers also point out that the activities that students engage in vary in complexity, and that 'provider commitment' (by the placement provider) is important (p. 113). Furthermore, although inter-professional learning has been researched substantially, evidence of inter-professional supervision is lacking. Following their small-scale study of inter-professional supervision, Yang et al. (2017) warn against the limitations of the activity. They found that, on occasion, students were supervised by a supervisor from another health profession who had not had adequate preparation for the role, which resulted in student dissatisfaction with the required practice learning; and, at times, inter-professional supervisors were chosen due to a shortage of supervisors in their own profession.

Moreover, in a study of students' experiences and staff perceptions of the implementation of placement development teams, Williamson (2009) reports that students indicate a need for more direct, personal organisational support, and better communication between university and placement areas. Additionally, research also suggests that the effectiveness of the learning supervision role depends on the level of the healthcare professional's motivation and interest in students' learning (e.g. Hallin and Danielson, 2009).

Having delved into and analysed key facets of practice learning supervision, the final section of this chapter concludes the concept and role by suggesting a model and framework for practice supervision based on previous research in the topic area.

Frameworks for Practice Supervision, and the Content of Supervisor Preparation Programmes

As noted earlier in this chapter, in addition to the supervision of students' learning in care settings during practice placements, supervision also has a range of other applications in health and social care. For the supervision of social workers in relation to child protection work, for example, Saltiel's (2017) research suggests that the supervision of qualified social workers enables further learning that consequently enhances care provision for service users, and thereby reduces child deaths.

Saltiel's research also acknowledges the 'complex skills' that experienced supervisors utilise, and which novice supervisors 'struggle to acquire' (p. 533) in the perceived current under-resourced work environment, and recommends a supportive learning environment for newly qualified social workers. The point highlighted in these findings is the recognition that recently qualified care professionals may not reach high standards in their work if they are not provided with educational, developmental and emotional support, because otherwise they rely only on their managers' instructions and their pre-qualifying education. Consequently, it is reasonable to suggest that if qualified care professionals have a need for supervised learning, then health and social care profession students need this mechanism even more so.

For pre-registration nursing and midwifery students, the NMC has succinctly stated the roles, responsibilities and educational preparation of practice supervisors. For the preparation of practice supervisors, Falender (2014) has previously suggested that competency-based supervision of learning does not refer only to the supervisee developing and achieving practice competencies, but also to the supervisor being provided with competency-based education for the role. This implies an educational preparation for supervisors of learning that is 'fit for purpose', and that there is growing consensus that competency-based preparation of supervisors should include addressing:

- the formation of a strong supervisory alliance
- the development of a supervisory/learning contract
- supporting the student with self-assessment
- providing constructive and positive feedback
- the identification and repair of strains in the alliance
- complying with the legal and ethical aspects of supervision
- evaluating service-user outcomes
- managing supervisees who are not progressing as expected.

The arguments presented above clearly suggest that the content of practice supervisor preparation programmes needs to be comprehensive so that it can benefit learners and supervisors, as well as, ultimately, care service users. However, as suggested earlier in this chapter, practice learning supervisors' readiness for the role needs to be ascertained beforehand, and they need to be motivated to fulfil this role.

The features of effective supervision, according to Kilminster et al. (2007), which essentially comprise a framework, incorporate the following:

- Supervision is aligned to the practice setting's and the care organisation's clinical guidelines, as well as being based on the student's HEI practice competencies.
- Direct supervision involves learner and supervisor working together and observing each other.
- Frequent constructive feedback is provided to supervisees.
- Supervision is structured, with regular timetabled meetings.
- The supervisory relationship is developed in conjunction with written learning agreements, and takes into account the assessment components, and maybe an appraisal for healthcare apprentices.
- Supervised learning includes elements of management of care, teaching and research, with structured reflective discussions, in addition to learning care interventions.
- The supervision process should be informed by a '360-degree perspective', which therefore includes service-user feedback, inter-professional supervision, together with reviewing written work by students, and records of supervision.

Research conducted by Finnerty and Collington (2013) on a model of supervision that was applied to supervising midwifery students' learning revealed that the model is beneficial, primarily because the model is consistent with coaching, which in turn entails role modelling, reverse role modelling and experiential learning. However, one model of supervision that has stood the test of time for some years now is Proctor's (2011), which comprises addressing the normative, formative and supportive aspects of supervision, as well as the restorative aspect.

In concluding this discussion on frameworks and models of supervision of practice learning, it is feasible to deduce the most relevant content of practice supervision preparation programmes. The two sets of items presented in bullet form above, comprise a very good starting point for the content of an effective practice supervision preparation programme, which should be complemented by incorporating the NMC's (2018a) clauses under 'Effective practice learning' and those under 'Supervision of students' in *Standards for Student Supervision and Assessment*.

Adapting Proctor's supervision alliance model into a framework for supervision of practice education

Although intended initially for peer-support-type clinical supervision, Proctor's model of supervision can be adapted effectively to practice supervision in nursing and midwifery and similar roles in other care professions to enable students to achieve their learning outcomes. In a little more detail, the model comprises:

- formative supervision: refers to the educational aspect of the placement, etc.
- normative supervision: refers to adherence to clinical guidelines and procedures that have been approved by the organisation, and therefore comply with the profession's code of practice, etc.
- supportive supervision: refers to allowing students time to learn and practise newly learnt clinical skills, etc.
- restorative supervision: reviewing student progress with practice objectives; re-establishing placement requirements following sickness or other breaks; managing under-achievement; etc.

NHS England (2017a) highly recommends the adaptation of Proctor's model to 'clinical midwifery supervision' for RMs. However, the model can also be reconstituted into a framework for the effective practice supervision of pre-qualifying healthcare students, as suggested in the box below.

Applying a Framework of Practice Supervision

Formative supervision:

- Identifying supervisees' practice objectives that must be achieved
- Facilitation of learning for acquisition of knowledge and skills
- Optimising incidental learning opportunities and relevant 'spoke' visits
- Instituting reflective practice

- Improving care intervention skills, resulting in improved care for service users
- Evaluating practice learning provision
- Formative assessment and contributing to students' summative assessment (discussed in Chapter 7 of this book).

Normative supervision:

- Adhering to the clinical guidelines and procedures that have been approved by the organisation
- Abiding by the profession's code of practice, and exercising **ethical competence** towards service users, colleagues and peers
- Evidence-based practice and changing practice
- Establishing supervisory relationships
- Negotiating and agreeing on a learning contract for the whole placement
- Enabling the supervisee to value the practice placement and the supervision mechanism
- Awareness of quality of care
- Supervisor's leadership.

Supportive supervision:

- Supervisor's positive attitude and skill in the relationship
- Allowing the supervisee time to learn and practise care intervention skills
- Acceptance of the student, and mutual respect
- Providing support and direct help in challenging situations
- Motivating the student to learn through feedback on progress with their practice objectives
- Creating a climate for learning in the care setting.

Restorative supervision:

- Managing under-achieving students
- Mid-placement review, or more frequent monitoring of progress
- Supportive teaching skills/facilitation of learning
- Using empathy
- Re-establishing placement requirements following sickness or other breaks
- Trust and rapport.

The examples identified under the adaptation of Proctor's framework in the box above provide a comprehensive backdrop for constituting a framework of your own for a practice supervisor preparation programme, which is done by taking into account the specific requirements of your own professional specialism. This can be done by populating Template 1.1. Furthermore, the template can then comprise a self-assessment tool for practice supervisor competence by grading the competence level on each item between 1 and 5, 1 being for non-competent and 5 for highly competent.

Template 1.1 Supervisor self-assessment using a framework for practice supervision

Practice Supervisor's Name:......................... Date of self-assessment:.......................	
Components	**Competence level and comments**
Formative supervision • .... • .... • .... • .... •	
Normative supervision • .... • .... • .... • .... •	
Supportive supervision • .... • .... • .... • .... •	
Restorative supervision • .... • .... • .... • .... •	

NHS England (2017a) endorses Proctor's (2011: 25) recommendation that the restorative function should be addressed first, because until the supervisee can relax, and is free of anxiety and stress, they might not be as fully receptive to formative and normative development. Examples of key components of the restorative function include:

• addressing the emotional needs of students and staff
• supporting the development of resilience
• creating space for reflective conversation, supportive challenge and open and honest feedback
• contemplating different perspectives
• processing any difficult emotions experienced by healthcare professionals through a supportive, confidential relationship.

However, it is argued that in terms of the supervision of learning for pre-registration students, the formative and normative functions take priority, but are underpinned by the supportive function to fully enable the student's progress towards achievement of the agreed placement objectives.

So, the relatively rich literature on supervision ultimately always tends to incorporate learning, and describes the features of effective supervision and the principles of supervision, which essentially comprise 'good practice' in supervision. What would you say, then, are the actions that supervisors of learning in your health or social care profession would take that constitute good practice? In the supervision of learning in care professions, identifying all actions that comprise good practice would result in a lengthy list of considerations and activities, and in addition to the features of effective supervision identified above, they include:

- ensuring a full endeavour to establish a strong supervisory relationship from the very beginning
- incorporating the agreed level of direct supervision with nominated supervisors, which entails learner and supervisor working together in service-user care situations
- the supervision process being enriched by input from multi-professional team members, which should be in written form and include mention of the student's learning activities and any assigned work
- informing those involved in supervision of any prior concerns about the student's learning requirements
- protecting supervisor–student interaction time, preferably without interruptions and definitely with privacy
- ensuring confidentiality, and abiding by all other relevant codes of practice set by professional regulators (e.g. HCPC's)
- ensuring that non-verbal messages match verbal statements
- … [add your own].

Make a note of your own perspectives on good practice activities as you feel appropriate. The supervision features and activities identified above can consequently be grouped under headings of a framework for effective practice supervision related to your specific profession. Kilminster et al.'s (2007) framework, detailed above, comprises an example of effective supervision.

Chapter Summary

This chapter has focused on practice supervision for enabling health and care students to develop competence in safe and effective clinical interventions, which is based mostly on research and other literature on supervision and mentorship, and has therefore addressed:

- relevant perspectives on the practice supervisor role, and definitions of and distinctions between the practice supervisor and various other learning facilitation roles, such as preceptor, clinical educator, practice assessor, practice education facilitator; all these roles are established with the aim of facilitating healthcare learners' acquisition of care intervention skills, knowledge and appropriate attitudes
- a number of reasons for requiring practice supervisors to support learning for healthcare students on preparatory education programmes during practice placements, and the necessary characteristics of practice supervisors
- effective practice supervision, which encompasses effective working relationships; and relevant supervisor–learner communication, which includes both generic and specialist communication skills
- research findings on the detrimental effects of poor, inefficient or adverse practice supervision, and ways of resolving these when they occur
- the use of different approaches, models and frameworks for the supervision of practice learning, good practice in practice supervision, and then a framework for effective supervision of practice-based learning.

Further Optional Reading

1. For an exploration of research and different perspectives on coaching in a wide range of settings in the UK and abroad and discussion on inherent issues, see:

   - Garvey, B., Stokes, P. and Megginson, D. (2017) *Coaching and Mentoring: Theory and Practice*, 3rd edn. London: Sage.

2. For an example of the application of coaching in healthcare, see:

   - Royal College of Nursing (2022) *Using a Coaching Model in Practice Supervision*. Available at: Using a Coaching Model in Practice Supervision | Practice-based learning | Royal College of Nursing (rcn.org.uk) (accessed 25 May 2022).

3. For research on how practice supervisors and learners develop trust in each other, see:

   - Hauer, K.E., Oza, S.K., Kogan, J.R., Stankiewicz, C.A., Stenfors-Hayes, T., Cate, O.T., Batt, J. and O'Sullivan, P.S. (2015) 'How clinical supervisors develop trust in their trainees: A qualitative study', *Medical Education*, 49(8): 783–795.

2

HOW LEARNERS LEARN

Introduction

As the treatment and care of individuals' healthcare problems are the main part of healthcare professionals' work, an appropriate proportion of their pre-registration education course is dedicated to students learning clinical skills and knowledge in practice settings. In a nursing pre-registration course, for instance, which amounts to a total of 4,600 hours of learning in three years, the NMC (2018e: 13; 2019a: 10) requires a minimum of 50 per cent of this learning time to take place in practice settings (of which a small number of hours of practice learning can be facilitated by 'simulation' in skills laboratories and in other education settings). Thus, learning in practice settings occupies a pivotal role in professional preparatory education, and indeed, learning is a career-long practice enhancement journey for all healthcare professionals.

Fundamental to learning patient care skills, is learning the associated knowledge base and values and behaviour. Accordingly, this chapter examines the wide choice of ways in which students learn, and Chapter 3 focuses on teaching and facilitation of students' learning. The NMC (2018a: 6) indicates that practice supervisors' duties include enabling 'students to learn and safely achieve proficiency and autonomy in their professional role'. Furthermore, the NMC's (2018b) and HCPC's (2016) standards of conduct indicate that registrants must support their students' learning, and also share their skills, knowledge and experience with their colleagues for the benefit of healthcare service users. Doing so incorporates ascertaining the learner's stage of learning, selecting appropriate learning opportunities for them, and enabling students to integrate learning from practice and academic settings.

The NMC (2018a) doesn't provide extensive detail of the practice supervisor role in the facilitation of learning, but does provide succinct guidance. Chapter 2 consequently draws on research on the multiple theories of learning, and focuses on ways in which healthcare learners learn the competence and knowledge required for providing care that is 'person-centred, safe and compassionate' and effective (NMC, 2018c: 7).

▬Chapter objectives▬

1. Identify the specific knowledge and competencies that healthcare students learn during their pre-registration education programmes, including different forms of knowledge and clinical skills.
2. Identify various reasons for learning by individuals, and the process of learning professional competence.
3. Analyse the prevailing major views and perspectives on learning, teaching and education.
4. Understand and critically analyse key theories of learning and indicate how they can be applied to ensure learning is more effective in practice settings.
5. Comprehend students' different approaches to learning, as well as their learning styles, and ways in which practice supervisors can adapt their teaching to match students' individual approaches and styles.

What do Healthcare Learners Learn, and Why?

The first section of this chapter begins by identifying the specific knowledge and competencies that healthcare profession students need to learn during their initial preparatory programmes, in order to become a competent practitioner by the time they gain their qualification and achieve registrant status.

Healthcare competencies

For nurse education programmes, in *Future Nurse: Standards of Proficiency for Registered Nurses*, the NMC (2018c) identifies the knowledge and skills that students have to acquire in order to become a registered nurse (RN). For midwifery, the required knowledge and competence are constituted in *Standards of Proficiency for Midwives* (NMC, 2019a). The HCPC's (2017) *Standards of Education and Training Guidance* provides recommendations for the content of pre-qualifying AHP education curricula, which is supported by specific standards of proficiency (SOP) for each of the 15 allied healthcare professions that it currently regulates. The SOP determine the professional competence that each profession's pre-registration students have to achieve for their name to be entered on the HCPC professional register. Consequently, the HCPC has published SOP for:

- arts therapists
- biomedical scientists
- chiropodists/podiatrists
- clinical scientists
- dietitians
- hearing aid dispensers
- occupational therapists
- operating department practitioners
- orthoptists
- paramedics
- physiotherapists
- practitioner psychologists
- prosthetists/orthotists
- radiographers
- speech and language therapists.

AHP students have to demonstrate competence in each of these SOP, en route to becoming a registrant in their chosen profession. The SOP also define the scope of practice for each profession at the point of registration, and therefore constitute areas of knowledge, skills, behaviour and values to enable the registrant to 'practise lawfully, safely and effectively' (e.g. HCPC, 2014a: 4).

For physiotherapists, for example, the SOP are detailed in *Standards of Proficiency – Physiotherapists* (HCPC, 2013). The SOP are based on the 15 generic statements identified by HCPC (2013), along with a number of profession-specific standards. Profession-specific standards for physiotherapists, for example, under generic statement 4, 'be able to practise as an autonomous professional, exercising their own professional judgement' (2013: 8), include:

4.1 be able to assess a professional situation, determine the nature and severity of the problem and call upon the required knowledge and experience to deal with the problem

4.2 be able to make reasoned decisions to initiate, continue, modify or cease techniques or procedures, and record the decisions and reasoning appropriately.

As you may have noted, all the above selected SOP are skills or competence areas that pre-registration student physiotherapists will have become proficient in by the time they become registrants with the HCPC. As for the paramedic profession, as another example, the specific SOP are detailed in *Standards of Proficiency – Paramedics* (HCPC, 2014a), and examples of profession-specific SOP for paramedics under generic statement 14, 'be able to draw on appropriate knowledge and skills to inform practice', include:

14.4 know how to position or immobilise patients correctly for safe and effective interventions

14.12 be able to conduct a thorough and detailed physical examination of the patient using appropriate skills to inform clinical reasoning and guide the formulation of a differential diagnosis across all age ranges.

━━━━━━━━ ACTION **POINT** 2.1 ━━━━━━━━

SOP for your allied health profession

Unless you have done so already, access the HCPC SOP for your allied health profession, and peruse them in detail to ascertain your understanding of them. Then think from the stance of the pre-registration student and ask yourself whether the student's understanding of these standards will be exactly the same as yours.

Professional standards are reviewed periodically, often every five years, after thorough appropriate consultation, and all HEIs currently offering pre-registration healthcare education programmes have to incorporate them into their pre-registration courses.

For nursing, as can be expected, the NMC provides comprehensive details of all areas of competence that students must achieve and demonstrate to be able to register their name on the NMC's register as 'registrant' in the relevant field of practice, these fields being: (1) adult nursing; (2) children and young persons nursing; (3) learning disabilities nursing; and (4) mental health nursing. The overall NMC's (2018c) SOP for pre-registration nursing education identifies course outcomes that are structured under seven 'Platforms', along with specific skills identified under two annexes: Annexe A – Communication and relationship management skills; and Annexe B – Nursing procedures. The seven platforms of outcomes are:

1. Being an accountable professional
2. Promoting health and preventing ill health
3. Assessing needs and planning care
4. Providing and evaluating care (see examples in the box above)
5. Leading and managing nursing care and working in teams
6. Improving safety and quality of care
7. Coordinating care.

For nursing associate students, the outcomes are specified in *Standards of Proficiency for Nursing Associates* (NMC, 2018f), but the overall roles and duties of nursing associates are published by HEE (2017); and for nurse apprenticeships by the Institute for Apprenticeships & Technical Education (2022a), which is currently based on the NMC (2018c) SOP. These standards documents are available free of charge on the internet. The General Medical Council (GMC) and other healthcare regulators publish their own corresponding standards.

Standards of proficiency are translated into specific practice competencies locally or in regional groups of universities, or reproduced verbatim in PADs, and students will have to become competent in them during practice placements. No doubt it would be useful for all practice supervisors to access a copy of the whole SOP document for pre-qualifying education (e.g. NMC, 2018c), and to refer to it as and when required.

In the standards of proficiency for nurse education, under 'Platform 4 – *Providing and evaluating care*', the NMC's (2018c: 17) related outcome is: 'The proficiencies identified below will equip the newly registered nurse with the underpinning knowledge and skills required for their role in providing and evaluating **person-centred care**.' A few examples of SOP under this platform are:

4.7 demonstrate the knowledge, skills and ability to act as a role model for others in providing evidence-based, person-centred nursing care to meet people's needs related to mobility, hygiene, oral care, wound care and skin integrity

4.11 demonstrate the knowledge and skills required to initiate and evaluate appropriate interventions to support people who show signs of self-harm and/or suicidal ideation.

In addition to the regulatory bodies' standards, each healthcare profession's collegial professional body, for example the Royal College of Nursing and the British Medical Association, tends to publish further guidance to facilitate implementation of the regulatory body's standards in professional preparation programmes.

Furthermore, every two to three years, one or more major organisational inquiry into nurse education publishes its findings and makes recommendations. Because of occasional reports of poor nursing care, mainly in the media, the Royal College of Nursing (RCN) (2012), for example, commissioned one such inquiry with the remit to explore the nature of 'excellent preregistration nursing education in the UK' and how it should be delivered. The recommendations of the inquiry, known as the Willis Report, include 'Nursing education should foster professionalism which includes embedding patient safety as its top priority, and respects the dignity and values of service users and their carers' (p. 6).

In relation to fostering professionalism, according to the NMC's (2017: 3) *Enabling Professionalism in Nursing and Midwifery Practice* publication, professionalism 'is characterised by the autonomous evidence-based decision making by members of an occupation who share the same values and education … Professional nurses and midwives demonstrate and embrace accountability for their actions'.

So, maintaining the safety and dignity of service users is a key concept in the Willis Report (RCN, 2012) recommendations, and clearly such recommendations directly indicate elements that pre-registration education should cover and that student nurses must learn – see also the section in Chapter 9 of this book under the heading 'Students raising concerns'. Furthermore, increasingly, healthcare regulators require healthcare education providers to incorporate service-user input into the planning and therefore content of pre-registration courses (e.g. NMC, 2018d, clause 1.12, 2.7), so that students gain a deeper understanding of service users' perceptions and perspectives from their 'lived experiences' of the care and treatment they received when they needed them for their own health problems.

The DH's (2013) *Education Outcomes Framework for Healthcare Workforce* is another prominent publication, whose recommendations have been instituted to influence the content of pre-registration programmes. The framework was developed as a component of the Health and Social Care Act 2012 (DHSC, 2012). When the Act was implemented in 2013, it triggered a radical change in the management of healthcare delivery in England, changes that are still in the process of being consolidated. In relation to the education and training of the healthcare workforce in England, the Act includes the establishment of Health Education England (HEE) for the overseeing and operationalisation of funding for education, although it is set to merge with NHS England/Improvement and NHS Digital in 2023.

Furthermore, for nurse education, in addition to SOP, an extensive range of specific healthcare skills that students must become proficient in are identified by the NMC (2018c), which are grouped under two headings:

- Communication and relationship management skills – which, under four sections, include communication skills for assessing, planning, providing and managing best practice, evidence-based nursing care; for working with people in professional teams, etc.
- Nursing procedures – which are under 11 sections, for example procedures for assessing people's needs for person-centred care.

The student's learning needs: knowledge and competence

In addition to the placement competencies that students are required to learn, as adult learners (Knowles, 2020) students are also likely to have their own aims and thoughts on areas of healthcare knowledge and competence that they would wish to acquire during specific practice placements. This should be encouraged and explicitly supported, as appropriate.

Students acquire knowledge in, say, human physiology, pharmacology and treatment methods, which are components of the NMC's (2018c) seven 'platforms'. The terms *competence* and *competency* are often used in relation to the skills that healthcare students learn. Different types of knowledge are discussed shortly but, first, what do the terms 'competence' and 'competency' mean?

Defining 'competence'

There are conflicting definitions of the terms 'competence' and 'competency' in the literature. As the term *competence* is often used rather glibly, it consequently has several definitions. Overall, in the context of healthcare professions, competence refers to the autonomous application of skills, relevant knowledge, appropriate attitude and values when engaged in service-user clinical care interventions that are safe and effective, and aim to restore, maintain and/or promote health.

However, Benner (2001) sees being competent as being only at the midway point in the 'novice to expert' stages of the skill-acquisition continuum. This is the point where the learner is deemed able to perform the skill safely and effectively unsupervised, but further learning is required to become 'proficient' or 'expert'. Learning beyond being deemed competent by an assessor is also consistent with Stacey et al.'s (2014) argument that learners should progress from being competent to being capable, with capability referring to performing interventions with accountability and having the ability to deal with unfamiliar patient situations. For a detailed analysis of the concept of clinical competence as related to nursing, see Notarnicola et al.'s (2016) article in the Further Optional Reading section of this chapter.

─Reflection point 2.1─

Being competent

Focusing on your own experience of working with colleagues in your healthcare profession, and of students approaching the end of their pre-registration course, consider what being competent means. For example, which pay band or what amount of practice and experience makes a healthcare professional 'competent'? Why does the NMC and HCPC refer to this level of practice as 'proficient'?

Benner (2001) also suggests that the term competence has different interpretations related to skilled performance, and it is described by its intent, function and meanings (as in competency statement). On the other hand, policy and research documents indicate that the terms *competence* and *competent* apply to the person, that is, to the professional's overall knowledge, skills and attitudes and their 'fitness to practise'. The term *competency*, on the other hand, applies to specific clinical skills, which in nursing also include the associated knowledge and attitude components; and from their concept analysis of the term, Axley (2008) deduces that competency is not merely the attainment of skills, knowledge and attitudes, as it also involves the healthcare professional's personal insightfulness, self-assessment, interpretive ability and consideration of team members' points of view.

Types of knowledge base associated with professional skills

The knowledge base required for clinical competence can be grouped in different ways. Schon (1995) notes that healthcare professionals have an accumulated repertoire of knowledge, with mastery over its applications. Benner (2001) identifies practical knowledge and theoretical knowledge, as well as tacit knowledge.

Benner suggests that novices – that is, healthcare professionals who are new to healthcare – are more inclined to use rules and guidelines, such as practical knowledge, while 'expert' healthcare practitioners also use their intuition.

Different types of knowledge that professionals use can also be viewed from Carper's 'patterns of knowing' perspective (cited in Thorne, 2020). They are:

- empirical knowledge: knowledge derived from research and scientific experiments, which therefore can be measured, tested and corroborated
- ethical knowledge: knowledge based on morals and philosophy, but which is usually difficult to test
- aesthetic knowledge: knowledge based on sensitivity or intuition, such as in the 'art of nursing'
- personal knowledge: knowledge of one's self and how it influences one's professional practice.

Each of these 'patterns' of knowledge is seen as being equally important for healthcare practice and for developing further knowledge. Therefore, in relation to physiotherapy and knowledge regarding hip replacement, for instance, empirical knowledge refers to all research evidence related to hip replacement operations, with the patient experiencing less chronic pain and a better quality of life afterwards. Ethical knowledge could refer to whether, say, an 80-year-old widow consents to such an operation – would it still be right to subject her to such a potentially traumatic experience?

Aesthetic knowledge refers to the expertise, extensive experience and intuition of the physiotherapist, for example, to enable the patient to mobilise fully after the operation. Personal knowledge refers to the physiotherapist knowing themselves as a person, their preferences and values, and the effect that these might have on their professional practice.

The learning supervisor's role towards the physiotherapy student would be to enable the student to acquire skills and practical knowledge, which is based on good insight into the student's level of scientific, ethical and personal knowledge. However, for registrants, although colleagues are often the more immediate source of information on which to base clinical decisions, they can also be a source of knowledge of research related to healthcare in the specialist area, and of useful networks. However, as for clinical managers, although the various decisions that they make are based on empirical knowledge, other decisions are often influenced by previous experience and intuition.

Major Views and Perspectives on Learning, Teaching and Education

What is learning?

How individuals learn has been researched and defined over a number of years, as can be expected. So, how do we define learning? How do you define 'learning'?

Generally, dictionaries provide a broad explanation of the term. For instance, to learn is to 'gain knowledge of something or acquire a skill' and 'gain knowledge or skill by experience or by practice' (Brookes and O'Neill, 2017: 525). More specific definitions have come from philosophers, educational psychologists and neuroscientists. They all generally agree that learning is a process that leads to a modification in behaviour or to the acquisition of new abilities or responses, and which is additional to natural physiological development, growth or maturation.

Accordingly, Gagné et al. (2005: 3) define learning as a process that leads to a change in a learner's disposition and capabilities that can be reflected in behaviour. This is a near universally accepted definition of learning that suggests that learning changes something in the person as a person and adds to the things they are able to do (mentally or physically). Then, after learning, the new disposition or capability persists over a substantial period of time.

Similarly, Curzon and Tummons (2013: 11) define learning as 'the apparent modification of a person's behaviour through his or her activities and experiences, so that his or her knowledge, skills and attitudes, including modes of adjustment, towards their environment, are changed, more or less permanently'. Furthermore, Barron et al. (2015) identify multiple definitions of learning (see more information in the further reading section), despite which the definitions tend to concur that:

- learning is reflected in changes in behaviour, physicality and attitudes
- learning occurs in day-to-day life experiences, in addition to planned formal education
- learning a psychomotor skill is permanent in nature in that the individual subsequently has the abilty to perform the skilled act at future points in time.

In healthcare professions, learning is a lifelong process of skill and knowledge acquisition, updating them through planned participation in focused reading and structured programmes of study. This is because specialist skills may 'decay' (e.g. become outdated) mainly due to such factors as changes in medical devices, social values and so on. Learning in the healthcare professions is about learning competence and knowledge, the nature of which was discussed earlier.

Perspectives on learning

Learning experiences are influenced by where the learner 'is coming from', as each person perceives new experiences in a different way, depending on how the new experience relates to the individual's past. However, two opposing views about formal learning are suggested by Ramsden (2003), who identifies learning as either: (a) a quantitative accretion of knowledge, i.e. facts and procedures; or (b) a change in the way in which people interpret and understand the world around them.

Moreover, according to Socrates (2000 years ago), education is not merely transferring knowledge of facts and procedures from 'teacher' to 'pupil'. Rather, it is 'an adventure, an activity of the mind, a pursuit demanding reflection, analysis and investigation, a social activity undertaken by equals freely associated to engage in dialogue' (Jeffs, 2003: 28). This adventure and activity is also referred to as the 'process' of learning.

Radical distinctions are also made by Freire (2005 – first published 1970), who argues that there are two contrasting perspectives on education and learning, which he identifies as the 'banking' concept of education versus 'problem posing'. On the one hand, the banking concept is the traditional mode of learning and involves the teacher helping a student fill their mind with knowledge, which is later 'cashed out' relatively unchanged, for example in written or verbal examinations. On the other hand, the problem-posing approach to education is education through dialogue, in which the facilitator and students meet and exchange ideas and experiences through critical discussions and debate. Neither the facilitator nor the students necessarily have the 'right' answer as there is room for 'multiple realities'.

Another perspective is provided by Peters (1966, 1973) regarding the differentiation between training and education. What distinctions would you draw between education and training, between nurse education and nurse training, for example? Peters (1966) notes that training means knowledge and skill development devised to bring about some specific end. However, the aims of education, he notes, are that:

- something of value is being passed on and learned
- the individual comes to care about the learning involved, to develop understanding and to achieve
- what is being learned must have a place in a coherent pattern of life, that is, relevance among other things in life.

Therefore, education 'implies that something worthwhile is being, or has been, intentionally transmitted in a morally acceptable manner ... The educated person is one whose life has been transformed by the deepening and widening of his understanding and sensitivity. To be educated is not to arrive at a destination; it is to travel with a different view' (Peters, 1973: 122).

These perspectives on learning correspond with the concepts of teacher-centred learning and student-centred learning, which are discussed in Chapter 3. So how do the definitions and these views on learning and education apply to, or compare with, the approaches taken in healthcare profession education curricula?

━━━━━━━━━ **ACTION POINT 2.2** ━━━━━━━━━

Different perspectives on nurse education

Discuss with a course or work-based peer your thoughts on how far Ramsden's (2003), Freire's (2005) and Peters' (1966, 1973) perspectives on learning apply to professional education related to your healthcare profession. Is there an equally well-researched perspective on learning that is more contemporary?

In nurse education, the difference between education and training is that the word 'training' is usually associated with developing the ability to take an approved set of actions to perform a certain clinical task. This is thought of as a convergent process of learning to complete a task competently. Education, however, is seen as a divergent process in that, in addition to initially learning the step-by-step actions needed to perform a task, the healthcare professional is also constantly reflecting on each action in the context of their deep knowledge-base background, principles, values, ethics and effect on the recipient individual.

Education does not stop at a predetermined point of attainment, but progresses further in the development of critical ability and, consequently, the individual remains open to learning new knowledge, principles and perspectives. Education facilitators should therefore provide an environment where students feel sufficiently supported to decide on areas and depth of learning, as long as the core curriculum aims are achieved.

Where do healthcare learners learn?

Naturally, learning does not occur only in university classrooms through lectures, workshops and books, as it also has to occur in work-based settings during healthcare service-user contact. Learning occurs in skill laboratories and in the ward teaching room or office. Furthermore, learning occurs in the trust's postgraduate or in-service training departments. In the practice setting, learning can be informal, gained from structured teaching sessions, or opportunistic.

Additionally, learning occurs in the university's student common room, in informal social meetings and even 'in car parks, in corridors, over tea as well as through unnoticed patterns of behaviour and interaction in the classroom itself' (Field, 1999: 12). This notion that learning can come from friends and peers and in a whole range of settings is referred to as 'social capital' (Gopee, 2002). A corresponding notion is 'human capital', which refers to the self-investment of time and effort by individuals through learning at university or in public libraries, as well as at home and in the non-traditional places suggested by Field (1999). Learning occurs everywhere, including, for example, in therapies. Learning contributes to progress, and notions such as the 'learning society' and 'learning organisation' (in that most companies have training departments, and foster learning from customer comments) have evolved.

Lately, other effective ways of 'social' learning have been recognised, such as 'communities of practice' and 'action learning sets' – the first being more informal and the latter more formal, but both are equally effective. Communities of practice refer to groups of people sharing a passion for something of interest, which they want to know more and more about or do, and learn by interacting regularly, as identified by Wenger (2000) and Webber (2017). The learning that ensues is not necessarily intentional, but is achieved by sharing information with each other, and building relationships that enable learning from each other (e.g. Morley, 2016) and by engaging within the community of practice.

The feasibility and benefits of students learning from each other are increasingly being recognised, as also noted, for example, by Nygren and Carlson (2017). Additionally, students studying for a specific subject have an overall common interest, but smaller groups of students may develop a 'passion' for specific sub-topics and meet informally to research and learn more and more about the sub-topic. The same may apply to health and social care professionals in relation to their specialist area (e.g. Leggat et al., 2014). Action learning sets are more formal classroom- or meeting-room-based discussions on pre-identified curricular topics, as confirmed by research (e.g. Walia and Marks-Maran, 2014).

Theories Underpinning Learning

There are a number of theories of learning that can underpin professional education programmes. Exploration of these theories has taken place over several decades. It has swung between theories of learning, models of learning, principles of learning and styles of learning, with theories and styles of learning being the more popular concepts at the beginning of the twenty-first century. This section examines the different published theories of learning, that is, different attempts to explain how people learn.

So, a theory tends to imply or endeavour to explain cause and effect, that is, if we do x, then y should happen; or y happens because we do x. For instance, if the Smiths send their child to an independent school, then they will have a better chance of securing a student place in a reputable university. That is a theory. According to the dictionary (Brookes and O'Neill, 2017: 970), a theory is a 'set of ideas based on evidence and careful reasoning, which offers an explanation of how something works, or why something happens, but has not been completely proved'.

Similarly, the Merriam-Webster (2022) dictionary defines a theory as 'a plausible or scientifically acceptable general principle or body of principles offered to explain phenomena'. Consequently, a learning theory, the humanistic learning theory, for example, is an organised view of a group of concepts that should result in a better understanding and explanation of how we learn, and therefore lead to more effective learning.

There are at least ten schools of thought, theories or models of learning, which have all created different definitions and incorporate a variety of concepts, but most of them have evolved from the three more robust learning theories, namely:

- behaviourist learning theories
- cognitive learning theories
- humanistic learning theories.

Behaviourist learning theories

Most learning theories belong to the field of psychology, which, in the earlier part of the twentieth century, used to be about introspection, that is, thinking deeply about how mental processes work. However, gradually there was a move away from this paradigm (see, for example, Nolen-Hoeksema et al., 2014) and it was suggested that psychology should be a science, and psychological theories should be based on observable and quantifiable data, that is, those manifested in changes in behaviour. Initially, psychologists worked with animals to observe behaviour changes, and later researched people's behaviour changes.

Behaviourist learning theories refer to learning through the response to particular stimuli, resulting in classical conditioning or operant conditioning. Classical conditioning refers to changes in behaviour through stimulus–response, whereby the desirable responses to particular stimuli, that is, newly learned behaviours, are rewarded. Operant conditioning is a subsequent development by Skinner (1971) and others, whereby approximations of desired behaviour are rewarded and thereby the target behaviour develops gradually. Being rewarded for new learning is also known as 'positive reinforcement' and can be external, in the form of verbal affirmations from the teacher – for example, using such statements as 'well done', or through material rewards; or they can be internal, received through self-satisfaction from the learning, for instance.

Behaviourist learning theory can be applied in healthcare professionals' education programmes. For instance, operant conditioning can be effectively applied when students with a weak academic background might achieve high levels in academia if earlier attempts are positively reinforced. Overall, healthcare learners are positively internally reinforced, by feeling a sense of achievement on being able to perform new healthcare skills, and externally through their practice supervisors acknowledging or recognising their newly developed competence.

Another example is that gaining praise for becoming competent at a particular clinical skill, or part-skills, towards the desired competent performance, can positively motivate the student and make them want to learn new skills. Thus, praiseworthy performances or approximations of competent practice or of part-skills by healthcare learners, are rewarded or positively reinforced.

Social learning theory builds on these early behaviourist theories whereby the individual observes the competent behaviour or skill performance of professionals, learns the behaviour and reproduces it, and if the attempt is positively reinforced then that behaviour or skill is likely to be adopted. It refers to the behaviour, attitudes and values of teachers or other role models that may be replicated by learners in the same way (Bandura, 1996), and thus learned in social situations, as discussed in Chapter 1.

Theories, sub-theories and inherent concepts of learning can be grouped in different ways by different authors, but such classification is mostly only an academic exercise. However, such groupings can disentangle the multifarious theories of learning, and therefore a tentative summary of sub-theories of learning and some inherent concepts emanating from the three main theories are presented in Table 2.1.

Table 2.1　Learning theories, sub-theories and some inherent concepts

Learning theories	Sub-theories	Some inherent concepts
Behaviourist learning theories	Bandura's social learning theory	Reinforcement for learning Operant conditioning Role model Vicarious and opportunistic learning
Cognitive learning theories	Gestalt theory of learning; Piaget's stages of intellectual/cognitive development	Insightful learning Discovery learning Constructivism The 'aha!' phenomenon Experiential learning Reflective practice Ripples model of learning
	Ausubel et al.'s assimilation theory	Information processing 'Flipping' method Situated learning
Humanistic learning theories	Alan Rogers' characteristics of adult education and andragogy	Andragogy or adult learning Self-directed learning Learning contracts Peer learning
	Carl Rogers' student-centred approach to learning	Student-centred teaching Experiential learning Problem-based learning Social capital
	Maslow's hierarchy of human needs	Learning for self-actualisation and growth
	Kohlberg's moral development (Sanders, 2018)	Stages of moral development

Cognitive learning theories

As just indicated, behaviourist learning theories initially constituted an attempt to make psychology more scientific and empirical. More recently, various education sectors, including nurse education, have incorporated aspects of behaviourist theories and social learning theory into their professional education programmes, for example through systematic feedback to students on their knowledge and competence, and through consciousness of being a role model for learners.

Subsequent to research by Piaget (1962), the work of Ausubel et al. (1978) and others led to the evolution of cognitive learning theories, which take the view that learning is an internal purposive action involving thinking, perception, information processing and memory. Cognitive learning theories include:

- the Gestalt theory of learning – entailing insightful learning, the 'aha' phenomenon
- Ausubel et al.'s assimilation theory – which incorporates information processing
- experiential learning – learning through engaging in practical activities, followed by reflection.

Cognitive learning theories were initially based on animal experiments by Kohler (1925), but all three above-mentioned theories can be applied to healthcare professional education programmes. They include learning by insight (or insightful learning) emanating from problem-solving situations, which overlaps with Gestalt learning theory, which in turn refers to seeing the whole picture, while insight is gained through the 'aha' phenomenon, that is the sudden realisation of a solution to a problem, or how various parts fit into a pattern, for instance the 'penny-dropping' experience.

The Gestalt theory of learning (e.g. Koffka, 1935) can be applied to professional education programmes by structuring learning so that learners are given problem situations to resolve (such as in problem-based learning), and through group discussions, analysing ideas and trial and error, whereby particular insights are gained. Thus, group discussions as well as project work, self-directed learning and peer learning can enable this process. Implementation of problem situations that can be used in teaching include, for instance, asking a small group of students to resolve a snapshot of a clinical situation, such as helping a patient with partial paralysis move from a bed to a chair safely.

To a notable extent, Bruner's (1960) discovery learning theory refers to insightful learning. It involves situations that are devised in such a way that the learner can discover principles and underlying techniques for themselves. It also involves the use of past experience and existing knowledge to form new insights. For instance, a student who witnesses a patient with asthma gain relief from distressed breathing by using their inhaler, can gain further insight into the specific functions of bronchioles and alveoli in oxygen transfer that they previously encountered in books or lectures.

Ausubel et al.'s (1978) assimilation theory is based on the view that most meaningful cognitive learning takes place as a result of interaction between the knowledge (cognitive structures) that the individual already possesses, and new information that the individual encounters. Thus, the single most important factor influencing learning is the knowledge that the learner already has. This forms the basis for the transfer of learning, in that, for instance, once the learner comprehends the principles of asepsis in hospital settings, the knowledge and comprehension can be adapted in community care settings.

Thus, Ausubel et al.'s (1978) assimilation theory refers to activating the relevant knowledge that the student already has so as to assimilate new knowledge into their existing mental structures. This also increases retention, and is therefore also relevant for adult learners, as they already have substantial knowledge prior to starting on an academic course.

For new information to be 'received and assimilated' or subsumed into an anchoring structure or schema, Ausubel and his colleagues suggest giving the learner prior reading or the opportunity to engage in particular activities in preparation for the teaching session (referred to as 'advanced organisers', and more recently as 'flipping'). The advanced organiser creates an anchoring structure for the new knowledge, like a scaffolding of the individual's existing knowledge on which to build what the student needs to know. For instance, prior to a practice placement with a physiotherapist, the learner could be advised to revise or learn about the microstructure of muscles, in readiness for learning how they are strengthened through exercises by a patient who has had a broken leg operated on.

Cognitive learning theory therefore involves learning by participation, and continually taking into consideration the person's previous knowledge and competence, such as clinical skills already learnt by the student on previous placements, and university skills laboratories.

Experiential learning refers to learning by doing, albeit supervised, rather than by merely being informed by teachers about a particular topic. It can be achieved by building simulation activities in teaching–learning sessions, for instance, as advocated by Kolb (2014), among others. Experiential learning is therefore a component of reflective learning.

─**Reflection point 2.2**─────────────

Learning from experience

Consider the question: Do we learn from all experiences we come across in our day-to-day activities?

In response to Reflection Point 2.2, you might have felt we can't be learning all the time, that is, all of our 16 waking hours each day, every day of the year. On researching how much we learn from all the situations that we encounter each day, minute by minute, Jarvis (2010) found that there are several situations in life that are non-learning situations, while other situations do present learning opportunities, but in different ways. Jarvis identified ten types of learning encounters, as briefly summarised in the box below. The list does not include self-directed learning, nor styles of learning, as they are concepts of learning that fall under humanistic learning theories.

Ten Types of Learning Encounters

Non-learning   When we encounter a situation that we have dealt with before, we respond to it in the same way as before (also referred to as presumption), and no new approach to dealing with the situation is required

Non-consideration   When we are presented with a new learning situation but we do not take it up, which may be because we are simply not interested in it, we are too busy, or the topic area feels too complex

Rejection   When we consciously or deliberately reject a learning opportunity, maybe because we have had negative experiences related to that situation in the past, or because we sense information overload

Ambivalence   Conflict between our thinking and our emotions can leave us undecided about whether to pursue a line of learning

Incidental learning   Also referred to as *pre-conscious knowledge learning*, we sometimes learn without realising we have; we also learn through our bodily senses, e.g. by the scent or look of something

Memorisation   Learning facts and recalling them without much thinking being involved, or learning them for short-term or longer-term use

Emotional learning   When we think about what we are learning which gradually becomes a part of our feelings and attitude

Action learning   Learning from participation in skilled activities, but may include learning by 'trial and error'

Discovery learning   When we find a solution to a problem that we are presented with, or by conducting experiments

Reflective learning   Also referred to as contemplation, learning by deliberately reflecting on a situation very soon after the event

Jarvis' types of learning acknowledge the reality that there are particular situations that do not lend themselves to much learning for each individual, that is, non-learning experiences. Learning by memorisation is also referred to as non-reflective learning and includes rote learning, and also temporary learning such as a telephone number for one-off use.

However, reflective learning focuses on the important part that experience and deliberate contemplation play in the learning process. Reflective learning refers to the learning that occurs as a result of systematic reflection on situations just encountered. Increasingly, healthcare students and registrants are using e-portfolios to record their reflections on course-related situations that they encounter, either during practice placements or when discussing health profession matters, either formally in classroom settings or informally at other venues (e.g. Tickle et al., 2022).

Consider Case Study 2.1 – a reflective recording in the portfolio of a student social worker, Sheila.

─Case study 2.1─

Sheila's portfolio recording

I visited Mr J while his care coordinator, who is also my practice supervisor, was on annual leave. At this time, Mr J expressed concern about his care coordinator and questioned her supportive abilities. My initial reaction to this problematic situation was to explain that different practitioners would use different approaches, and I advised him to raise the issue with the care coordinator. In a further conversation by telephone, Mr J reiterated the issue but in a more agitated manner and asked me to speak to the care coordinator. His care coordinator suggested that we visit Mr J together to question him about what he actually wanted from the service and what type of support he felt she should offer. She felt Mr J didn't always engage with services (he frequently missed appointments), and that his drug-addiction problem was the issue he most needed to address, but which she did not specialise in. Mr J was receiving services from the drug team but, again, he didn't always attend his appointments. However, it was clear Mr J felt he needed more support. As a result, we discussed a referral to an agency which provided outreach support specifically for people with a history of offending and drug/alcohol abuse problems. Mr J was keen to accept this support.

I deduced from managing Mr J's situation that the negotiated line of care and treatment can be more effective than prescribed routes, and it is also consistent with person-centred practice that treats the service user as an individual with his own thoughts and preferences.

Reflective recordings from clinical situations provide an essential learning vehicle for students. Case Study 2.1 demonstrates the purpose of reflection, which is learning from the situation or 'incident', despite being only a brief account. Kolb (2014), for instance, suggests that learning can be conceived of as a four-stage learning cycle that involves identifying the immediate concrete experience or an incident as the basis for observation and reflection. Out of this cycle arise new concepts for hypothesis and theory building. Implications of these are considered in new situations and then theory is confirmed, adjusted or advanced.

This form of learning is widely used in general and professional education programmes. Individuals are encouraged to learn from problematic new situations or 'critical incidents' that they encounter, to analyse them in the context of published literature and to record them systematically in their portfolios. These can also comprise assessed work components of their programme of study.

The rationale for reflective practice in healthcare is that it is also a means of constructing or generating knowledge from incidents. The origins of reflection on incidents go back to times when, for instance, techniques for dealing with aggressive behaviour in mental health nursing were minimal. When clinical staff met after such incidents to discuss the situation, they started realising that if cues and signs of potential violence were identified in the individual patient before the disruptive incident actually occurred, they could take certain actions to prevent it from happening in the first place. This was formalised and seen as a therapeutic means that could be used, step by step, to prevent the disruptive incident, and also to gain a better understanding of the service user's thinking. This also constituted constructing knowledge from clinical practice.

Similar 'concrete experiences' have led to changes in clinical practice, such as use of the triage system in Accident and Emergency departments, and to ensuring that normal saline solution is at room temperature or above, prior to using it for wound cleansing. Some of these examples are noted in Chapter 6, in the context of practice development.

Kolb's (2014) four-stage learning cycle, from the initial concrete experience or incident, through to exploring the experience retrospectively so that it leads to new learning, generalising from the new learning, to applying new learning to similar new situations, is presented as a closed circle with the fourth stage (applying new learning) leading to the first (the initial concrete experience). However, it is likely that the new learning may not be fully effective when applied to similar new situations, or even to identical new incidents, and therefore it becomes another new experience or incident to learn from.

Consequently, the experiential learning cycle can be presented more meaningfully as a spiral that shows that applying new learning to similar situations must be undertaken with an open mind, as further learning might ensue in the light of new evidence and evolving social changes, as well as possibly research (see Figure 2.1).

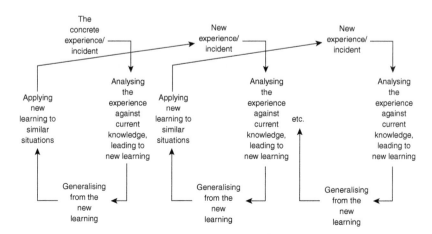

Figure 2.1   The experiential learning spiral

Adapting (i.e. making small changes) to published models and frameworks in one's teaching and learning is not uncommon, and can in fact be recommended as they are applied to specific groups of people or activities. This is also because Kolb's model of learning has its critics. For example, Bergsteiner et al. (2010) thoroughly examined Kolb's learning cycle and argue that the graphics of the model are flawed, and suggest changes. Rogers and Horrocks (2010) argue that since learning from new experiences requires 'critical reflection', all learning cycles need to be adapted in the search for new principles before new conclusions are reached.

Nonetheless, teachers and students can utilise alternative models of reflection, such as Johns' (2017) model of reflective practice, which involves (1) description of the incident; (2) reflection on what the professional was trying to achieve; (3) influencing factors; (4) alternative strategies; and (5) learning from the experience.

For instance, when the student reflects on a clinical intervention that they encounter for the first time during a practice placement, they can afterwards describe the experience in detail. This could take place in their professional portfolio or in a structured setting, maybe with support from a peer or a senior member of staff in a climate of mutual support. Next, the student can reflect on the aims of the intervention and how the student felt during the procedure. They can then think about the clinician's 'internal and external factors' that determined their actions. Thereafter, they have to explore the alternative actions that could have been taken, and learning ensues from them.

Thus, the student develops and generates further insight into the new experience. However, to benefit from this concept, the scheduling of the reflection process should ensure that time is made available during practice placements, or on return to university, for structured reflection, consolidation and evaluation.

Constructivism

Also increasingly popular as a further development of cognitive learning theories, is the 'constructivist' learning theory. As a concept that was pioneered previously by Berger and Luckmann (1967) as the 'social construction of reality', constructivism refers to how individuals construct new thoughts, images, concepts and theories from structured and new or incidental experiences, that are 'scaffolded' onto the individual's existing current and past knowledge. A further evolving ensuing term is 'constructionism', which refers to specific instances of creation of knowledge from life experiences and encounters with learning situations.

Constructivism is founded on the premise that, by reflecting on our experiences, each one of us constructs our own unique understanding of learning encounters, and in the quest for meaning, we construct our own mental images and models of reality. Thereby, the student does not accept verbatim all knowledge presented to them, but assimilates it in the context of their prior knowledge and their current social surroundings. Research findings on constructivism, as a basis for effective learning, include those of a study by Duane and Satre (2014) that supports the uses of this theory.

Furthermore, Choe et al. (2014) conducted a study examining the effect of two constructivist teaching strategies, namely action learning and 'cross-examination debate', and concluded that both strategies enable active interaction among students which can enhance their adaptability in practice settings and self-knowledge. Problem-based learning is another teaching strategy that can incorporate the principles of constructivism.

Humanistic learning theories

A third group of theories that have been developed with regard to how learning occurs are humanistic learning theories, which include:

1. Alan Rogers' characteristics of adult education and andragogy
2. Maslow's learning as self-actualisation
3. Carl Rogers' student-centred approach to teaching.

Humanistic learning theorists claim that the preceding theories omit aspects of human existence such as feelings, attitudes and values, and thereby overlook the more holistic perspective that incorporates attitudinal components of learning. They suggest that learning should be concerned with personal human growth. Students can therefore learn concepts, theories, models and propositions (i.e. 'propositional knowledge') from books and other learning resources, and spend more classroom time on experiential learning activities, which include thinking processes that also incorporate an exploration of values, attitudes and feelings.

Healthcare profession students as adult learners

In the context of the more holistic humanistic theories of learning, adult learning, which is often referred to as andragogy, is one that has been well-researched, and includes self-directed learning and student-centred teaching.

―――Reflection point 2.3―――――――――――――――――――――――――――

Students as adult learners

Consider the question: Should ways of teaching adults be different from ways of teaching school children or college students? That is, what is different about adult students in contrast to school or college pupils? Think of reasons for your answer.

Both Knowles (2020) and Rogers and Horrocks (2010) suggest various ways in which teaching adults, or adult education, is different from teaching children.

A prominent underpinning assumption about the preferred way of learning by adult learners is that they are competent at self-directed learning. Teaching adults includes teaching university students on generic or professional courses. Some of the differences, as suggested by nurses on post-registration courses, are identified in Table 2.2.

Table 2.2   Differences in the ways in which adults and children learn

How children learn	How adults learn
• Children have a shorter attention span, and therefore a variety of learning activities is needed, including starter activities. • Teaching children is pedagogy, e.g. imparting knowledge to them. • Children are more open to new ideas. • There is a need to reinforce information over time.	• Adults are (usually) self-motivated to learn. • Adults may have relevant (or faulty) professional and life experiences. • Open discussion is more feasible in adult groups. • Lesson content can be adjusted based on ongoing evaluation of learning needs.

However, in both instances, an effective student–teacher relationship is important and has to be based on mutual trust. Different teachers may have their own repertoire of different teaching techniques and styles when teaching adult students. Rogers and Horrocks (2010) conclude by identifying the characteristics of adult students or learners as individuals who:

- define themselves and have a self-image as adult students
- are in the middle of a process of growth, not at the start of the process
- bring with them a package of experience and values
- come to learning with intentions
- bring with them expectations about the learning process
- have competing interests
- already have their own set patterns of learning.

Moreover, from adult educators' professional perspectives, adult education (or andragogy) also requires a consideration of whether the adult student is merely biologically adult or merely of legally adult age, or is also a psychologically and socially responsible adult.

──**Reflection point 2.4**──────────────

Adult education in healthcare courses

How far is the adult learning approach relevant or applicable to education of healthcare students?

The above-mentioned characteristics of adult learners suggest that adult students' learning can be facilitated more effectively within an ethos of self-directed learning. Practice supervisors tend to build self-directed learning into practice placement programmes for learners by allocating time for consulting relevant learning resources or exploring further relevant clinical experiences.

One of the aims of adult education is to enable individuals to realise that they are the initiators of their learning. Accordingly, although substantial knowledge and skill are acquired after becoming a registered nurse, it is up to the individual professional to decide which areas of learning they need to participate in. This learning could be instigated by specialism-based experiences, and the self-direction becomes career-long.

Self-directed learning (SDL) is a key feature of adult education, and research tends to support this mode of learning, indicating that students who actively engage in SDL undergo a transformation from initial negative feelings such as confusion and frustration, culminating gradually in a sense of self-confidence and skills for lifelong learning. From a qualitative study that explored midwives' perception of SDL, Embo et al. (2014) concluded that midwives do benefit from SDL, although it needs to be supported by a feedback culture for enhanced effectiveness. In another study, Phillips et al. (2015) used a 'Self-directed Learning Readiness Scale' to ascertain student nurses' readiness for SDL, and found that first-year students show less readiness for SDL than more senior students, while those with a previous first degree show higher readiness.

However, another side to SDL in adult education is highlighted by Hughes (1999), who indicates that this approach is not necessarily 'emancipatory' as it can be a 'repressive instrument', in that it can marginalise the benefits of group and peer learning in education settings. Hughes suggests that governments might misuse SDL by arguing that less central funding is required when applying SDL in student education.

However, from their research on SDL, Du Toit-Brits and Van Zyl (2017) concluded by identifying the characteristics of effective self-directed learners, which include: self-determination to learn, assertiveness, self-discipline, being organised, perseverance, a high degree of self-motivation, inquisitiveness, and being goal oriented, that facilitators of learning should help learners develop or strengthen in themselves.

─Reflection point 2.5─

Characteristics of self-directed learners

Consider the characteristics of self-directed learners identified by Du Toit-Brits and Van Zyl, and reflect for yourself on whether you already have these characteristics. Which of these characteristics do your students tend to portray or exercise?

Specific competencies are required for facilitating effective SDL, according to Knowles (2020). In light of the above-mentioned general characteristics of adult learners, and the required teacher competencies, it can be concluded that in healthcare:

- Adult education constitutes collaborative activities between teachers and learners (and can include use of a learning agreement).
- Teaching should build on learners' professional experience.
- Learners should participate in identifying their learning needs, setting learning outcomes and evaluating learning.
- The role of the teacher is that of a facilitator.
- The outcome of the teaching and learning encounter should be to enable the individual to develop into a responsible autonomous learner.

The implications of the above examination of SDL for practice supervisors is that it cannot be assumed that, even as adults, students are necessarily competent or willing to be self-directed learners, and therefore several may need guidance on which areas of knowledge and skills they should pursue to enhance their learning during practice placements.

Using learning contracts

During practice placements, practice supervisors usually make their facilitation of learning even more effective by the use of learning contracts, a mechanism that is very much a feature of adult education, and involves negotiated and self-directed learning (e.g. Knowles, 2020) between teacher and student. As the word contract implies, a learning contract is a written and signed agreement between teacher (practice supervisor in this case) and student, resulting in the latter's active involvement in decisions over practice objectives and other areas of related learning. Therefore, learning contracts are usually an essential feature of practice placement learning, with each party's responsibility in the achievement of the objectives identified.

The agreed set of objectives in learning contracts of course includes the learning outcomes of the course curriculum, and because the learning contract affords the student some control and responsibility over their learning, it also motivates them to engage more widely with the placement experience. Further, it is a medium for identifying the student's pace of learning, to explore the means of theory and practice integration, and can be supported by ascertaining the student's preferred learning style.

A learning contract section or template is usually already included in the student's placement competencies document, and the practice supervisor and student discuss and agree on how learning will take place, and precisely how they will know that their objectives have been achieved. These are usually written down by the student and, when agreed, both practice supervisor and student sign and date the contract. Learning pathways based on patient journeys can be incorporated as a strategy for achieving particular objectives. An example of a learning contract is presented in Template 2.1.

Template 2.1   A learning contract

Name of student:			Cohort:	
Placement:			Practice supervisor's name:	
Learning needs	Objectives	Resource and strategies	Target date	Evidence of achievement
What do I want to learn? – Topic area	What do I want to have achieved at the end of this learning? – Specific outcomes	How will I learn, and who will support me?	Date of achieving the objectives	How will I know I have achieved my intended learning?
1. Assessment of a new patient	Able to assess the health and care needs of newly admitted/ referred patient/service user	Practice supervisor, dietician	30-05-2023	Practice supervisor reviews and agrees with my assessment and care plan
2. Teach patients	Able to teach a type 2 diabetic patient how to adhere to their dietary plan	Practice supervisor, dietician. Consult diet sheets, guidelines. Read up on type 2 diabetes	30-05-2023	Practice supervisor observes my teaching and signs me as competent in this skill
3.	...			
Agreed contract				
Signature of student:			Date:	
Practice supervisor's signature:			Date:	
Name of academic link lecturer/practice education facilitator:				
Comments on achievement of contract objectives:				
Signature of student:			Date:	
Practice supervisor's signature:			Date:	

Crucial components of the learning contract include the specific resources (human and material) that are required to enable the student to achieve the agreed objectives and also the specific dates by which each objective will have been achieved. An alternative to a learning contract is a 'learning agreement' (RCN, 2017; University of St Andrews, 2022), which has similar features but might not include the signatures of those involved, nor rigid 'achieve-by' dates.

After both parties have signed the learning contract, the achievement of the outcomes should be constantly monitored to gauge the student's progress with them. Furthermore, learning contracts should not be seen as a chore, nor as a mere formality, because they constitute an effective vehicle for integration of theory and practice in the practice setting for social work students, for example, as noted by Boitel and Fromm (2014). They suggest that the learning contract requires the student to think about the relationships among the classroom-taught application of learning, the practice placement experiences, and the competencies that need to be achieved, and does so with efficacy.

The practice supervisor will have developed knowledge and understanding of the use of learning contracts as part of the practice supervisor preparation programme, along with how they can deliver these functions in the context of other roles that they have to fulfil. Moreover, Rogers and Freiberg (1994) indicate that learning contracts endow the student with some freedom to learn aspects that they wish to learn and pursue areas that they find particularly interesting. A learning contract is also a medium for resolving any doubt that there may be about specific purposes of the learning experience. It clarifies the activities that the student would engage in and provides motivation and reinforcement through the achievement of objectives.

Learning and self-actualisation

Another humanistic learning theory focuses on individuals' need for self-actualisation, which, according to Maslow's (1987) theory of a hierarchy of human needs, is the highest-level need, other ones being our physiological needs, safety needs, the need for belongingness, and our self-esteem needs. It could be argued therefore that the goal of education is to assist individuals to achieve self-actualisation, to help the person to become the best that they are able to become with the resources that are accessible.

Consequently, teachers and practice supervisors normally have some awareness of the student's basic needs, such as the need to belong to the team, or of anything that the student might be preoccupied with. Maslow also observed that there are a number of characteristics of individuals who achieve self-actualisation, which include them:

- demonstrating acceptance of self and others
- accepting problems as learning opportunities
- demonstrating democratic character

- having a philosophical, non-hostile sense of humour
- showing creativeness
- seeming to transcend any culture.

Student-centred teaching

Renowned thinkers and researchers on how students learn, including Carl Rogers (1983), have, over the years, argued that teaching may be an overrated activity, and that the focus should be on learning instead. To shift the focus to effective learning, Rogers and Freiberg (1994) have advocated the use of empathic understanding, genuineness and being non-judgemental in learning situations. These activities are helping skills that have been successfully transferred from therapeutic counselling activities to student learning situations. The teacher consequently becomes the facilitator of student-centred teaching, as is also advocated by Freire (2005) and Knowles (2020).

Consequently, the facilitator achieves student-centred teaching by creating an appropriate environment and identifying the required resources for learning, and thereby empowers students to become responsible for their learning, to develop self-awareness and to think of alternative answers to questions posed by the teacher. Student-centred teaching is also examined in Chapter 3.

Teachers and practice supervisors tend to apply the above-mentioned theories of learning as appropriate, and student-centred teaching with particular groups of students. However, on reviewing the main prevailing theories of learning, Race (2014: xii–xiii) observed that most theories are worded in academic technical language used by educational psychologists that the majority of readers find cumbersome and not easy to comprehend. He therefore constituted his theory of learning using much simpler words, which he termed the 'ripples on a pond' model of learning, which in turn identifies seven fundamental factors underpinning successful learning, namely:

- wanting to learn
- taking ownership of the need to learn
- learning by doing
- learning through feedback
- making sense of what is being learned
- verbalising or speaking – to deepen learning
- making informed judgements – assessing.

The ripples model of learning is a more recent further development of experiential learning and is therefore rooted in 'learning by doing'. Race argues that the seven factors underpinning learning occur in sequence, with each factor (or stage or ripple) interacting with those next to it, much like a pebble falling into a pond and creating ripples, with each stage moving in backward and forward directions. It is presented as concentric circles. It is interesting to note that the first three 'ripples' tend to represent learners' motivation and the actions that they take to learn, which constitute factors that are crucial for effective learning.

Race's ripples model of learning can be incorporated in educating healthcare profession students by ensuring that each factor is achieved, by supporting and reinforcing the student's motivation to learn, creating the medium for 'learning by doing', by giving feedback and creating opportunities for students to teach others.

Learners' approaches to learning and learning styles

In addition to the perspectives on learning explored at the beginning of this chapter, and different learning theories, learning is also influenced by the different approaches to learning adopted by individuals, and their styles of learning.

Students' approaches to learning

Students' specific alternative approaches to learning have been identified through extensive research on how students learn. One of the main proponents of approaches to learning is Ramsden (2003), which is also further analysed by Biggs and Tang (2022). Ramsden's research, which builds on the findings of previous researchers, identified individuals who take a deep approach to learning, those who take a surface approach and those who take the strategic approach. Students tend to adopt one of these three approaches, depending on the level of individual commitment to particular episodes of learning. The defining features of each approach are presented in the box below.

Deep, Surface and Strategic Approaches to Learning by Students

Deep approach

- Engages with full interest with the course content
- Examines logic and argument, and does so cautiously and critically
- Relates ideas to previous knowledge and experience
- Checks evidence and conclusions drawn
- Looks for patterns and underlying principles

Surface approach

- Studies without reflecting on the knowledge presented
- Treats the course as unrelated sections, with bits of knowledge
- Memorises facts and procedures in relation to assessments
- Experiences difficulty in making sense of the new ideas presented
- Feels undue pressure and worries about coursework

Strategic approach

- Puts consistent effort into studying
- Ensures the conditions and materials for studying are appropriate
- Manages or organises time and effort to greatest effect
- Is alert to assessment requirements and criteria, and pays attention to cues about marking schemes
- Gears learning to the perceived preferences of lecturers

Whether a student takes the deep or surface approach to learning might also depend on the stage of development of the subject area. Social sciences and arts may warrant a deep approach, while parts of science subjects such as biology, and law might be perceived as only requiring surface approaches, at least in the earlier stages, because they often constitute factual, single-answer knowledge. Newer and less factual subjects might also warrant a deep approach.

Approaches to learning also relate to the quality of the learning undertaken. Ramsden (2003) reports that if someone treated learning as an external imposition and concentrated on memorising facts, then that person was taking a surface approach to learning, and this would result in poor knowledge and understanding of the subject. Alternatively, if they intended to understand, and interacted conscientiously with the content of the knowledge presented to them (a deep approach), they stand a better chance of getting the author's or teacher's message and arguments. As for adapting to the student's approach to learning, the practice supervisor would prefer the student to take a deep approach but, during very busy times, strategic and surface approaches might temporarily be relevant.

Major learning styles

In contrast to learning theories and students' approaches to learning, learning styles refer to the unique but habitual ways in which individuals tend to, or prefer to, respond to learning situations so that they acquire the targeted skill or knowledge. For example, do they accept new learning instantly, or do they prefer to reflect on it before accepting it fully? Do they question first whether the learning has practical applications, or do they accept new learning at theoretical levels?

Learning styles (or learning preferences) have been researched over a number of years, and Honey and Mumford's (Mint Human Resources, 2022) classification of styles of learning is one that has been most widely published. An individual student might prefer to learn by attending a course or lecture, that is, in formal teaching situations where new information is presented. Others may prefer to learn by doing one of the following:

- watching professionals and seeing the end-product first
- trial and error, generally through experimentation
- reading and other forms of personal study such as distance learning
- discussion with others.

Another well-accepted proponent of learning styles is Kolb (2014), who identifies another set of learning styles manifested by students, namely the converger, the diverger, the assimilator and the accommodator. Honey and Mumford suggest that individual learners' style of learning may be in the mode of activist, reflector, theorist or pragmatist. Jarvis (2010: 86) suggests yet another learning style that comprises focusers, scanners, impulsivity and reflectivity. The main learning styles inherent within these categories are summarised in the box below.

Popular Learning Styles

Converger vs Diverger   Convergers are individuals who tend to use abstract thinking, progress to active experimentation and generate a single correct solution; divergers tend to start from concrete experiences, they then generate ideas, and afterwards speculate on broader perspectives.

Impulsivity vs Reflectivity (similar to *Accommodator vs Assimilator*)   Using the 'impulsive' style means the individual tends to respond to new knowledge first, at times spontaneously (is accommodating), and reflect later; those who use reflectivity tend to reflect first (assimilate) and respond subsequently.

Activists vs Reflectors   Individuals who are activists tend to involve themselves fully in new experiences; reflectors, on the other hand, ponder on experiences from different perspectives, thoroughly analysing them before participating in the experience in practice.

Theorists vs Pragmatists   Theorists are individuals who start from observations and develop or synthesise them into theories; pragmatists tend to consider the practical application of new knowledge first and consider theories afterwards.

Focuser vs Scanner   Focusers are individuals who examine the whole problem and develop solutions from them; scanners tend to solve one aspect of the problem at a time and assume that it is the correct one unless it is disproved.

Holistic vs Serialistic   Individuals using the holistic approach tend to prefer to see a phenomenon as a whole; while serialists prefer to identify its components and their roles as part of the whole phenomenon.

Visual, Aural, Read-write or Kinaesthetic (VARK)   VARK distinguishes between students who like to be shown the correct way of performing a task (visual), or prefer to be instructed (aural), or prefer to read and take notes, or prefer to learn by doing.

━━━━━━━━ ACTION **POINT 2.3** ━━━━━━━━

Learning style self-assessment

Locate the 16-item VARK questionnaire (VARK Learn Limited, 2022) on the internet (vark-learn.com) and print out a copy. Subsequently, perform a self-assessment and look at the results to identify which learning style you tend to veer towards.

An alternative learning style self-assessment questionnaire is offered by Honey and Mumford (Mint Human Resources, 2022) who designed the 80-item Learning Style Questionnaire (LSQ), which is also available on the internet. The main benefits of the learning style self-assessment questionnaire include:

- the identification of areas in which an individual's less effective learning processes can be improved
- the development of ways in which specific learning skills can be improved, for example reflective learning.

Consequently, it is generally recommended that teachers and supervisors of learning should adapt their teaching style to accommodate students' learning styles. However, logically, in teaching in academic or practice settings, whenever we are teaching more than one student, it is difficult to adapt to all students' learning styles at the same time. Furthermore, research on learning styles (e.g. Ng, 2014) almost always indicates that students do not choose and use only one fixed style of learning, as they use different styles or a combination of styles during different learning events.

Additionally, identifying and adapting to each student's particular style of learning might have only limited practical value as it is educationally limiting, in that it suggests narrowing down approaches to teaching, according to Power and Farmer (2017). Moreover, individuals might also consciously change their learning style according to the situation because students could develop their ability in all styles of learning and change or adapt them as new knowledge and skills are encountered. Style may also change through new experiences and at different stages of maturation.

Accordingly, Ng (2014: 484) suggests that lesson plans for teaching practical skills should use a blend of activities that stimulate the visual, aural and verbal as well as kinaesthetic senses to enhance learning effectiveness because the majority of students possess 'multimodal' learning styles. Nonetheless, in practice settings where practice supervisors work on a one-to-one basis with the student during practice placements, identifying learning styles could well enable the practice supervisor to adapt their teaching to the student's style of learning more fully.

A potential problem is that, for example with the learning style 'Impulsivity vs Reflectivity', a learner who leans towards impulsivity may be a fluent or quick learner, or probably a 'surface' learner who participates in learning superficially.

The learner who tends to use the reflectivity style may either be a 'deep' learner or one who takes time to consider alternatives, and therefore can be indecisive.

Furthermore, on examining the literature on learning styles, An and Carr (2017) recommend considering individuals' behavioural or personality differences such as fluency in learning, the learner's attitude to the topic area, or their temperament. They also recommend adopting a wide range of teaching styles so that learners can understand their learning weaknesses and can thereafter decide whether to work on their weaknesses and rectify them.

Consequently, it is arguable that, where feasible, the practice supervisor should endeavour to assess their student's learning style and approach to see if they can adapt to them in order to make their teaching more effective. This could make the achievement of practice objectives easier and more efficient.

An example of the adaptation of the 'Theorists vs Pragmatists' style of learning is as follows. For instance, if the practice supervisor finds that a particular student has leanings towards the pragmatist style for any particular component of learning – that is, they immediately want to know how the learning applies to actual patient care situations – then the practice supervisor can first focus on the practical application of the learning and subsequently move on to the underpinning theories. The practical knowledge can follow immediately afterwards and the theoretical knowledge later. The 'theorist' student may wish to acquire all necessary theoretical knowledge before engaging in its practical application.

Another example of the application of learning styles is when students have to improve their drug calculation skills, as a few students struggle to become competent at drug calculation. Consequently, there has recently been a proliferation of books and e-learning packages on drug calculation, and many universities also have a mathematics support department to help students who need to refresh their calculation skills.

Practice supervisors are in a suitable position to help their students or supervisees learn these skills during practice placements where drug calculation applies directly to the service user in their care. During drug administration, the practice supervisor might seize the opportunity to ascertain their student's drug calculation skills. So, if the learner is more of a pragmatist than a theorist (or leans towards the 'visual' style), then the practice supervisor can show the learner step by step how patient X's medication dose is calculated, preferably long before they learn to administer the medication. It is a competency that simply has to be mastered (e.g. NMC, 2018c, 2019a).

Principles of learning

Based on the views, theories, styles and approaches to learning discussed in this chapter, there are certain fundamental principles of learning that underpin effective learning, effective from the standpoint of both facilitators and learners. Partly derived from Gagné et al.'s (2005) and Knowles' (2020) research, these principles are:

- Whatever a student learns, they must actively learn it themselves – no one can learn it for them.
- Each student learns at their own chosen pace, as this varies depending on their particular circumstances, mental abilities and various other factors.
- A student learns more when each step is immediately reinforced or corrected.
- Full, rather than partial, mastery of each step makes the total more meaningful.
- When given responsibility for their own learning, students are more likely to become more highly motivated and likely to learn and retain more.
- The teacher as manager of learning should assume that McGregor's (1987) theory Y prevails, that is, learners are self-motivated to learn, and they seek out learning opportunities for themselves (theory X implies learners have to be directed or coerced to learn).
- Students who come to education expecting to be passively fed information and knowledge should be eased into andragogical principles of learning and teaching soon after.

Chapter Summary

This chapter has focused predominantly on the 'what' and 'how' of learning professional knowledge and competence, addressing major views, theories, approaches and styles of learning, and has therefore explored:

- What healthcare learners learn, and why, in the context of the student's learning needs and the different types of knowledge associated with professional skills.
- The definitions of competence and healthcare competencies, and issues related to them.
- Major views and perspectives on learning, teaching and education, which include what learning is, and where and how individual healthcare learners learn.
- Theories underpinning learning, in particular behaviourist learning theories (including Bandura's social learning theory), cognitive learning theories and humanistic learning theories, such as andragogy and self-directed learning, the student-centred approach to teaching, learning as self-actualisation and the use of learning contracts.
- How learners learn healthcare skills, which included an examination of students' approaches to learning, such as deep, surface and strategic approaches, and the major styles of learning, and how the practice supervisor can adapt their teaching activities to students' individual approaches and styles.

Further Optional Reading

1. For an extensive analysis of different perspectives and definitions of 'learning', see:

    - Barron, A.B., Hebets, E.A., Cleland, T.A., Fitzpatrick, C.L. and Hauber, M.E. (2015) 'Embracing multiple definitions of learning', *Trend in Neurosciences*, *38*(7): 405–407.

2. For a detailed analysis of clinical competence related to nursing, see:

    - Notarnicola, I., Petrucci, C., De Jesus Barbosa, M.R., Giorgi, F., Stievano, A. and Lancia, L. (2016) 'Clinical competence in nursing: A concept analysis', *Professioni infermieristiche* (an Italian journal), *69*(3): 174–181.

3. For a detailed discussion on 'vicarious learning' in relation to social learning theory, see:

    - Roberts, D. (2010) 'Vicarious learning: A review of the literature', *Nurse Education in Practice*, *10*(1): 13–16.

3

FACILITATING LEARNING

Introduction

Having explored comprehensively the requirement and application of supervision of learning during practice education in Chapter 1 and ways in which practice learning supervision is practised by healthcare professionals, and then in Chapter 2 the different major perspectives on learning, which include learning theories, approaches and styles, this chapter concentrates on principles and methods of teaching and facilitation of learning that practice supervisors engage in during students' practice placements.

The chapter therefore considers the various professional groups of learners whose learning healthcare learning supervisors facilitate; whether to teach or to facilitate learning; systematic ways of facilitating learners' acquisition of practice skills and knowledge; as well as ways of managing any issues related to the facilitation of learning in practice settings.

―Chapter objectives―

1. Identify a wide range of students and learners whose learning is facilitated by qualified healthcare professionals.
2. Differentiate between teaching and facilitation of learning, and the different contemporary perceptions of, and approaches to, teaching and learning.

(Continued)

3. Evaluate a number of ways in which practice supervisors and other educators can enable healthcare students to acquire health and care skills, the steps involved in effective planning for skills teaching, along with the underpinning knowledge base.

4. Demonstrate knowledge of structured and systematic methods of teaching that can be implemented by practice supervisors to enable students and learners to acquire health profession skills and knowledge; and to manage issues related to the facilitation of learning.

5. Evaluate various methods of teaching and the teaching aids that can be selected for effective teaching for all categories of learners, including students with a disability or with neurodiversity.

Whose Learning do Healthcare Professionals Facilitate and Why?

━━━━━━━━━ ACTION **POINT 3.1** ━━━━━━━━━━━━━━━━━

Who do healthcare professionals teach?

To start exploring the facilitation of learning, first make a list of all the groups of people who nurses and other healthcare professionals teach in both healthcare settings and in the wider health and care sites. Having done this, add the exact healthcare topic areas that they are likely to teach to the different groups of individuals.

The healthcare professional's role includes a substantial teaching component and you might therefore have felt that Action Point 3.1 was rather simplistic. However, it does reflect the reality of the extent of teaching that RNs, RMs and registered AHPs undertake, and, in response to the activity, you might have mentioned the following:

- Nurses teach student nurses (first, second and third year), healthcare support workers on national vocational qualification courses, student nursing associates, students on nurse apprenticeship programmes, patients/service users, patients' relatives/carers, and junior doctors and other qualified colleagues.
- Midwives teach women/service users, for example new mothers and fathers, how to care for a new baby.
- The practice nurse teaches primary (and secondary) level ill-health prevention, for example how to quit smoking, lose weight, expectant mothers regarding their diet, and relaxation for those with high blood pressure.
- SCPHNs teach mothers with different needs, such as single teenage mothers or those in different age groups.

AHPs and doctors have a direct teaching role towards healthcare service users and often also teach other healthcare staff.

Why do Healthcare Professionals Need to Know How to Facilitate Learning?

On a day-to-day basis, the healthcare professional's role focuses largely on attending to healthcare service users' health problems. Teaching activities generally tend to be more sporadic and are engaged in at required and opportune moments, in addition to any scheduled work-based teaching of students. Nonetheless, there are several reasons why healthcare professionals teach and facilitate learning. First, in addition to teaching colleagues and juniors being a job requirement for most healthcare professionals by virtue of their contract of employment, teaching also constitutes one of the four essential components of healthcare professionals' groups of duties (HCPC, 2016: 1), the other three being clinical practice, management of care, and research. Alternatively, six categories of healthcare professionals' duties are identified by Gopee (2022: Chapter 1) as:

- organising care for the span of duty and beyond
- care and treatment activities
- managing staff and other resources within their areas of responsibility
- teaching and educating colleagues, students and patients
- engaging with research and the evidence base for practice
- leadership.

Correspondingly, the NHS KSF (DH, 2004; CIPD, 2021b) notes under 'personal and people development' (which is one of the six categories of all healthcare professionals' work) that healthcare professionals' duties include contributing to the development of others during ongoing work activities by structured approaches, and informal and ad hoc methods, and demonstrating and sharing skills and knowledge.

Similarly, teaching usually forms part of healthcare professionals' codes of practice, which stipulate that they must be willing to share skills and experience. For instance, the NMC's (2018b: clause 9) and HCPC's (2016: clauses 2.5 and 2.6) codes of practice specify that registrants 'must' share their skills, knowledge and experience for the benefit of their colleagues and service users, and also support their students' learning. This form of teaching includes teaching new skills to registrant colleagues, for example in the use of new medical devices such as a new glucometer, how to conduct a patient assessment using a new form, applying a new wound care ingredient, or using the national early warning system (NEWS-2).

Developing teaching skills is also an integral component of healthcare professionals' pre-registration education programmes, as identified by the NMC (2018c: 30), which, under the heading '*Communication and relationship management skills*', for example, states: 'Demonstrate effective supervision, teaching and performance appraisal', providing 'clear instructions and explanations when supervising, teaching or appraising others'. Under 'Platform 5 – *Leading and managing nursing care and working in teams*' (NMC, 2018b: 20), clause 5.8 reads 'support and supervise students in the delivery of nursing care ... and documenting their performance'.

Furthermore, some time after registration with the regulatory body, specialist RNs and other healthcare professionals are, at times, required, or invited, to do small-group teaching on specific aspects of their specialist areas of work within the healthcare trust, or in classroom teaching on specialist university-based courses. Moreover, research by Campbell and Evans (2016) confirmed that managers have a central role to play as facilitators of workplace learning, particularly so if they adopt a coaching approach and act as a role model for teaching and learning.

Additionally, healthcare professionals might also seek out opportunities to teach merely to advance their own teaching or presentation skills that they have previously acquired to varying degrees. They could thereby also start to develop public speaking skills. For more experienced practice supervisors, teaching provides them with an opportunity to apply the principles of teaching and learning, and experiment with new teaching techniques. Furthermore, practice supervisors have to teach because of only variable levels of success in joint education–trust roles such as lecturer-practitioners and the clinical teaching role of nurse lecturers.

Facilitating Learning or Teaching

At times, we hear the statement, 'John (or Jane) is an excellent (or a born) teacher', but, as with most skills, teaching can be regarded as an 'art' and a 'science'. This means that although someone may appear to have a natural knack for teaching, it is also a skill that can be learned by applying research-based teaching techniques. Teaching courses such as *Taking Teaching Further* (Education and Training Foundation, 2022), offered at colleges of further education, and the Postgraduate Certificate in Education, are specifically designed for this purpose.

After several years of teaching experience, eventually the skill becomes so well developed, refined and mastered that it appears akin to an artistic talent. However, thinking about some of the concepts discussed in Chapter 2, such as self-directed learning and reflective learning, consider the question: Should practice supervisors teach students and juniors, or facilitate their learning? Both concepts are suggested for contemporary practice learning supervision activities.

Approaches to teaching and learning

Dictionaries tend to define teaching as 'to tell or show someone how to do something' and 'to give instructions (or lessons) to students' (Brookes and O'Neill, 2017: 959). Such definitions tend to signify teaching as one-way traffic, that is, the teacher controls what the learner will learn, the volume of the teaching content and the sequencing of the content, and they reflect one of the earlier approaches to teaching. However, various other approaches to teaching and learning have evolved over the years, so much so that Joyce et al. (2009) indicate that there are more than 22 models of teaching, some of which are well researched while others still need rigorous testing.

An underlying trend that figures clearly in all these approaches and models of teaching is the transition from the rather unpalatable term 'teacher-centred' teaching to 'student-centred' teaching. Three stages of evolution of approaches to teaching can be identified, which are as follows:

1. In the earlier stage, teaching was seen as the teacher imparting selected and predetermined knowledge and skills to students as they were the expert in that subject area. In such approaches, students in turn are passive recipients of the instruction, but this can result in students feeling inhibited from exploring alternative perspectives on the topic area.
2. In a gradual change in attitude towards teaching and learning, teaching was viewed later as enabling active learning, an approach in which teachers structure learning activities for students so that the latter actively engage with the subject matter and explore various aspects of specific topic areas in the curriculum or syllabus. Thus, the teacher leads students to conclusions by enquiry and questioning.
3. In the third and current stage, teaching is viewed as 'facilitating learning', whereby teachers work in partnership with students and jointly determine their learning needs in the overall context of the curriculum and the means by which those learning needs will be met. The teacher creates the conditions for learning and does not control all learning outcomes, thus allowing the student a substantial degree of choice in what to learn, and providing scope for creativity.

These three stages of development in ways of teaching therefore reflect an evolving trend from the earlier one, implying a teacher-centred approach to the latter as much more student-centred, and therefore progressing from teaching to the facilitation of learning, that is, shifting the focus from teaching to learning by students. The approach chosen of course depends on several factors such as the particular student group's motivation to learn, the teacher's own beliefs about teaching and learning, and the subject matter, or a deliberate combination of these as the teacher feels appropriate.

The three teaching approaches can also be categorised as didactic, Socratic or facilitative, respectively. Contemporarily, Ramsden (2003) refers to these approaches as theories 1, 2 and 3. However, Biggs and Tang (2022) interpret these three approaches as three 'levels of thinking about teaching' and note that at stage (or level) one, if the student does not 'absorb' the knowledge and skills imparted to them, because they have not got either the ability or the motivation to do so, then the teaching is unlikely to be as effective.

At level two, in addition to the ability to impart knowledge and skills, the teacher needs additional skills such as those required to structure learning activities and to negotiate student learning so as to ensure the curriculum's learning outcomes are met. Yet further skills are required at the third and current level of thinking about teaching, which is the facilitation of learning, as this is based on the student's own learning needs and is about enabling students to engage with their learning more actively. The earlier approaches were also reflected in the method of assessment applied by educators, which had negative effects on students' learning and achievement (see Chapters 7 and 8).

The trend in moving away from teacher-centred to student-centred approaches was suggested several years ago by Bruner (1960), for instance, who advocated 'discovery learning' theory, indicating that this approach can make learning more effective as it is an active process that is stimulated through student curiosity about the subject area. The teacher therefore devises situations, poses problems or questions, and creates a medium for the student to discover the structures and principles underlying the situation or topic area.

The discovery learning approach feeds into currently advocated methods such as problem-based learning, which is an instructional method in which students work in small groups or individually to gain knowledge from simulated problem situations and acquire problem-solving skills at the same time. In turn, learning by simulation is a proven effective method of teaching healthcare students, as found by Kandola et al. (2022) and Taylor et al. (2021), among others (see Chapter 4 of this book for detailed analysis of the facilitation of learning by simulation).

Practice supervisors apply the facilitation of learning approach in addition to the instructional teaching of clinical skills. Problem-based learning, for example, can be implemented in the form of self-directed learning in clinical practice, in, for example, management of a staff conflict situation, or management of a new illness or syndrome encountered for the first time by the student, and so on. Problem-based learning, however, must conclude with reflection on the learning that ensued, especially to ensure no erroneous conclusions have been drawn by learners. The teacher must also ensure that the learning is directly linked to students' practice competencies identified for the placement, module or course.

Current definitions of teaching take these evolving learning philosophies into account. For example, according to Curzon and Tummons (2013: 20), teaching is 'a system of activities intended to allow learning to happen, comprising the deliberate and methodical creation and control of those conditions in which learning does occur'. The definition reflects student-centred teaching, as distinct from one-way information-giving.

Learner-centred approaches

Teacher-centred teaching approaches, as just specified, have some advantages in that they are economical, and with their expert knowledge of the subject the teacher can maximise the allocated time by selecting and focusing on the most significant areas of the topic.

Drawing on theories underpinning patient or service-user-centred therapy for people with psychological problems, Rogers (1983) formulated the student-centred approach to learning, which formed a major defining shift in approaches to teaching and learning, which comprise of the following:

- Human beings have a natural potentiality for learning.
- Much significant learning is acquired through doing.
- Learning is facilitated when the student participates responsibly in the learning process.
- The most socially useful learning in the modern world is the learning of the process of learning, a continuing openness to new experiences and the process of change.

═══════════ **ACTION** **POINT 3.2** ═══════════

Teacher-centred or student-centred teaching

To follow up on the aforementioned approaches to teaching, identify a number of factors that you consider to be the strengths and weaknesses of teacher-centred and student-centred teaching methods in healthcare professional education programmes.

Jarvis (2010) notes that using teacher-centred methods of teaching reinforces hierarchical social relationships between teachers and learners (or practice supervisors and students), and thereby replicates models of authority in which the teacher might be seeking to control and mould individuals to fit into social systems. Rogers (1983) suggested earlier that such approaches cause learners to become dependent on teachers and thereby compromise their growth and development. The possible weaknesses of teacher-centred methods or strategies include the following:

- They assume that students usually lack discipline and are irresponsible.
- They disregard experience as a resource for learning.
- The orientation to learning is subject-centred rather than building on the individual student's existing knowledge.
- The motivation to learn is external, for example for merely gaining a qualification.
- They can suppress the individual's creative powers.
- The student's opinions and questions tend to be largely overlooked.

Consequently, pivotal to the effective facilitation of learning is the relationship between individual learners and the facilitator. Rogers sees the teacher as a facilitator of learning, a provider of resources for learning and someone who shares feelings as well as knowledge with learners. The prerequisites for being an effective facilitator of learning are awareness of self and being oneself in the teaching situation, through (as mentioned in Chapter 1 in relation to building an effective working relationship):

- Genuineness – the facilitator demonstrates full honesty and willingness to declare their strengths and the areas in which they are lacking, where appropriate. They remain a real person and are not drawn by the image of a distant and authority-vested teacher.
- Trust and acceptance – the facilitator must be able to gain and retain the student's trust, and vice versa, and overtly accept any limitations that students might have.
- Empathic understanding – the facilitator consistently endeavours to see situations from the learner's viewpoint.

Rogers contrasts the kind of learning that is concerned solely with cognitive functioning such as acquiring knowledge, with that involving the whole person. The learning naturally needs to be guided by the approved curriculum for the course the student is on to be able to obtain the relevant award (i.e. qualification). Rogers suggests that it is possible for the teacher to build into a programme this freedom to learn. This can be done by using students' own experiences and problems so that the relevance is more obvious, and by identifying relevant resources – both material and human – for their students. The goal of education is therefore to enable the student to become a fully functioning person as a whole (Rogers and Freiberg, 1994).

In healthcare learning, the student-centred approach is reflected in the andragogical approach to facilitation of learning, as advocated by Knowles (2020) (and discussed in Chapter 2), and with 'learning by insight', that is, 'a perception of a whole group of relationships ... a suddenly occurring re-organisation' of one's thoughts (Curzon and Tummons, 2013: 62). Additionally, following a concept analysis of facilitation of learning, Burrows (2008) concludes that the four critical attributes for effective facilitation of learning are: genuine mutual respect; a partnership in learning; a dynamic, goal-orientated process; and critical reflection.

Case study 3.1

Facilitating Izzy's practice-based learning

Izzy is a 34-year-old ex-schoolteacher who is now a first-year midwifery student. Izzy is a graduate, who, after initial teacher training, soon found the job easy but had no wish to take on management responsibilities. The job was soon becoming too routine when she realised that in fact she had always wanted to be a midwife instead. Izzy is also raising her own family and has remained an active member of the Parents and Teachers Association.

Consider the ways in which Izzy's practice supervisor, Emily, can take a learner-centred approach to learning facilitation during the practice placement. Make some notes, taking into account Izzy's previous vocation.

Practice supervisors can consider ascertaining and adapting their facilitation of learning role to the learner's previous knowledge of health and their preferred styles and approaches to learning, as noted in Chapter 2. Izzy's age, responsibility and discipline as a qualified teacher and a mother can be taken into account when taking a learner-centred or person-centred approach to placement learning. A self-directed approach to learning, in collaboration with Izzy and with guided study if required, can be warranted to make learning more meaningful and complete for her.

Despite these benefits of the student-centred approach to teaching, there may also be drawbacks, some of which are identified in the box below.

Arguments for, and Possible Drawbacks of, the Learner-centred Approach to Teaching

Arguments for:

- It motivates, as the aims and objectives are clear and relevant.
- Learning is meaningful.
- It encourages divergent and critical thinking through dialogue.
- It allows autonomy and creativity.

Drawbacks:

- Can be time-consuming if emphasis is on the nature or process of learning, rather than how much of the curriculum is covered. Rogers (1983) was aware of this and suggested that there should be freedom within a system of constraints.
- Structure and guidelines may suffer.
- Timetables and deadlines might not get adhered to.
- There is an assumption that everyone is capable of self-directed learning.

Despite likely weaknesses, the student-centred approach to the facilitation of learning is preferred as it entails more active involvement in learning. This is also consistent with Biggs and Tang's (2022) assertion in relation to the senses and remembering, in that, in general, learners learn 80 per cent of what they do as learning activities, 50 per cent of all they see and hear, but only 10 per cent of all they hear.

In experiential learning, as a way of adapting learning theories to methods of teaching, students need to be given opportunities for 'doing', that is, applying or using the knowledge or skill. For example, most healthcare pre-registration courses include the topic 'moving and handling patients'. This is an apt example that lends itself to both problem-based learning and experiential learning, in that having been exposed to the knowledge base (e.g. principles of moving and handling), students can then learn by doing. This can occur in university skills laboratories under close supervision of the facilitator. Students can be given problem situations to solve, which may enable them to make the topic their own and internalise it.

A concluding suggestion on the facilitation of learning is that, in the context of the current-day vehement push towards efficiency, practice supervisors and their learners need to seize learning opportunities as they arise, which is also referred to as opportunistic learning or teachable moments.

Facilitating Learners' Acquisition of Clinical Skills

Healthcare professionals' clinical activities are founded on skilled healthcare interventions, and therefore their pre-registration education programmes are designed to enable individuals to become competent at performing a comprehensive range of specific clinical actions to improve patients' or service users' health. Competence is a different concept from skill, in that it comprises of skills as well as an extensive knowledge base, as discussed in Chapter 2. A skill therefore signifies having expertise in an activity that has been developed as the result of training under the supervision of an expert, or is self-taught, that enables the individual to perform the particular task adeptly, and also flexibly. Skills require mind and muscle coordination and effective movement that end with the desired result. The features of a skilled activity include physical and mental dexterity, the ability to respond quickly, and the capacity to attend to a number of requirements more or less simultaneously in contemporary care settings.

The process of learning clinical skills

Progression with learning and mastering clinical skills can be placed along a continuum that identifies early attempts at learning a skill to becoming proficient. A widely used framework for categorising levels of psychomotor skill development and testing in healthcare courses is that suggested by Steinaker and Bell (1979) in a taxonomy of experiential learning. The term *taxonomy* broadly refers here to levels of learning, that is, learning from lower levels to higher levels. In Steinaker and Bell's model, skill development progresses from lower-level exposure, through participation, identification and internalisation to dissemination.

Experiential learning refers to learning that involves going through the experience of engaging and actually doing the skill. Competency or skill development through the different levels occurs over two, three or five years of further learning and enhancement of the skill. Steinaker and Bell's five levels of learning and the likely interpretation (or criteria) related to a clinical skill are presented in Table 3.1.

Table 3.1 Taxonomy levels and criteria

Levels	Criteria
Exposure	Have some knowledge of equipment, methods and concepts used for the skill
	Show willingness to participate
Participation	Perform clinical activities under supervision
	Explain the rationale for each activity when questioned
	Interact well with patients/service users
	Cognisant of implications of practices
Identification	Perform the clinical activity without having to be prompted or supervised
	Apply theory to practice
	Demonstrate awareness of situations
Internalisation	Consistently apply theory to practice in a range of settings
	Compare and contrast different approaches to practices
	Solve problems by analysis and evaluation
	Show willingness to share experiences
Dissemination	Use opportunities to teach service users and families
	Share experiences with peers and others
	Able to accurately teach the skill, and aware of any management issues

Consider a mental health student who has to demonstrate a certain level of proficiency in helping or counselling skills by the end of their third year of professional education:

Exposure – refers to the student observing the practice supervisor helping or counselling appropriate service users and becoming aware of the preconditions and specific helping skills being used by the practice supervisor.

Participation – refers to when, under supervision, the student attempts to use selected helping skills, e.g. low-level self-disclosure.

Identification – is when the student starts to feel competent at some of the helping skills and this is acknowledged by their practice supervisor.

Internalisation – can be difficult to achieve within the constraints of the pre-registration course, as this implies that the learner is so proficient at these skills that they see them as part of themselves as a person.

Dissemination – refers to being so knowledgeable and competent in the skill that the person can have specific and valid opinions about the skill, can explain them to learners and colleagues, and even teach them, which is rarely achieved during pre-registration programmes.

Teaching competencies at the appropriate level entails careful planning by the teacher after careful assessment of the student's existing abilities and motivation to learn. Another well-established model of learning a clinical skill is Benner's (2001) stages of skill acquisition, which is based on a framework initially deduced from how trainee pilots learn their vocation and eventually become an expert in flying aeroplanes. These stages are novice, advanced beginner, competent, proficient and expert, in this sequence, and they relate to longer-term activities on expertise development as they progress from initial cruder attempts to a more refined performance, with a substantial associated knowledge base.

Fitts and Posner (1973) earlier on identified three phases of learning most skills – the cognitive phase, the associative phase and the autonomous phase:

Cognitive phase – concerned with the learning of the procedure, but the more complex the skill, the longer the learning will take.

Associative phase – engaging in skilled performance of part-skills or in whole practical skills, with interfering responses eliminated.

Autonomous phase – in the long term, the skill becomes automatic and can be performed without the student thinking much about it.

The three phases are not completely distinct, as they overlap, with one phase leading to the next, and by the end of the pre-qualifying preparation programme (and as NQHP), the individual reaches the 'competent' stage (Benner, 2001), the 'internalisation' level (Steinaker and Bell, 1979) and the 'association' phase (Fitts and Posner, 1973). Further detailed information on levels of learning are elicited in the QAA's (2014) framework for higher education qualifications.

Teaching and learning a specific psychomotor skill

A significant component of the practice learning supervisor's role is to teach learners clinical skills. However, on and off, PEFs have complained that the previous mentor courses didn't adequately equip course attenders with teaching skills, a major limitation noted by Jayasekara et al. (2018) as well.

━━━━━━━━━━━ ACTION POINT 3.3 ━━━━━━━━━━━

Skill acquisition and maintenance

Think of, and list, all factors that the practice supervisor as a teacher needs to consider, and all preparations that they need to make to teach a particular clinical skill in the practice setting. Then list all the factors that might affect enabling the efficient acquisition of one specific psychomotor skill in the practice setting. Finally, list all the factors that might affect maintenance and performance of the clinical skill at the same or a higher standard.

There are several factors that need to be considered when preparing to teach a clinical skill. Those required for teaching blood glucose monitoring using test strips and blood glucose monitors, for instance, include:

- which patient?
- the specific condition requiring it
- the equipment needed
- being fully conversant with the approved procedure for taking a blood sample
- gaining the patient's consent
- factors affecting the reading of results
- ensuring there's enough blood on the test strip
- safety aspects
- own knowledge
- the student's knowledge base – practical and theoretical
- reading the result – up/down/normal
- recording the result, and taking any necessary action
- opportunities to practise
- the frequency of measurement
- testing the equipment and cleaning it after use
- evaluating, observing, supervising
- what if?
- the time allocated
- recording the learner's competence.

A list of factors that need to be considered for a particular clinical activity, like the one above, is rarely fully prescriptive as there are other variables that need to be taken into account in relation to the individual health service user's health problems or needs, and the equipment and other resources that are available.

Teaching a clinical skill requires, first of all, a skills analysis. Generally, the trust's procedure for the clinical action constitutes a very good basis for structuring a lesson plan for the skill. The practice supervisor can also consider how the task is performed or executed, step by step, by those who are recognised as expert at the particular clinical intervention. These are discussed shortly. Such a detailed analysis of the clinical skill also constitutes its performance or assessment criteria, which is discussed in Chapter 7.

For a systematic approach to teaching a clinical skill, Peyton's (1998) model of teaching and learning clinical skills has been widely advocated. The model comprises of a four-step process to effective teaching: (1) demonstration of the skill; (2) deconstruction of the skill; (3) comprehension; and (4) performance. When applied to teaching the clinical skill step by step, several specific sub-steps have to be taken and decisions made by the teacher, and in the systematic review and meta-analysis of Peyton's model, Giacomino et al. (2020) conclude that the model is effective in teaching small groups of students, but are unsure of its effectiveness if the teaching is performed by peer students or by student tutors.

Consequently, the principles and process of teaching a clinical activity comprise of the following:

1.   Initially, demonstrate the skill in its entirety as a fully integrated set of operations, that must be demonstrated at mastery level. The correct movements that go to make up the skill must be in evidence throughout.
2.   Break the skill down into its component and subordinate activities (deconstruct), so that each action demonstrated is accompanied by clear step-by-step commentary, and its rationale provided (comprehension). The relation of separate activities to one another and their sequences that make up the skill are explained.
3.   Ensure skill acquisition through supervised performance by the student, with all correct actions reinforced, and more practice opportunities provided later. By experiencing and repeating the essential movements of the activity, the learner discovers the kinaesthetic cues of successful performance.
4.   Provide swift, continuous and accurate feedback to the learner, as delayed feedback on performance can make the feedback less effective, and include praise as positive reinforcement.
5.   Formatively assess part-skills or the whole skill regularly and in work-related realistic conditions, if required.

This process and sequence of actions are generally fully applied when teaching a skill in skills laboratories but can be easily adapted by the practice supervisor when teaching in the practice setting. The sub-steps that would form part of the process include the learner's awareness that they lack (or are deficient in) the skill to perform the clinical intervention, because if the individual feels that they are already competent (rightly or wrongly) in that skill then they might not be fully open to learning it. Either way, for effective learning of the skill, the learner has to be motivated to learn it, and feel that they will gain from having that skill.

Furthermore, before demonstration (step 1), the teacher might ask the learner to look through the approved procedure or clinical guideline for the intervention; and/or to read up on the anatomy and physiology of the body system related to the clinical intervention. Additionally, when the learner is performing the clinical skill, the teacher is also formatively assessing how competently the learner is performing each part-skill, and also may have to intervene if the learner is about to make a mistake. Patient safety needs to be assured at each step of the clinical activity.

An example of a 'lesson plan' for teaching a clinical skill to a learner is presented in the following template, with a few dotted lines for completion depending on the learner group being taught. It provides details of the sequence of activities involved in teaching skills effectively, by providing an example of a lesson plan for teaching a clinical skill, which, in this instance, is manual measurement of blood pressure (MMBP) (see Template 3.1). Very briefly, this comprises five steps: introduce the skill > demonstrate the skill > explain the key actions taken > re-demonstrate and give the rationale for each action > skill performance by learner (which is akin to Peyton's four-step approach).

Template 3.1 Steps in lesson planning for teaching manual measurement of blood pressure (MMBP)

Date:	Cohort:	Number of students: ....
Title of the course & module:			
Subject of lesson (clinical skill being taught): Manual measurement of blood pressure			
Lesson aim(s):			
Lesson learning outcomes: 1. .... 2.			

Duration of the lesson: 1 hour 50 mins		Classroom:	
Time (minutes)	**Lesson content**	**Teaching method**	**Teaching aids**
2	State and explain lesson topic, aim and learning outcomes	Verbal exposition (VE)	ppt slide
5	Ascertain students' existing **knowledge** of MMBP, and rationales	Questions & answers (Q&A)	--
5	Explain the clinical skill, and the **rationales** for performing them, including recapitulation of related anatomy and physiology	Q&A	ppt slides
5	**Demonstrate** MMBP at normal speed	Demonstration	Equipment & student volunteer
10	**Explanation**/overview of rationale for each step	VE	
15	**Demonstrate** the skill at slow pace, explaining/ascertaining rationales for each step	Demonstration	Equipment & another student volunteer
30	Supervise students handling equipment and **practising** MMBP on each other	Supervision	Sets of equipment
3	**Recapitulation**, and invite and respond to any question	VE & Q&A	---
3	Indicate location of paper or electronic copies of clinical **guidelines** or procedure for performing MMBP	VE	ppt slide
20	Repeated **practice** of MMBP by each student	Practice	Sets of equipment

(Continued)

Template 3.1   (Continued)

10	**Test** each student (if required), or evaluation of session	Test/evaluation	MCQ/gapped handout papers
2	**Evaluation** of session and announce title of next clinical skill session	VE	Time-table slide
ppt = PowerPoint; MMBP = manual measurement of blood pressure; Q&A = questioning students and responding to their answers; Equipment = includes sphygmomanometer and stethoscope			

The template may need to be adapted according to whether the skill being taught is in a skills laboratory (at university or a healthcare trust), to the number of students being taught (which can be from 1 to 30), to the availability of extra lecturers to supervise each learner practising the skill, to whether each student has to be summatively assessed, and so on.

Integrating skill acquisition with other domains of learning

In addition to skill acquisition, healthcare profession students are required to acquire extensive knowledge as well as develop the appropriate attitude towards service users. Precisely which areas of knowledge and competence do healthcare students learn on their pre-registration courses? Naturally, comprehensive knowledge of human physiology, pathophysiology, pharmacology for example, are essential knowledge bases. However, each clinical activity comprises three domains of activity: psychomotor (skill), cognitive (knowledge) and affective (attitude) (e.g. Bloom, 1956). The affective domain is often incorporated in guidance documents, for example NMC (2018c: 3, 9), and worded as compassionate and sensitive care.

The psychomotor domain refers to motor, muscular and coordination skills; the cognitive domain refers to the use of knowledge and information; and the affective domain refers to attitudes, behaviour and values. The three domains equating broadly with skills, knowledge and attitudes, also equate largely with doing, thinking and feeling, respectively, and they are integrated essential components of each competency and not distinct and separate activities. All healthcare interventions incorporate these three domains and therefore learning the clinical skill must also incorporate all three components.

────── ─Reflection point 3.1─ ──────────────

Psychomotor, cognitive and affective domains of competencies

Consider any two clinical activities (e.g. an intramuscular injection) and ascertain the exact skill, knowledge and attitude components for each clinical activity.

──────────────────────────────────────

The sequence of events that both teacher and learner should engage in during skill acquisition is summarised in Table 3.2. It captures the principles of teaching and facilitation of learning of a psychomotor skill or competency, with the cognitive and affective domains being key components. The five essential elements of the affective domain to be achieved by the learner are: *receiving, responding, valuing, organising* and *characterising* (Anderson, L.W. et al., 2014).

Table 3.2 Skills teaching sequence integrating the psychomotor, cognitive and affective domains

Psychomotor domain	Cognitive domain	Affective domain
Awareness that learner lacks the skill or is deficient in it ↓	Establish learner's existing 'practical knowledge' base underpinning the skill	Receiving – i.e., ensuring learner realises that it will be beneficial to learn the skill
Ensure the learner is motivated to learn the skill ↓	Permit learner to be active in seeking all related practical knowledge	Responding – learner is willing, and takes action to learn the skill
Analysis of the step-by-step procedure/components of the skill ↓	Have clear learning outcomes for learning the skill	Responding – learner understands the step-by-step procedure
Prepare equipment, etc., to teach the skill ↓	Assemble appropriate equipment/devices and materials	Responding – have knowledge of equipment and materials required at every step
Demonstrate the skill at normal speed ↓	Enable learner to observe and assimilate all details of the procedure	Responding – appreciates the manual dexterity required
Discuss each step just performed; re-demonstrate part-skills as required ↓	State rationale for each action; emphasise important points; discuss safety points; encourage learner to ask questions	Valuing – the rationales for each step taken; learner is willing to participate in performing the skill or part-skill
Allow learner to perform whole skill/part-skills ↓	Select components to work on, and actually 'doing' the skill, i.e. experiencing it	Organising – mental rehearsal of each skill component, with rationales; asking questions when unsure
Allow learner to perform the skill under supervision ↓	Observe in silence, and with confidence in the learner; correct any mistake	Organising – positive approach to the clinical activity by learner

(Continued)

Table 3.2 (Continued)

Psychomotor domain	Cognitive domain	Affective domain
Praise and review ↓	Give feedback on performance; Reward progress	Organising - reinforcement and sense of achievement, confidence
Allow to apply/repeat the skill under supervision ↓	Using the learning in real situations. Assess progress and knowledge of rationales	Characterising - accepting the procedure is the correct way of performing the skill

'Practical knowledge', which is also referred to as 'knowing how', is one of two types of knowledge associated with skills teaching, the second being theoretical knowledge (i.e. more in-depth 'knowing that'). Healthcare courses involve the acquisition of both types of knowledge, and students are assessed on them at different academic levels or stages, as detailed shortly in this chapter. After practising the skill on several occasions, a summative assessment of competence will be performed by the practice assessor and, if the learner is deemed competent, they are usually permitted to practise the skill without direct supervision. One of the key purposes of Table 3.2 is to highlight how the cognitive and affective domains of learning are integral components of learning any clinical activity.

As a general guide, for 25 per cent of the teaching time the teacher demonstrates the clinical activity, 15 per cent of the time is for verbal explanation, and 60 per cent for guided practice. Other factors that are essential for effective and efficient acquisition of the activity include:

- the complexity of the skill
- individual differences in speed of learning, and the background knowledge of the learner
- the teaching situation – environment, light, space, room temperature
- the quality of instruction
- knowledge of progress
- the availability of practice opportunities
- the availability of the necessary equipment – checking it beforehand, describing it
- getting feedback on skill performance
- a positive approach
- a running commentary, if appropriate
- a true-to-life setting
- allowing time for questions
- time for practice – with positive reinforcement
- its transferability to different real-life settings.

Template 3.1 can be adapted as an effective step-by-step lesson plan for teaching any clinical skill. Alternatively, see Gagné et al.'s (2005) *Principles of Instructional*

Design for a comprehensive detailed analysis of skills teaching. As for applying Peyton's (1998) four-step model of teaching a clinical skill (e.g. Ng, 2014), it is noteworthy that oversimplifying a task in this way can mask the complexity of the clinical activity in terms of the numerous mini decisions required during the activity, and the extensive knowledge base. Additionally, not stating clearly the SMART learning outcomes of the lesson (SMART stands for specific, measurable, achievable or agreeable, realistic or relevant and time-bound), or not ascertaining the learners' existing knowledge, can result in the session being less effective.

So, all teaching sessions must have clearly stated objectives or learning outcomes. Learning *objectives* are different from learning outcomes, in that objectives are more teacher-centred, i.e. the teacher/instructor's objectives for the session, while outcomes specify the learning that the learner should achieve by the end of the session, and is therefore learner-centred. For instance, chapter objectives are specified at the beginning of this chapter, but not learning outcomes, which is because the emphasis is on the knowledge that the author intends to convey rather than specifying the observable learning that the reader must achieve.

Learning outcomes tend to follow the aim(s), which succinctly state the overall purpose, but learning outcomes are there for students in clear, simple language that tell the student the specific knowledge, skills, behaviours and competencies, that they should acquire from the session/course. How to identify the aims and learning outcomes of the lesson and the format in which it is conventionally written, is presented in the box below.

Aims and Learning Outcomes for a Lesson on Attending to an Individual who has Collapsed and Might Need Cardio-pulmonary Resuscitation (CPR)

Aim of Lesson

To assess an individual who has collapsed, check whether they are breathing and perform CPR, if required.

Learning Outcomes

At the end of the session, the student will be able to:

1. Assess and identify whether the person is breathing normally (cognitive)
2. Demonstrate how to place an unresponsive casualty in the recovery position (psychomotor)
3. Initiate and perform cardio-pulmonary resuscitation using a mannequin (psychomotor)
4. Demonstrate how to safely use an automated external defibrillator (AED) (psychomotor).

Note that the 'Aim' starts with the word 'To', and the objectives and learning outcomes always have a stem stating the knowledge or competence that the student 'will be able to' perform and explain in relation to a practical skill such as cardio-pulmonary resuscitation; and then the items of outcomes always start with an action verb, such as 'demonstrate'.

To constitute learning outcomes, educators often use frameworks or classifications, such as those identified in Bloom's (1956) taxonomy, which was later adjusted by Anderson, L.W. et al. (2014), for example, and which is explored later in the next section in relation to knowledge acquisition. Both Steinaker and Bell's (1979) levels of clinical skills learning in an undergraduate programme and Bloom's (1956) levels of knowledge, skills and attitude development, can be juxtaposed or considered in conjunction with QAA's (2014) *Frameworks for Higher Education Qualifications* for cross-checking or validation of levels of learning over different years of the programme the student is on.

Facilitating Knowledge Acquisition

Despite the current paradigm shift away from teaching to the facilitation of learning, formal teaching also has its place in professional preparatory programmes. The knowledge component of many clinical activities is best imparted to learners directly through formal teaching. There will be times when the practice supervisor will have to conduct short, structured teaching sessions, probably in a room in the practice setting that has some teaching facilities such as flipcharts and a computer with a projector and screen. These sessions are generally quite short or last an hour or so, delivered to very small groups of learners or colleagues. Therefore, a good insight into how to structure and deliver a teaching session is a useful component of the practice supervisor's armoury of capabilities.

Effective teaching requires careful and thorough planning. The lesson needs to be fully structured, with flexibility built in, depending on whether it is a colleagues' workshop or being delivered to students.

Planning a structured session for teaching a knowledge base

The deliberate logical designing of a teaching session constitutes lesson planning, an example of whose components is presented in the box below.

Steps in Lesson Planning

1. Identify the topic and parameters of the lesson.
2. Research the subject.
3. Consider the students' previous knowledge.

4. Write down the aims and learning outcomes, or objectives.
5. Jot down as many points as possible in keeping with the objectives; then select, prune, sequence and structure these points.
6. Select the appropriate teaching methods.
7. Screen the activities against the learning outcomes.
8. Write the lesson (include teaching aids).
9. Prepare aids, equipment and classroom.
10. Give the lesson.
11. Evaluate the lesson.

Each step presented in the box requires specific attention in its own right. For instance, the third step requires the teacher to consider the knowledge that the students in the group already have, as well as any prior reading that was suggested before the teaching session. This accords with the use of appropriate learning theories such as Ausubel et al.'s (1978) assimilation (cognitive) theory (discussed in Chapter 2). It is also consistent with Bruner's (1960) notion of linking new learning to previous knowledge; and with the contemporary 'flipping' method of teaching.

As to the sequencing of lesson content and teaching methods (steps 5 and 6 in the box above), this is partly based on Herbartian (Encyclopaedia Britannica, 2022) rules (or approach) for lesson presentation, which has stood the test of time and is also referred to as 'traditional rule' to gain the students' attention and keep them engaged with the lesson content. It involves proceeding from:

The known to the unknown – link new concepts to what is already known by the learner (e.g. water to blood, water pipes to blood vessels).

The concrete to the abstract – demonstrate a link between visible or tangible materials with invisible concepts (e.g. aspirates or infusion to acidity versus alkalinity).

Observation to reasoning – from how things are done to why.

The simple to the complex – simple explanations to increasing levels of complexity (e.g. diffusion of a substance from one side of a jar to another – to movement of oxygen and CO_2 between alveoli and alveolar capillaries, or to the intra- and extra-cellular movement of potassium).

The particular to the general – use specific examples to illustrate general theories (e.g. the theory that giving information reduces anxiety, as people generally have a need to know what is happening).

The whole view, to the parts, then return to the whole view – the subject matter as an entity, analysis of component parts, return to the overall view.

Step 6 in the box above suggests selecting the appropriate teaching methods. A range of teaching methods is available to the teacher (see the box below). The teaching method(s) selected for the session must be based on principles of teaching and on learning theories. The appropriateness of the method depends on the teacher's level of knowledge of theories and principles and their values, research and verbal skills, and facilitative skills, and on the aims of the lesson, for instance.

Most Frequently Used Teaching Methods

- Lectures
- Buzz groups/work in sub-groups
- Seminars
- Skills demonstration
- Guided study or self-directed learning on a specific topic
- Role plays
- Problem-solving games/exercises/workshops
- Case study/patient-centred discussions
- Simulation
- Video recording of student presentations, for playback and self-assessment
- Tutorial - individual/small group
- Free-flow idea exercises (previously known as brainstorming), e.g. concept-mapping
- Questions and answers
- Dissertation or project supervision
- Online learning, e-learning and distance learning (or blended)
- Using apps and 'usable learning objects'
- Group discussion
- Team teaching.

Each of these methods has its advantages and disadvantages that are examined later in this chapter. The eighth step in the box titled 'Steps in lesson planning' is to 'write the lesson' and includes identifying the teaching aids to be used. An example of a lesson plan for teaching a clinical skill was presented in Template 3.1 earlier in this chapter.

In relation to steps 8 and 9 in the box titled 'Steps in lesson planning', or the use of an appropriate range of teaching aids such as whiteboard/flipchart or PowerPoint slides, some of these will be explained briefly and their advantages and disadvantages will also be explored later in this chapter.

In planning the lesson, the teacher needs to consider any likely constraints such as class size (for instance, is it 10 students or 200 students?), the number of copies of worksheets, if any, to be used, and the accessibility of articles that will be recommended as further reading. The teacher's aim in a lesson is to motivate, stimulate and communicate, to hold the class's attention and to achieve the defined objectives, and therefore further essential considerations by the presenter are the following:

1. The lesson must be appropriately pitched.
2. SMART learning outcomes must be clearly identified.

3. Exposition must be ordered, simple and clear.
4. Development must be logical and sequential (flow coherently).
5. Presentation must be based on the essential 'social character' of the lesson (e.g. laboratory work or lecture).
6. Presentation must involve a variety of media.
7. Presentation must be carefully adjusted in the light of fluctuations in class attention.
8. Appropriate body language should be used.

Furthermore, a well-constituted presentation requires a clearly defined structure, the elements of which will normally include:

•   an introduction, a main part and a summary
•   a logical sequence in the main parts
•   regular sign-posting – this is what we have covered so far, this is what we will explore next, and these are what we will address afterwards
•   key learning points or main headings
•   built-in monitoring and review – checking that the main learning points are being understood.

Appropriate communication and delivery skills are crucial. The presenter's role is also to engage with the audience, to challenge, to enthuse, to support, to motivate and to clarify. The next step is to give the lesson based on the lesson plan, and to evaluate it at the end of the lesson. The evaluation of the lesson can include use of an evaluation form, or the students can be asked to write three things that they liked or found most useful about the session, aspects that they felt were weak, and suggestions for improvement (see Chapter 9 for more on evaluation).

Levels of theory acquisition

The objective of many a teaching session is to impart knowledge and understanding of the designated topic area and, depending on various factors, it can cover application, analysis and synthesis. These concepts are largely enshrined in the cognitive domain of Bloom's (1956) taxonomy of learning, which follows six hierarchical levels, which has only minimally been modified since the initial publication. The first or lower level of learning is the acquisition of knowledge, followed by the higher levels – comprehension, application, analysis, synthesis and evaluation, in this sequence, as illustrated here:

1. *Knowledge* – refers to knowledge of the topic area and content.
2. *Comprehension* – refers to understanding of the knowledge gained, such as why things work the way they do.

3. *Application* – refers to how the knowledge and understanding gained can be applied to general and specific care settings, for example.
4. *Analysis* – refers to analysis of all components of knowledge and application; and consideration of alternative perspectives.
5. *Synthesis* – refers to utilisation of the knowledge and comprehension, and alternative perspectives, to arrive at solutions to problems.
6. *Evaluation* – refers to evidence of knowledge and competence (e.g. research findings related to the knowledge on the topic).

Knowledge is the most basic level of learning, in which the student shows a recall of specific facts, classifications, categories and sequences or methods in the topic area. It is a significant component of student assessment, as when the student has to demonstrate knowledge of human biology or of research methods. Comprehension refers to understanding and interpretation of the topic area, and can be shown by the student explaining why certain actions are taken, or why certain things happen, and their possible implications and consequences. Application occurs when the student applies knowledge and understanding to 'real-life' situations such as patient care.

Analysis entails the ability to break down theories and concepts into their component parts and explain the relationships between elements and the whole. It considers strengths and weaknesses, and alternative explanations or actions. *Synthesis* requires the individual to recombine various components of the topic area, and to reconstruct a whole new concept after analysing them. The student thereby utilises creativity in producing something unique, for example a plan, a design or a proposal. *Evaluation* implies the ability to make judgements regarding the value of the knowledge and competence learned, preferably research-derived.

A simple and brief example of levels of learning related to 'the heart and blood pressure' is presented here to illustrate how cognitive levels of learning (Bloom, 1956) apply to learning in healthcare:

*   Knowledge – knowing the anatomy and physiology of the heart and that pressure is exerted on the blood vessels each time the heart pumps a certain volume of blood through them.
*   Comprehension – understanding that the reason for the heart beating rhythmically at approximately 60 beats every minute, generating a blood pressure (BP) of approximately 110/70 mm Hg, is to ensure that essential ingredients such as glucose and oxygen are transferred to every tissue in the human body, and continuously.
*   Application – awareness that the above BP reading can change for a variety of reasons, which might include diseased organs, and its significance for patient care.
*   Analysis – when a person is seen to have high BP, the nurse needs to consider the whole range of possible reasons for this.
*   Synthesis – designing, and advising the individual on, a set of actions to take to reduce their BP, and explaining the effects of unstable or high BP based on their own unique aetiology and perceptions of high BP.

- Evaluation – ascertaining the value of the above set of actions, the skills and compliance of the patient in relation to them, and any research evidence on which the recommended actions are based.

The analysis of the cognitive domain of learning is essential as it can be extended to critical analysis, which, as already noted above, entails breaking down information and exploring alternatives. Critical analysis involves the use of critical thinking, whereby we:

- examine all the component parts of a situation
- identify what existing knowledge or information we have, related to the situation
- distinguish relevant information from the irrelevant
- challenge generalisations, assumptions and rituals
- imagine and explore alternatives and then choose the appropriate options.

From their research into students' academic writing skills, Gopee and Deane (2013) conclude that because some students struggle particularly with critical analysis in their academic writing, universities should strengthen their writing support department, as well as their student peer-collaboration facilities. As for the whole of Bloom's (1956) level of knowledge acquisition, Anderson, L.W. et al. (2014) recommended a refinement of the taxonomy whereby the synthesis and evaluation sequence are reversed into 'evaluate' and 'create', as illustrated in Figure 3.1.

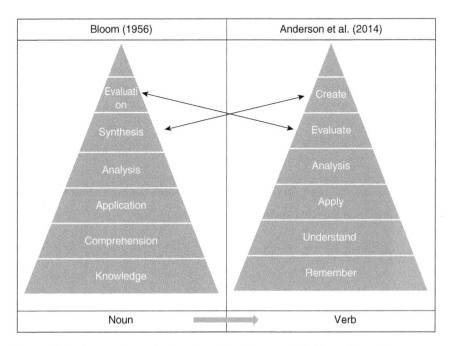

Figure 3.1 Comparison of Bloom's and Anderson et al.'s hierarchies of knowledge acquisition

So, Anderson, L.W. et al. reverse the fifth and sixth levels of Bloom's levels of learning, which is no doubt useful for identifying educational objectives, except that, as with any novel framework, it requires further work in its applicability to education programmes for the healthcare professions.

Teaching Methods and Teaching Aids

For structured lessons on clinical skills or knowledge acquisition, effective teaching requires choosing and applying the appropriate teaching methods and aids, which are selected based on such factors as the aims and learning outcomes of the session, class size, the students' existing knowledge levels, and so on. A number of teaching methods were identified in the box presented earlier titled 'Most frequently used teaching methods'.

Teaching methods – their advantages and disadvantages

Lectures remain an efficient teaching method for imparting knowledge and comprehension of a selected component of a subject area. A lecture is economical in that the knowledge can be imparted to hundreds of students by one lecturer during a particular teaching session, and also presented by video link live to other lecture theatres in other universities, in the same or other countries.

However, only a limited level of application and analysis can be achieved, as, in very large groups, it is difficult to cite examples of application to each student's field of interest. Moreover, it is easier for students to let their minds wander off the subject, which they generally cannot do in smaller groups. Discussions, workshops and group work to explore application, analysis and synthesis of components of the lecture, should therefore always follow lectures. Similarly, the advantages and disadvantages of other teaching methods also need to be appreciated.

━━━━━━━━━━ **ACTION POINT 3.4** ━━━━━━━━━━

Teaching methods – advantages and disadvantages

Taking an analytical approach, the strengths and weaknesses of each of the examples of different teaching methods listed in the box titled 'Most frequently used teaching methods' can be identified. Consider these different teaching methods, feel free to add any others of your own, and identify as many advantages and disadvantages as you can for at least three of these methods.

You should have been able to identify one or two advantages and disadvantages of each of the aforementioned teaching methods. With *skill demonstration*, for instance, the advantages include immediate visual display of the clinical activity being performed. It reinforces any previously acquired knowledge of the clinical activity, activates many senses, enables procedure-directed practice, correlates theory and practice, and is economical with time. The disadvantages could be that the learner might be left-/right-handed related to the positioning of equipment, the skill might involve movements that are too complex, and too much information might be given. As learning and mastering a skilled clinical activity can take time, there is also a danger that the learner might be expected to perform the demonstrated clinical activity at similar speed to the skilled demonstrator too soon.

The advantages of using *case studies* or *patient-centred discussions* as a teaching method are that there is active participation by students, they are useful in the application of theory to practice and they present an opportunity for structured problem-solving. These improve the following: understanding the situation, diagnosing the problem, creating alternative solutions and predicting outcomes or implications. The disadvantages include having insufficient information about the patient and the extent of relevance perceived by each student.

For e-learning modes of facilitation of learning, this has been strongly encouraged over the years, and even whole courses are available by e-learning, and more recently by online learning; and during the coronavirus pandemic at the start of the 2020s, a vast number of courses were delivered online. The benefit of this mode of delivery was that students were able to continue with their studies, with teaching delivered online using Zoom, Microsoft Teams and other similar technological facilities. Some were delivered by 'hybrid learning', that is, a combination of face-to-face and online teaching. However, despite teachers receiving the appropriate training to deliver teaching through these facilities, the weaknesses of online learning soon became obvious as the technology occasionally failed. At important meetings when using this mechanism, learning technologists had to be present throughout the meeting, which obviously meant double the staff time was required.

Presentation and teaching aids

There are several types of presentation aids that the teacher can utilise to make their teaching sessions more effective, to add emphasis to aspects of the session, and, at the same time, to vary the session and thereby to retain the audience's attention. These aids include:

- flipchart and pens
- whiteboard
- PowerPoint slides
- video recordings

- plastic models of body parts/objects
- gapped handouts
- simulated materials or liquids
- visualisers.

The purpose of teaching aids is therefore to introduce variety into the teaching process, to extend visual and other sensory perceptions, to give meaning to abstractions and to assist in the conceptualisation of complicated issues. The choice of visual aids involves a consideration of appropriateness to the context or message, their cost-effectiveness, their availability and their suitability for your style of presentation. Each teaching aid requires a good understanding of how it works.

━━━━━━━━━━ **ACTION POINT 3.5** ━━━━━━━━━━

Strengths and weaknesses of different teaching aids

Consider the strengths and weaknesses of the different teaching aids listed earlier, add other ones that you know of, and discuss with someone who has had some experience of classroom teaching what the strengths and weaknesses of each of these aids might be.

The PowerPoint presentation is a highly favoured method of presenting the knowledge base of a topic area to a small or large audience. The advantage is that it is prepared in advance and can be made very lively and interesting, using pictures, cartoons and short films for greater impact. The likely disadvantage is that too many words are put on each slide, or if the slides are presented at a high speed, this may not allow time for the audience to take the content in properly, or the equipment (computer, video links, etc.) may fail.

Facilitating learning for students with a disability

In addition to theories and individual styles of learning, facilitators of learning should also heed the special educational needs of individual students with a disability (e.g. Department for Education & DHSC, 2020, updated). The number of students disclosing that they have a disability is increasing (e.g. Olofsson et al., 2015), including those who are students on healthcare profession courses. Universities have an obligation to comply with legal requirements, such as the Equality Act 2010 (Advance HE, 2020), and practice supervisors have to be aware of this obligation towards students with disabilities as well under the Act.

The QAA (2010: 7) prefers the term 'disabled student' but the definition of disability in the Equality Act 2010 (Advance HE, 2020: 19) is 'a physical or mental impairment, which has a substantial and long term adverse effect on [someone's] ability to carry out normal day to day activities'. The above-mentioned Act also identifies a list of different impairments that constitute a disability, including dys-lexia, autism, dyscalculia, and severe mental health problems.

Consequently, the above Act indicates that organisations must provide 'reason-able adjustment' facilities to support students with a disability with their learning and with their course assessments. Almost all organisations concerned with the education of healthcare profession students, including the RCN (2022b) and the QAA (2010), prepare their own written statement on how they make 'reasonable adjustments' for students with a disability. The RCN's (2022b: 9) guidance on how such adjustments may be made in the practice setting for students with a disability or neurodiversity, includes the following:

- placement closer to home and adjustment to working hours
- the use of coloured overlays to assist in reading text on white paper
- allowing additional time to read and complete a task
- provision of a quiet area to write up notes, or for when specific tasks require intense concentration
- use of a voice recorder for handover
- use of a calculator
- use of apps for reminders
- giving verbal rather than written instructions
- giving instructions one at a time, slowly and clearly, in a quiet location
- reminding the person of important deadlines and reviewing priorities regularly
- using a wall planner and creating a 'to do' list.

For advice and support on how to make adjustments for students with a disability, practice supervisors can consult various named individuals and departments such as the partner university's lecturer(s) who specialises in this topic area, Occupa-tional Health services and student unions. Furthermore, other than in the context of policies related to disabilities, there is also an abundance of research and other literature on the topic area. Scullion (2010), for instance, identifies the two most prominent perspectives on disability: the medical model and the social model. The medical model, as the term implies, endeavours to enable people with disabilities to function to their maximum by rectifying the problem as far as they can at the pathophysiological level. The social model, on the other hand, tends to view those with disabilities as individuals who should not be stereotyped and stigmatised; rather, adjustments should be made to their social environment to enable them to function to their maximum, and for barriers to be removed. Scullion indicates that, as a strategy to challenge discrimination, healthcare professionals should promote and enhance the social model of disability through 'social advocacy'.

Research on the extent to which the needs of students with a disability are met, includes that by Olofsson et al. (2015) and Lavender (2017). Olofsson et al.'s (2015: 346) study found that almost half of students with dyslexia need a longer period of study than other students, while Tee et al.'s (2010) study revealed that disabled students require 20 per cent more contact time with lecturers than non-disabled peers, and they therefore recommend the appointment of a 'student practice learning advisor' for extra support. Additionally, Lavender's (2017) study of modes of learning by paramedic students with dyslexia concluded by reinforcing the need to allow students with disabilities planned extra time for their learning in practice settings.

‐Case study 3.2‐

Students with disabilities

Student nurse Vicky informed the pre-registration course director during the first week of the course that she has been told previously when she was at college that she might have dyslexia. The course director advised the student to attend the Student Welfare Department of the university for an assessment of her particular difficulties, and to determine the adjustments that should enable her to undertake her course activities with more ease. Consequently, Vicky was issued with the following facilities and advice, some of which should help in academic settings, others in the practice setting:

- provision of notes from the lecturer on coloured paper, if possible, or use of coloured overlays
- use of coloured overlays for reading text on white paper
- a spell checker, or a specialised computer with a built-in spell checker, etc.
- permission to have a person take notes for Vicky at lectures or to use a tape recorder to audio-record lectures
- visual diagrams to explain things
- the allowance of additional time when taking written examinations
- the allowance of extra time to complete nursing tasks in the practice setting
- the giving of instructions one at a time, and allowing requests for clarification or double checking of instructions
- use of pocket books to write words or instructions to remember during a clinical shift
- use of checklists
- the allocation of a quiet, uninterrupted area and additional time to write up nursing patients' progress notes.

Vicky was understandably apprehensive about how quickly she was going to be able to adapt to activities in the practice setting during practice placements, and, on the other hand, although her practice supervisor had attended sessions on students with disabilities both during practice supervisor preparation and at an update session some months earlier, she hadn't actually anticipated that one of her students would have dyslexia problems. At the initial individual interview with the student, when the student mentioned her disability, and also indicated that she had been able to use certain contraptions to cope with university lectures and simulation activities, the practice supervisor remembered that, in the course of her normal duties, she had to adjust to people with various individual differences, and did not pursue this aspect of the conversation too far at that point in time.

However, by the end of the second shift with the student, the practice supervisor had investigated various ways in which students with special needs or disabilities could be supported in practice settings, including the Royal College of Nursing's (2022b) guidance on neurodiversity (which includes dyslexia), and noted continuing use of the term 'reasonable adjustments'. Giving the student extra time with clinical activities and extra support was deemed essential by the supervisor, as well as asking Vicky how she normally managed her particular dyslexia problems. The practice supervisor also consulted the university's learning support department, and discussed the adjustments required by Vicky with other practice supervisors in the team. By the end of the practice placement, the student had achieved all her practice objectives and passed her first placement.

Universities have their own published declaration on ways in which they meet the learning and assessment needs of students with disabilities. Although all seems to have ended well for student nurse Vicky in Case Study 3.2, it also highlights the need to inform the practice placement setting beforehand if a student with a disability is due to be on placement with them, so that appropriate reasonable adjustments can be made and put in place well before the student starts on placement. For quality assurance purposes, the NMC (2022b) requires universities to provide evidence of this being the case.

In the context of disability discrimination, it is noteworthy that, in May 2022, a judge ordered a UK university to pay a substantial sum in damages to the parents of a student with 'social anxiety disorder', because the court found the university guilty of discrimination by ignoring her social anxiety, which had led the student to commit suicide (Wace, 2022).

Issues With Facilitation of Learning in the Practice Setting

The practice supervisor's duties includes teaching learners on a one-to-one basis, and at times in small groups in the practice setting. In both situations, the practice supervisor needs to have full knowledge of various components of the session, for example the content and sequence of the lesson, in order to ensure that the learner gains an orderly, systematic understanding of the topic or clinical activity. However, the problematic situations that might arise when facilitating student learning may present challenges to practice supervisors.

For a variety of reasons, in practice settings it cannot be guaranteed that a teaching session will go ahead as planned, although most do go to plan. Urgent need to cover for sickness, emergencies such as cardiac arrest, or the patient not consenting to student involvement, are some of the reasons. However, many care-provider settings now have dedicated teaching areas, which can help focus attention on teaching sessions.

Furthermore, there can be confusion in the interpretation of students' 'supernumerary status' during placements, in that the student might (erroneously) claim that they are there only to observe clinical activity, while the practice supervisor believes that they should participate as well as observe. Supernumerary status can be manipulated by some students to the extent that they take excessive time off from practice settings as study time, to the detriment of learning hands-on care and clinical skills, as many practice supervisors claim that healthcare delivery is learned by doing, not by merely knowing about it.

Chapter Summary

This chapter has focused on the practice supervisor's role in the facilitation of learning, both formal and incidental, and has therefore examined:

- Whose learning healthcare professionals facilitate, and why; the various reasons for teaching; and the definitions and different perceptions of teaching, along with why healthcare professionals need to know how to facilitate learning.
- General perspectives on learning, indicating a move away from teaching to the notion of facilitating learning, and to student-centred approaches to teaching and learning.
- Facilitating the learning of clinical skills, teaching a psychomotor skill, levels of psychomotor skills and stages of skill acquisition, and the domains of learning.
- Facilitating knowledge acquisition, including undertaking planned and structured short teaching sessions, either on a one-to-one level or in small groups of learners or peers.
- The types of knowledge associated with skills, such as practical knowledge and theoretical knowledge, along with levels of theory acquisition, and levels and stages of skill acquisition (taxonomy levels).
- Step-by-step planning of teaching sessions, including the utilisation of different methods of teaching and teaching aids, and an analysis of how they might be used effectively.
- Strategies for facilitating the learning of students with disabilities, and some of the issues that might surface in the facilitation of learning in practice settings.

Further Optional Reading

1.   For much more detail on how to teach, see:
     - Curzon, L.B. and Tummons, J. (2013) *Teaching in Further Education: An Outline of Principles and Practice*, 7th edn. London: Bloomsbury Academic.

2. For updates on the current provision for students with disabilities and detailed guidance on how to support learning for students with disabilities, see:

    •   Quality Assurance Agency for Higher Education (2010) *Code of Practice for the Assurance of Academic Quality and Standards in Higher Education, Section 3: Disabled Students*. Available at: https://nadp-uk.org/wp-content/uploads/2015/02/2010-Code-of-practice-for-academic-qual-standards.pdf (accessed 28 April 2022).

3. For further discussion on the facilitation of learning, see:

    •   Warburton, T., Houghton, T. and Barry, D. (2016) 'Facilitation of learning: Part 2', *Nursing Standard*, 30(35): 41–48.

4

APPLICATION OF SIMULATION TO HEALTHCARE STUDENTS' LEARNING

Natasha Taylor

Introduction

Simulation is used widely in healthcare learning to develop the ways in which students and other healthcare learners communicate and interact with, and assess and treat, patients/service users. This type of experiential learning encompasses a whole range of approaches and techniques, and is therefore not one tool or one technology; and it might not involve any technology at all. Simulation is used to simulate real-world situations and the term comes from the Latin word *simulare*, meaning to imitate. This type of learning is intended to enable health profession learners to develop specific knowledge and competence, behaviours and confidence.

Simulation means different things in other fields such as computing and mathematics, but healthcare simulation means to replicate and be involved in an imitation or a role-played healthcare situation. This doesn't necessarily mean a clinical situation, as it can be used for exposure to many real-life encounters. This can include peer or colleague interaction simulation, taking place nowhere near a clinical environment, or it can be in a traditional hospital or clinic or other healthcare setting.

Up to almost a quarter of the minimum amount of clinical skills' learning hours required during the pre-registration programme can now be achieved by simulation, according to the NMC (2021a), provided doing so is justified and certain mechanisms are put in place to facilitate them. Sometimes, the term medical simulation is used interchangeably with healthcare simulation, and they are pretty much the same approach, just used in different healthcare (or medical) cultures. Occasionally, discipline-specific simulation terms, such as nursing simulation, paramedic simulation or surgical simulation, are used. However, the approaches are mostly the same, the techniques are the same, the structure and governance and even the validating standards are (mostly) the same. The term simulation-based education (SBE) has become increasingly popular as a title.

──**─Chapter objectives─**──────────────────────────────

1. Develop a basic overview of healthcare simulation and its application to contemporary healthcare curricula.
2. Advance the application of healthcare simulation research, frameworks and standards to one's own discipline or specialism.
3. Show awareness of the basic ways to formulate, deliver and evaluate simulation learning.
4. Acquire knowledge and understanding, and develop critical evaluation skills in healthcare simulation.

Why do we Use Simulation?

Simulation is 'an artificial representation of a real-world practice scenario that supports student development and assessment through experiential learning with the opportunity for repetition, feedback, evaluation and reflection; (an effective) simulation facilitates safety by enhancing knowledge, behaviours and skills', according to the NMC (2018d: 14). Thus, simulation, as an educational activity, is most useful in such a critical area as healthcare, where decisions truly count, but solutions can be discovered in practice scenarios replicating the individual's health problems.

━━━━━━━━━━ **ACTION POINT 4.1** ━━━━━━━━━━

Benefits of learning by simulation

As a healthcare professional, you are likely to have met, been involved in or learned clinical interventions and skills by simulation (as per the explanation of simulation given above
under Introduction, and the NMC's explanation). You may also have encountered simulation as a registrant, maybe when attending an in-house advanced life support course, for
example. What are the potential benefits of learning and being assessed by simulation,
would you say?

From a meta-analysis of simulation-based learning, Chernikova et al. (2020: 499)
(as an example of benefits of simulation in healthcare) conclude that '(1) simulations are among the most effective means to facilitate learning of complex skills
across domains; and (2) different scaffolding types can facilitate simulation-based
learning during different phases of the development of knowledge and skills'. Overall, examples of learning by simulation include:

- advanced life support
- a chest model used to simulate choking, or a pneumothorax
- use of **haptic gloves** to interact in a computer-generated scene or surgical
  intervention
- inter-professional simulation, where different disciplines work together
- role-play – with people acting the part of a patient.

Most of these examples are referred to in context later in this chapter. The most
popular areas of research on learning healthcare by simulation, according to Wang
et al.'s (2022) bibliometric analysis, are: (1) inter-professional simulation in patient-
care teams; (2) patient simulation in psychiatric nursing education; (3) virtual reality simulation in midwifery and nursing education; (4) simulation in critical care
nurses' continuing education/training; and (5) simulation in paediatric resuscitation education. There are many reasons for applying simulation to learning healthcare intervention skills, and these include the following.

A range of easily accessible learning opportunities

One of the benefits of simulation is that it offers scheduled, valuable learning experiences that would be difficult or unethical to obtain in real life, such as simulations involving children or vulnerable people. How difficult would it be to undergo
traumatic or intrusive simulations? How much more difficult would these be for
particular people or groups?

In addition, students can address both behavioural (behaviours) and cognitive (mental processing) skills, including knowledge-in-action, procedures,

decision-making and effective communication by simulation. Critical team-work behaviours and collaborating under stressful conditions can be taught and practised by simulation. If the simulation is created and evaluated correctly, these can be observed and subsequently their effectiveness evaluated so that improvements can be made.

The freedom to make mistakes and to learn from them

Another benefit of learning by simulation is that working in a simulated environment allows for any mistakes that students might make, and without the need for immediate intervention to stop causing harm to the patient (or student). In real life, practising on a person, even with their informed consent, can be harmful. Students would have to get it right, immediately. This is not consistent with theories of learning, because we learn in stages. Although there are many different theories of learning, the concept of *scaffolding* (e.g. Chernikova et al., 2020) – learning in small, manageable steps and making mistakes and learning from them to achieve a goal – is especially pertinent in simulation education.

By seeing the outcome of their mistakes, students can gain powerful insight into the consequences of their actions and the need to get it (more) right when caring for real patients. That's not to say that simulation is always without harm – it can be harmful to both students and facilitators – which is one of the reasons why simulation needs to follow a set of guidelines or standards. This helps to lessen the potential harm that can be caused in such emotive and emotional situations.

The learning experience can be customised

Simulation can accommodate a range of students from novices to very experienced experts. Absolute beginners can gain confidence for parts of tasks because this allows them to focus on the more demanding parts of care. Additionally, some complex procedures and rare diseases don't present enough opportunities for practice, and therefore simulation enables the situation to be customised for practising, an experience that also enables consistency of occurrence. Consider a standard clinical placement during a course of study. Students have very different exposure levels, even if they go to the same clinical or non-clinical placement. It's a question of chance which patients/service users, skills, assessments, management and care each student will get exposed to. This leads to an inherent inequity between students, one that can be rectified by simulating some 'must see' experiences. It is not suggested that simulation can totally replace some actual experiences or skills, merely that simulation can support learners to fill a gap.

The learning experience can be replicated

Perhaps the most innovative aspect of simulation, as mentioned above, is that it allows students equity of access. All learners can experience all clinical contacts equally, rather than rely on the clinical contacts that are available at a given time in practice settings. Consequently, virtual placement is truly equitable.

Additionally, because any clinical situation can be portrayed at will, these learning opportunities can be scheduled at convenient times and locations for or by learners, and repeated as often as necessary. They can be carried out synchronously, where students need to login or take part at set times, or asynchronously, where students can take part any time, usually within set boundaries such as within a day or a couple of days. This allows students that may struggle, due to other pressures, or those that are neurodiverse, to take part in a learning experience that may have been off limits to them previously.

Detailed feedback and evaluation

Real events and the pace of actual healthcare activities such as emergencies do not allow time to review and learn about why things took place, or how to improve performance. Real events in healthcare are often high-speed, especially for the novice, and can seem confusing, with multiple complicated occurrences happening all at once. How do learners know what to 'unpick' in a real-life event, if they do not know what they are looking at, or when they are receiving multiple visual and audio inputs during placement? This is where controlled simulation constitutes another benefit of SBE, as the simulation event can be immediately followed by audio-visual supported (in other words, video-recorded) debriefings or after-action reviews that richly detail what happened, and why specific actions were taken.

We can even use advanced technology in simulation, that can gather data about what the learner is doing and when. These performance maps and logs provide an essential feedback mechanism to students and help facilitators target where improvement may be needed.

Healthcare simulation thus not only enables students to be better prepared for the actual encounters that they experience in the workplace, but can also be part of ongoing learning, as it ensures best practice is followed. Healthcare is dynamic and changes constantly, so that changes in practice can be rehearsed or imitated to ensure that they can be embedded in the system. In addition, and just as importantly, simulation can be used as a primary research tool. Patient safety is at the heart of what we do, and simulation ensures increased patient safety both before and during actual practice. This connection of research and standards also encourages connections between students and clinicians. Learning with each other and from each other can help to drive healthcare disciplines forward, both as individual disciplines and in working as inter-disciplinary healthcare teams.

A Brief History of Healthcare Simulation

As we've already found out, simulation is a technique, not a technology, which can be applied to replace or even amplify (add details to) real-life experiences. Simulated guided experiences are intended to conjure up or even replicate entirely real-world healthcare events. To better understand how and why simulation works so well in healthcare, a look back at the very long history of this technique is useful. Although aviation or nuclear industry simulation are often held up as the originators of systematic, widespread, safety-conscious simulation, these are only as old as aviation and nuclear power itself. The early and mid-twentieth century certainly showed the birth of simulation in these areas, but we need to look back several millennia to pinpoint the earliest use of healthcare simulators.

Historically, simulation dolls or body parts (simulated or real) date back to antiquity, with some earthenware teaching models being found. Unsurprisingly, women's anatomy or physiology, including obstetrics, often makes up most historic simulation models. We know that there is still a gender gap in women's health outcomes compared to men's, as there is less research on women's health issues compared to men's health, and the gender bias that is still prevalent was widespread in previous centuries. This, along with general distaste in women's health and anatomy by male clinicians in previous centuries, mean that actual women's anatomy would not have been appropriate to learn from. This then led to the use of clay or pottery, and later cloth, simulation models for teaching purposes.

Certainly, by the eighteenth century, simulated body parts were complex and often used to prevent the significant mortality associated with childbirth. Dr William Smellie is often given credit for his mechanical labour device. However, the mechanical labour device is thought to be based on an earlier model created by a French midwife called Louise du Coudray. Madame du Coudray manufactured hundreds of her version of a birthing model to teach midwifery (to other midwives) in the mid-eighteenth century. Thereafter, healthcare simulation models and body parts changed little, except for the change from cloth to plastics, ensuring greater wear and cleanability. However, an exponential explosion of technological advancement in the late twentieth century meant greater fidelity and realness in models.

Models and parts that moved, that could play simple sound files, for example, meant that not only could situations be closer to real life but, also, obsolescence occurred more often. This takes us to the first quarter of the twentieth century and the rise of innovative technologies which may have paved the way for the healthcare simulation of the future. Where we are now and where we may be going in the future with healthcare simulation, form the basis of the rest of this chapter.

How Does the Simulation Methodology Work?

As has already been briefly discussed, simulation isn't one tool or technology; it is more of an approach or a methodology. This means that there is a set of rules, methods or procedures which should be followed. Regardless of what the simulation is for, whether it uses a dummy or is online, or involves a real person acting the part of a patient, there are typical ways in which simulation needs to be done. The process is generally intended to be fully immersive – in other words, the student needs to get absorbed entirely in the situation and it must have a beginning (the pre-brief), middle (the interaction with the patient, clients, user or colleague(s)) event and end (the debrief). These phases of simulation will be explored further later in this chapter.

To ensure this beginning, middle and end are useful for the student and done in the best possible way, evidence-based frameworks can be used. It doesn't necessarily matter which of these frameworks, approaches or methodologies are used, just one that has good, solid evidence to support its use (e.g. Watts et al., 2021). This technique of healthcare simulation is a useful, evidenced way to develop students working in a range of health disciplines. However, like any learning and teaching, it needs proven approaches and frameworks to ensure it is effective and robust, and that students find it useful and, therefore, the patient/service user benefits too.

To better understand what these approaches to healthcare simulation are, this chapter outlines some significant components of simulation-based learning. The chapter isn't intended to develop simulationists from clinicians, it is intended to set out some of the major aspects of healthcare simulation to whet the appetite of those reading. To better understand healthcare simulation, there are some excellent postgraduate courses at many universities. These range from postgraduate certificates to master's degrees and even doctoral study opportunities. (For further information, contact a university you have a link with or the author of this chapter.)

Types and Tools of Healthcare Simulation

The next section of this chapter gives an overview of the types of different simulators (or simulations) there are, except just some main types are included. For a fuller list of simulators, see the Society for Simulation in Healthcare (SSH) (2022) dictionary, which is a free resource that can be found online (a link is given in the further reading section at the end of this chapter). This section therefore explores the utilisation of mannequins, skills or **task trainers**, simulated patients and virtual and extended reality.

Mannequin/Manikin

This is the name given to the part- or whole-body artificial (usually made from plastic or fibreglass) model used in traditional simulations. The two terms and their spellings are often used interchangeably. However, there is some thought that if a model is used for medical purposes or for a life artist, then the word manikin is the appropriate term; and if a model is used in a shop, say for hanging clothes on, or in a window display, then the word mannequin is more correct. Manikin comes from the Dutch term *manneken*, which means little man, with the French form of the word *mannequin* used in English to mean artificial man.

However, and this is where these terms become contentious, the term mannequin is used for robots or artificially intelligent models. With the rise in high-fidelity, smart models in healthcare, the term manikin or mannequin can be applied interchangeably. Regardless of the spelling used, most people in healthcare will know what you mean. Therefore, to prevent confusion and for ease of reading, the word mannequin will be used from here on.

The first contemporary mannequin that we would recognise was designed in the early 1960s, the ubiquitous Resusci Anne, also often called Resusci Annie. This was manufactured by a Norwegian toy manufacturer, working with a couple of physicians who discovered and published research on the style of cardiopulmonary resuscitation (CPR) we know today. The mannequin was used and developed to teach people how to perform CPR and remains a mainstay of resuscitation teaching today.

Although these mannequins are now far more advanced than earlier models, with baby to child to adult to older adult (and even resuscitation animals) available, the fundamental principles remain. This is to allow people to practise in a safe environment, without causing harm to others. These advances are needed to allow for full interaction with the simulated patient if anything other than basic CPR is to be taught. Current high-fidelity mannequins can simulate emotions, can absorb or release fluids, can simulate facial expressions or movements, and can even speak via sound file or streamed external sound.

These mannequins can be used in different areas as they are generally (relatively) portable. The more complex the mannequin, generally the less portable they are and the more they will need specialist knowledge to set up and make ready. This is why high-fidelity mannequins tend to stay where they are most often used, which is on a trolley or patient bed. The simulation can take place *in situ*, meaning in the actual place where people work, the actual clinical environment. This is not an area made to look like a clinical environment, such as a simulation centre or simulation room in a hospital or clinic, but to truly be in situ, the simulation needs to take place in the actual setting.

As an example, an in situ intensive care simulation would need to take place in the actual intensive care unit and not another clinical space within the hospital that can simulate the intensive care space. However, as you can imagine, carrying out a simulation in an actual intensive care unit can be frightening for patients who may see or overhear the simulation being carried out. It can also be unwieldy and difficult to carry out, and therefore it doesn't form the majority of healthcare simulation. Most healthcare simulation is carried out in physical environments created to look as close to real life as possible without being in those environments.

Mannequins tend to be used for whole-patient assessment and management, where audio and visual clues from the mannequin, such as baseline observations (or vital signs), can be observed. Some mannequins can accept fluids and medication, and electronically note what was given and when, and can be made to respond to interventions. These mannequins can even have moulage applied, such as make-up used to simulate injuries or skin discolouration. Clothing and wigs can be added, and skin colour can be changed using overlay masks. There are times though when parts of that patient assessment or management need to be practised. For this, whole-body mannequins are superfluous, and therefore only an arm or the chest, for example, can be used, as the focus is on only one skill or task. There are parts of the mannequin that can be purchased separately for the simulation of patient care purposes.

Skill or task trainers

Another type or tool for healthcare simulation is task trainers or skill(s) trainers. The two terms are often used interchangeably and comprise of models designed to help learners to practise specific healthcare procedures by simulation. The parts of the body are however often more complex than merely a part of a whole-body mannequin, and are often made to simulate a specific skill (or a related set of skills). Thus, a chest used to simulate choking is also very different from a chest used to simulate a pneumothorax.

Although the mannequin is invaluable for whole-patient, whole-body simulations, 'task trainers' (body part simulators) allow for the development of fine motor skills in isolation – in other words, they are specifically for the skill(s) that can be carried out on that task trainer. Task trainers also allow students to repeat these skills again and again before they perform them on real patients. Moreover, these skills or task trainers can be useful for even experienced clinicians, to ensure that muscle memory is maintained, especially in skills not encountered very often.

In addition, as we've already found out, mannequins can be difficult to transport, are bulky and often hugely expensive. For the cost of one full-body mannequin, several task trainers can be purchased, allowing for a greater number for student access. Maintaining a task trainer is also considerably easier than the high-fidelity mannequins. That doesn't mean that the mannequin and the skills/task trainer is an either/or requirement, as often a hybrid of both is used and the simulation switches between the two. Although task trainers are more cost-effective, some can be incredibly realistic and complex, with a functional structure under a lifelike skin, with fluid absorption and generation, if required.

━━━━━━━━━━━━ ACTION POINT 4.2 ━━━━━━━━━━━━

Types of models used for training learners

As a practice supervisor, which 'plastic' or technological models are you aware of, which you might have seen or have been mentioned by students? Which skills or tasks are initially learnt by students via simulation before they encounter them with real patients during practice placements?

Technological or plastic models, however lifelike, are inanimate objects, and they therefore cannot simulate complex human interactions, especially complex communication scenarios. For this, actual human beings are, at the moment, the most efficient and effective way of simulating interaction (see e.g. the quasi-experimental study by Noh and Park, 2022). This use of a person is discussed in the next section.

Standardised or simulated patient

The terms standardised patient (SP) and simulated patient which are often used interchangeably refer to a person carefully recruited and trained to take on the characteristics of a real patient. Standardised patients are particularly useful for complex communication, such as presenting their history and complaint, and answering when probed further with follow-up questions.

However, generally, only a very limited physical assessment can take place and often the SP does not have the same physical parameters as the patient being simulated. For example, if we want to simulate a hypertensive patient and we use an SP who is normotensive, then if the effort to prompt a hypertensive outcome is unsuccessful, this could be confusing and distracting for the student. Therefore, occasionally, a hybrid of these different types may be more appropriate to use.

Standardised patients can also receive moulage, make-up and so on, that simulate certain injuries and are strongly supported by service users who have been consulted for the use of SPs. The use of appraised ethnically or culturally representative SPs is also essential, with much controversy over the use of insensitive make-up or mask-type systems to simulate a different age or ethnicity than the SP. Some simulation centres hire the services of professional standardised patients, while some work with service users, and others work with volunteers, peers or colleagues as SPs. Regardless of who is an SP, standard frameworks need to be used to ensure the 'patient' is standard for every single learner. This means that all SPs need specialist training, pre- and post-briefing and, in some cases, they take a full and equal part in the simulation team.

Utilising the services of humans as standardised patients is well-researched, and much have been written about SP frameworks, one of these being the 'Simulated Patient Common Framework' (Manchester Metropolitan University & Health Education North West, 2015), that can be applied. However, the use of frameworks and SPs for training is a specialist skill that cannot be learnt just by trial and error, and therefore needs guided professional development of prospective facilitators. In general, better simulations apply a combination of mannequins, skill or task trainers and standardised patients.

Extended reality

Another tool for healthcare simulation is 'extended reality', which can take the form of virtual reality (VR), augmented reality (AR) or mixed reality (MR). Very briefly, VR is a computer-generated environment, featuring healthcare patients, which the student can interact with. Although VR has a relatively long history, with very primitive VR-type uses in the mid-twentieth century, it was the rise in home computing in the 1980s that saw the use of the term virtual reality, and which became accessible to most people. One quasi-experimental pre–post design study wherein student nurses participated in a 45-minute interactive simulated VR dementia experience, found that there were statistically significant increases in student awareness, knowledge and sensitivity of Alzheimer's disease, and the researchers anticipated that this would translate into improved care for individuals with dementia (Campbell et al., 2021).

Augmented reality is an interactive activity that combines real-world environments with computer-generated programmes, in which a smart phone is usually used, and the phone screen superimposes images, sounds, and even smells, over the actual environment. The use of AR as an overlay to a mannequin face allows the student to point a smart phone at the mannequin and 'see' an actual patient face, giving the student better cues and more information. Perhaps the best-known use of AR is Pokémon GO, which is a game that uses the player's smart phone and clock to detect where, and when, the player is in the game. Augmented reality can be and is used in healthcare simulation, often to good effect. As we have found out, high-fidelity mannequins, although somewhat moveable, look like mannequins (at the moment).

Mixed reality is like an advanced AR, whereupon the virtual and the real world can interact. As we saw in AR, the real world and the computer-generated world are different layers. The computer-generated world often sits over or in front of the real world. Mixed reality combines these two layers, for example the use of haptic gloves to interact in a computer-generated scene. This exciting innovation deserves a section of this chapter to itself, and therefore it is examined further under 'Evaluation of digital education technology'.

═══════ ACTION **POINT** 4.3 ═══════

Using appropriate simulation tools

You now know a bit more about some of the tools used for healthcare simulation. Think of some of the learning activities and tools that are used for in-house training by health service providers, and those that you might use for teaching learners in your clinical specialism. Which patient care activities can be learnt effectively by simulation? What are the pros and cons of your choice(s)? Here are a few possible examples:

- Advanced Life Support
- Breaking bad news
- Intravenous cannulation
- Head-to-toe assessment.

There is no right or wrong answer, as Action Point 4.3 is intended to make you consider and decide which tools would be most appropriate for teaching and learning in your specialism. For example, which tools might be used by paramedics to simulate a road traffic collision? Thinking of occupational therapists, which tools could be used to simulate a post-stroke patient? How about a physiotherapist – which tools might be used to simulate respiratory patho-physiology?

Process of Teaching and Learning by Simulation

As already noted, the process of effective teaching and learning by simulation comprises pre-briefing students, the simulation event itself (contact or interaction between facilitator and learner/others) and, in the end, the debriefing. Before the simulation event and even before the pre-brief, the facilitator has to identify the aims and learning outcomes or objectives of the event so that the purpose of the whole event is completely clear, and, therefore, like any learning activity, simulation needs to have its aims and outcomes and/or objectives identified. These terms are often used interchangeably but are very different in educational (and simulation) terms.

The aim(s) of a learning by simulation event, or even a whole course, is simply a way to combine everything we want the student to achieve during that learning event/course. Generally, a whole course will have multiple aims, whereas a short simulation event may just have one or two, and they should reflect the overall purpose and intention of the event. As an example, the aim of this book chapter is to provide an introduction to healthcare simulation for students, and how we do that is by setting objectives, which are then set out in the chapter objectives.

━━━━━━━━━━ ACTION **POINT 4.4** ━━━━━━━━━━

Identifying the aims and outcomes of the simulation event

Consider the content of the above two paragraphs on the aims and outcomes or objectives of a simulation event, and if needed, revisit the section in Chapter 3 entitled 'Identifying the aims and outcomes of the session', where an analysis of these concepts is presented. Then think about the following simulation learning outcomes: Which ones would you say are good and which are not so good? Which components of which outcomes would you keep, and which words would you change?

Example 1: Understand the principles of CPR

Example 2: Demonstrate CPR

Example 3: Demonstrate cardiopulmonary resuscitation on a simulated adult patient, according to RC(UK) 2021 adult basic life support guidelines

Example 4: Perform cardiopulmonary resuscitation on an adult mannequin, according to RC(UK) guidelines.

When the simulation event has been planned in full detail, including the learning outcomes, then the pre-brief for the event can proceed at an agreed point in time, with both learners and any co-facilitator.

Pre-brief

Pre-briefing is conducted before the actual simulation contact event, and is an essential part of the whole simulation activity. Simulation should not be conducted without a pre-brief (and debrief), although there is currently no set framework available, nor a way that has been shown to be better than the inclusion of pre-brief and debrief, as noted by Abulebda et al. (2022), for example.

In patient contact simulation events, pre-briefing is conducted before the 'action' part of the simulation when the student interacts with the simulated patient, whether a mannequin, standardised patient or virtual patient, and prepares and orientates the learner to the purpose of the activity. This is needed for many reasons, perhaps the most important being to set out the 'how and why' of the whole simulation event, and it allows everyone involved to have detailed knowledge of the whole process and of what is expected of them. It creates a safe environment, one in which the student feels fully part of the process, which can also help the student feel less anxious.

Pre-brief therefore gives the student an overview of the whole process, except that patient outcomes are not given to the student at this stage, as there can still be challenging components in the briefing. It is more about the 'rules' of how the simulated event will occur, a familiarisation with the environment, the learning outcomes and what is expected of them. This creates a much better learning environment, so that students can get more from the simulation if they know the boundaries and what they will learn during the simulation. The pre-brief should also include an idea of what form the debrief will take.

Although there is no set pre-briefing framework, generally there are three fundamental aspects:

1. It is crucial to state the aim(s) and learning outcomes of the simulation event, and, as we've discovered already, the aim(s) and outcomes need to be clear, simple, measurable and have appropriate learning verbs. The pre-brief enables the student to familiarise themselves with the environment and any equipment being used, and informing the student of how and when the debriefing will occur is essential. This setting of boundaries is useful for everyone involved in the simulation, not just the student. It is not wrong to be transparent with what is expected, and even when using simulation as a traditional assessment, the student needs to know the process that they will engage with. However, the vast majority of simulation is applied to develop learners, albeit at times it is used for traditional assessment, such as an objective structured clinical examination (OSCE).

2. Students need to know the logistic details of the simulation, such as how long the event will last, timings of breaks, and where to find toilets, refreshments, etc. This information can be communicated to the student way before the event, via email or even on the day. Where students are on a course of study, they may know this already, but it is always useful to be really clear about locations and timings.

3. The student, facilitator and anyone else involved (e.g. a standardised patient) should commit to respecting both each other and the process. If the goal is to create a safe learning environment, then respect between everyone involved, including appropriate behaviour boundaries, is necessary.

Debrief

Debrief is as important as pre-brief and is as essential as any other part of the simulation. Like pre-briefing, although numerous research-based frameworks on debriefing are available, no one framework or guidance is definitively recognised (Sawyer et al., 2016). However, also like pre-brief, there are key components that make for a good debrief. As we have seen with pre-brief, some aspects are generally carried out immediately before the contact part of the simulation, while some may happen a while before the student starts. The same happens with debriefing, as generally it's easier to debrief immediately after the event; but there are certain types of debrief that call for multiple or gap debriefing, which is where a set time occurs between the simulation event contact and the debriefing.

However, there are three general principles of debriefing that most frameworks contain, and that should be adhered to for more efficacy, as illustrated in Figure 4.1.

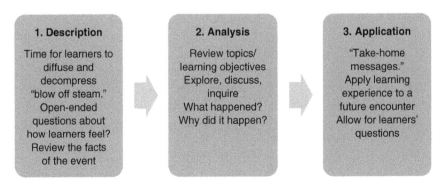

Figure 4.1 Three general principles of de-briefing following the simulation event

There is no set time for, or set way of, debriefing, as it depends on the framework used, but it is important to use a framework and inform the student of this during the pre-brief.

From their questionnaire-based research on the perceptions and satisfaction of mental health nursing students after learning specific specialist skills via clinical simulation, García-Mayor et al. (2021) indicate that participants in their study expressed a high degree of satisfaction with learning by simulation and with the OSCE procedure, and recommend that this method should be implemented more frequently. Participants also indicated that debriefing comprises a vital contribution to the learning process, although they also pointed out that they did experience some stress and anxiety during their OSCEs. However, it is important to consider that assessments are generally inherently a stressful process for students.

Contact part of the simulation event

The contact part is the section of the simulation that people often regard as 'the simulation' but, as we have seen, the pre-brief and the debrief are essential components of it. There is a reason for presenting this component third in this section. This is to make it very clear that all simulation events must have a beginning (pre-brief) and an end (debrief), in addition to the middle or contact part. All three parts are as important as each other and cannot be called simulation if the contact part is conducted in isolation.

For the contact part of the simulation, there needs to be one or more facilitators, which can be an academic, a clinician, even another student, or indeed anyone who knows the principles of healthcare simulation, as discussed in this chapter. Everyone has an equal role to play in the simulation event – the facilitator(s) is just one member of the team as is any student who forms part of the simulation team.

It is important to consider the facilitator–student power dynamics, as it can be very challenging to be a student when there is a facilitator watching their every move. This is where clear pre-briefing helps, but a consideration of how and where the facilitator stands and interacts might be needed. This will also help to normalise the simulation event and ensure the facilitator doesn't interfere with the overall event. This is especially important when using verbal challenge (usually questions) during the simulation. By allowing the student to steer and lead, rather than the facilitator doing so, the student can explore issues, make mistakes and learn from them, and progress in their learning. Of course, if the student is about to make a critical error that would put any member of the team at risk, then immediate intervention is needed by the facilitator.

Furthermore, simulation often brings up a plethora of emotions, for everyone in the simulation team, including the facilitator. Therefore, it is essential to provide a safe space for managing emotions before, during and after the event. Additionally, support systems need to be signposted because the effects of the simulation might not be felt until well after the event, which nonetheless needs addressing. Giving students a space to process their emotions is useful for all learning activities but especially so in simulation. Moreover, it might not be the obvious healthcare simulation that was the cause of issues, because simulation emotions are personal to each individual, and therefore what may seem a simple, non-critical event, could mobilise potentially difficult underlying feelings.

Inter-professional simulation

As we know, the way we deliver health services is changing. This previous silo working was also seen in simulation, when nurses did simulation with other nurses, paramedics with paramedics, physiotherapists with physiotherapists, and so on. In some cases, this accurately reflects real-life working but often healthcare interventions are inter-disciplinary (or inter-professional). Consequently if, for example, a patient contact requires both an occupational therapist and a dietician, then the simulation should include both an occupational therapist and a dietician.

This way of working, as well as learning together between different healthcare disciplines, is referrred to as inter-professional education (IPE). Inter-professional education is integral to undergraduate education and should be part of healthcare simulation, where it reflects real-life practice. However, uni-professional simulation is appropriate where it reflects actual practice, but IPE is needed when two or more different disciplines work together, as also noted by Velásquez et al. (2022).

There are, though, issues with IPE simulation and these are mainly due to logistics. It can for instance be difficult to organise multiple professionals to take part in a specific simulation event at the same time. This is where asynchronous simulation can be useful. Asynchronous just means not at the same time. Take, for example, a virtual simulated patient, whereupon the patient can be set up to have a group of students from different disciplines work together but not at the same time. Most systems can be set up so that the student can access the patient within a certain time frame, for example any time between 9am and 5pm on a set day, with the time frame being longer or shorter. In this way, groups of students who may have conflicting responsibilities can still work together.

Simulation Governance and Guidelines

In order to ensure that the simulations we provide are useful for our learners, we can apply published governance standards and simulation organisation guidelines. Governance assures the reliability of simulations, and we want students to get the most out of simulations, especially as they are often quite time-consuming, personnel-heavy and expensive.

National and international standards are generally the result of a collaboration between simulation education experts, using the latest evidence base, and working within, and with, simulation networks. The standards used may be by choice but may also be a requirement of the organisation or the validating body. Health Education England (HEE) (2018), for instance, which is the organisation that oversees the education, training and workforce development for healthcare, offers a framework for simulation-based education (SBE), which in turn comprises of: quality outcomes, leadership and governance, a strategic approach and resource allocation, faculty development and quality assurance – see box below for details.

HEE's Framework for Simulation-based Education

1. *Quality outcomes*: the delivery of safe, effective care through workforce development – SBE investment is aligned with the delivery and continuing improvement of high-quality, safe, effective care and with enhancing the learner experience.
2. *Leadership and governance*: leadership in SBE is clearly defined, and the appropriate governance model and processes are explicitly applied.
3. *Strategic approach and resource allocation*: each local area's strategic approach to simulation is aligned with national and regional approaches in order to ensure consistency. Where applicable, SBE is multi-professionally delivered and arrangements for resource allocation modelling are shared and understood.
4. *Multi-professional faculty development*: multi-professional staff development in SBE occurs across all areas, and sharing best practice is encouraged and supported widely.
5. *Quality assurance*: there is a well-defined method for quality assuring the content and delivery of SBE based on the HEE quality framework for education and training and other national standards as deemed relevant for the simulation activity.

Source: HEE (2018)

Research on the application of SBE (e.g. by Rossler and Tucker, 2022) suggests that SBE is effective in enhancing students' clinical judgement related to the provision of care. Standards or guidelines for SBE are varied but mostly overlap in approach, and therefore standards can be adapted according to local SBE needs. As an organisation, it is useful to have standards relevant to one's unique needs. Most organisations' healthcare simulation standards tend to be based on those of larger standard-setting bodies, which is valuable when collaborating with students, service users, key stakeholders and funders.

Evaluation of digital education technology

Even before the COVID-19 pandemic, digital education by simulation was increasingly being used in healthcare to support and advance students' learning. Digital education, which is sometimes referred to as e-learning, uses digital technologies for learning, which means education that students can access via a screen, such as a laptop, tablet or smart phone. Digital simulation, on the other hand, is a catch-all term that can mean different approaches and uses, such as virtual simulated placement, serious gaming, machine learning, avatars, and so on. The technology itself and the many educational concepts behind it are generally well researched (e.g. Hamilton et al., 2016).

Furthermore, the Substitution-Augmentation-Modification-Redefinition (SAMR) model (e.g. Hamilton et al., 2016), which is a useful, four-level approach for selecting, using and evaluating technology, can be integrated into simulation events. The SAMR model can also help to map which technology is needed for which type or component of learning for particular student groups. The model consists of (see also Figure 4.2):

Substitution – suggests that technology is just a tool substitute, with no functional change.

Augmentation – indicates that technology still acts as a direct tool substitute, but with functional improvement.

Modification – indicates that technology allows for significant task redesign.

Redefinition – is when technology allows for the creation of new tasks previously inconceivable.

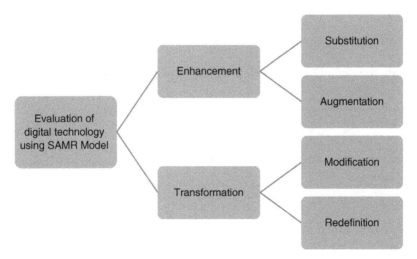

Figure 4.2   SAMR model for evaluating technology for simulation-based education

Simulation that is within the substitution or augmentation stages can be said to enhance learning, whereas activities that are within the modification or redefinition categories are said to transform learning. Using the SAMR model, alongside the learning verbs in the outcomes of the simulation event, can help steer the simulation facilitator to use the most appropriate technology for the event.

Digital technology is embedded in most of our lives, and digital or virtual simulation has increasingly been incorporated in healthcare curricula in recent years (e.g. Taylor et al., 2021). However, technology, by its nature, rapidly evolves and sometimes the student (and facilitator) in digital simulation is left behind. Therefore, when considering digital simulation, it's important to consider the digital literacy of those using it. Digital literacy has been identified as an issue in the workplace anyway and simulation activity is no exception. We know that digital capabilities correlate with improved outcomes, so increasing the digital literacy of students (and facilitators) can ensure an improvement throughout the whole healthcare system.

Chapter Summary

In conclusion, healthcare simulation is an exciting, innovative, valid and evidence-based way of supporting learning, and it is embedded widely in most healthcare curricula. Healthcare simulation has a long history and the types of technology and tools that are available for use are seemingly endless. However, there are certain standards and principles that run through all simulation, regardless of approach.

One of these principles is the way the simulation event is carried out, regardless of which technology or tool is used. The principle of beginning, middle and end (pre-brief, contact, debrief), for example, is essential, and well-written aim(s) and outcomes make these so much easier and more effective. This chapter has therefore addressed:

1. An overview of healthcare simulation and its application to contemporary healthcare curricula, and an assessment of the evidence base of effectiveness of learning by simulation in healthcare.
2. Advancing the application of healthcare simulation research, frameworks and standards to one's own setting.
3. Awareness of basic ways to formulate, deliver and evaluate simulation learning.
4. Developing knowledge and critical evaluation skills in healthcare simulation.

Further reading on healthcare simulation is recommended, and some suggestions are provided next, and also in the publications cited in this chapter. Happy simulating!

Further Optional Reading

1. For the most up-to-date standards of application of simulation, see:
   - Association for Simulated Practice in Healthcare (ASPiH) (2021) *ASPiH Standards for Simulation-Based Education (SBE)*. Available at: https://aspih. org.uk/standards-framework-for-sbe/#:~:text=The%20Association%20

for%20Simulated%20Practice,use%20across%20the%20UK%20and (accessed 22 May 2022).

2. For the HEE Framework for Simulation-Based Education (SBE), see:

- Health Education England (2018) *National Framework for Simulation Based Education (SBE)*. Available at: www.hee.nhs.uk/sites/default/files/documents/National%20framework%20for%20simulation%20based%20education.pdf (accessed 22 May 2022).

3. For the most up-to-date version of a comprehensive dictionary on simulation, see:

- Society for Simulation in Healthcare Dictionary – version 2.1 (2022) Available at: www.ssih.org/Portals/48/v2_1-Final.pdf (accessed 22 May 2022).

5

HEALTHCARE SETTINGS AS EFFECTIVE LEARNING ENVIRONMENTS

Introduction

Having explored the supervision of practice-based learning in Chapter 1, theories, perspectives and styles of learning in Chapter 2, the facilitation of learning in Chapter 3, and teaching and learning through simulation in Chapter 4, this chapter focuses on the factors that make healthcare settings effective learning environments for health profession students, as well as for qualified staff. Ensuring that the practice setting has an effective learning environment and culture is an essential responsibility of workplace student placement providers.

In the *Standards Framework for Nursing and Midwifery Education*, under 'Student empowerment', the NMC (2018d) states that HEIs together with their healthcare provider partners must ensure that all students have opportunities to learn from a variety of practice placements in healthcare settings. Under 'Learning culture', it indicates that students must be supported and supervised in practice settings that are 'conducive to safe and effective learning ... and where ... inter-professional learning and team working are embedded' (p. 5); and that the setting has a learning culture that is fair, impartial, transparent, and fosters good relations between individuals and diverse groups.

This chapter therefore examines ways in which practice settings constitute effective learning environments; healthcare professionals' involvement in creating, maintaining and monitoring their learning culture; associated educational policies; and issues related to student practice placement.

—**Chapter objectives**—

1. Clearly identify the various reasons for healthcare students being required to undertake practice placements.
2. Recognise the reasons for ascertaining students' previous clinical experience before identifying their learning needs, as well as their hopes and expectations with regard to the placement.
3. Identify how a functional learning culture can prevail or be created in the practice setting based on an organisational culture that values education and training, and which supports inter-professional learning by conducting regular education audits of practice placement settings.
4. Analyse the benefits of, and issues related to, workplace learning and identify ways in which the utilisation of learning pathways can enhance the student's learning.
5. Identify guidelines, policies and standards for clinical learning environments, and how practice settings can become learning organisations.
6. Recognise the likely problematic aspects of practice placements, such as the integration of theory and practice, and supernumerary status and 'supported learning time', and the likely solutions to these.

Why are Practice Placements Required for Health Profession Students?

This section of the chapter explores why practice placements are required for students on healthcare profession courses, students' hopes and expectations in relation to each practice placement, practice objectives and research on students' clinical experiences on placement.

The first reason for students requiring practice placements is that healthcare professions comprise skill- or competency-based activities, and these skills are acquired predominantly in practice settings. Several hundred student nurses, numerous AHP and medical students start their pre-registration or pre-service courses each year, and each student requires practice placements in practice settings to learn patient care skills directly, or to consolidate and extend their learning from university skills laboratories. Due to recent increases in the volume of students and in the variety of healthcare profession courses, most suitable practice settings in local trusts and the independent sector are used for placements, and the placement for all these students is usually jointly arranged by the education institution's placement department and PEFs or placement co-ordinators based in the placement provider organisation.

The terms practice placement and placement-based learning refer mostly to health profession students, and are also known as clinical placement, work placement, work experience, internship, work-based learning, posting, and so on, in the UK and other countries. The benefits of placement-based learning, according to Moroney et al.'s (2022) research, are that it enables students to:

- perform assessments of service users' health problems
- integrate theory with practice
- discuss and evaluate care with others inside the practice setting
- develop self-confidence and critical thinking skills
- build skills in time management and in prioritisation of care
- consider their future nursing role
- feel that they are a member of the healthcare team
- build skills in communication and empathy.

Each practice setting is advised in advance of which students are starting on placement with them and when. Students arrive on placement with a document containing practice competencies that the student must achieve during the placement, which takes into account the specific clinical skills and knowledge that the particular setting can offer.

Pre-registration education requirements so far include those identified in the Directive 2013/55/EU of the European Parliament and of the Council (EU Directives in short) (Legislation.gov.uk, 2020), which is currently being reviewed by the NMC (2022a). Based on the EU Directives, the NMC (2018e: 13; 2019a: 10) states that for nursing or midwifery qualifications, the duration of learning in practice settings must comprise at least one half of the minimum duration of their education programme, that is, half of a total of at least 4,600 hours. It also indicates that learning environments comprise of any space where learning takes place, along with the system of shared values, beliefs and behaviours within these settings. Furthermore, the HCPC (2017) indicates that practice-based learning must take place in an environment that is safe and supportive for both learners and service users (clause 5.4).

Another reason that practice settings need to be learning environments is the fuller appreciation of practice-based or work-based learning (WBL) which clearly recognises the wide occurrence and value of learning professional skills in work settings, in addition to learning in HEIs. Work-based learning is also one of the most prominent features of nursing associate training programmes (e.g. HEE, 2017: 23) and of apprenticeship-based programmes.

Work-based learning (or workplace learning) is a term that applies to learning in the workplace in all skill-based professions, and is equivalent to the term 'practice education' in nursing and midwifery, and to 'internship' in some university-linked programme such as business studies. Thus, WBL is an overarching term, which has been defined by several researchers, including Barr (2003), who indicates that WBL is learning that takes place at work, or learning that takes place away from work with the objective of improving performance at work. The definitions of WBL imply that, in addition to apprenticeship-type learning in workplaces, learning is supplemented by planned classroom-based lessons or skills-laboratory-based learning.

When WBL or practice-based learning is a component of a university-based programme, then it also consists of credit points, or credit accumulation and transfer scheme (CATS) points, the number depending to a good extent on the duration of the placement, such as whether it is for four weeks, eight weeks, 12 weeks or year-long. An extensive study of WBL by Moore (2010) revealed that managerial support in workplace development is crucial for WBL to be successful as a learning activity.

The beneficial effects of WBL in midwifery, for example, are documented by Marshall (2012) who reports that it enables practitioners to improve multi-professional collaboration and consequently the development of maternity services within the healthcare trusts. It is efficient and cost-effective for both employee and employer, and serves to strengthen the link between higher education and the workplace. It also helps to integrate theory–practice, which ultimately benefits healthcare students as well as service users.

However, when ineffectively managed, WBL can become associated with training, and too focused on short-term solutions at the expense of quality education, according to Lester and Costley's (2010: 561) research, but 'well-designed work-based learning programmes are both effective and robust'. Furthermore, from their systematic review of qualitative studies on WBL in healthcare, Nevalainen et al. (2018) conclude that appropriate workplace culture, physical structures, as well as interpersonal relations are essential preconditions for effective WBL. Further 'guiding principles' on effective WBL are provided by the Quality Assurance Agency for Higher Education (QAA) (2018) (see further reading section at the end of this chapter).

However, in general, various research studies have in the past revealed some weaknesses of practice settings as learning environments. Consequently, for learning to occur, the practice setting must embody an ethos that nurtures and supports learning, and does not deter it. Research carried out by Hamshire et al. (2019), for example, to explore the factors that enhance course completion rates by student nurses, suggests that clinical placement experience is the most common cause of student attrition from pre-registration nursing courses.

Furthermore, in their qualitative study of student experience during practice placements, Brook and Kemp (2021) report that flexible rostering of students during practice placements impacts positively on student attendance and attitude, and reduces student attrition. Others add targeted student support especially for first-year students, campus-based support (e.g. the Student Union, a text message from a lecturer) and managing student expectations to reduce students dropping out of their programme (Hamshire et al., 2019).

Practice education for paramedic students during practice placement

Related to paramedic students' practice-based learning, for instance, paramedicine as a profession is relatively new. Until the beginning of the twenty-first century, 'ambulance drivers' followed an apprenticeship-type model of learning, with teaching occurring while carrying out emergency duties with a more experienced member of staff. However, with the increasing evidence supporting more invasive procedures and pharmacological interventions, a greater need for better educated out-of-hospital practitioners was deemed necessary, which culminated in more involved educational preparation for paramedics in higher education, and led to the registration of paramedics with the HCPC.

All paramedics in the UK must achieve the SOP set out by the HCPC (2014a). Student paramedics pass the programme's formative and summative assessments on their journey to (and beyond) registration. These encompass a wide range of cognitive, psychomotor and behavioural learning, both in the university setting and during practice placements. Of course, most of the practice placement learning that a student paramedic undertakes is in the ambulance environment.

There are, however, no specific national standards required for supervising paramedic students and the literature on paramedic student supervision is scant. Although the need for standardised and qualified practice educators is outlined, no standard currently exists, as observed by Lane (2014), for example, and as noted in the HCPC's (2017) standards of AHP education.

Depending on the ambulance service, the student's learning may be supervised by:

- a named, qualified practice educator or mentor for the duration of the placement hours
- a named, qualified practice educator or mentor for some of the placement hours, with some hours working with a qualified member of staff
- a qualified member of staff, but not a qualified practice educator or supervisor, for the duration of the placement hours.

It is accepted that there are difficulties in the out-of-hospital supervision of practice learning because unlike other health professionals, ambulance staff typically work as a two-person team, in a mobile ambulance, with few or no base station visits. This means that the practice educator or supervisor of learning must go in an ambulance with a student, away from a base except ambulances are constrained for spaces to work in, with little room, and therefore any additional staff reduces the space available in the back of a vehicle for attending to the service user.

Students' perspectives, hopes and expectations

A number of practice settings have well-established welcome and orientation pro-grammes for students starting practice placement with them, which students work through and record in their PAD; and they have an induction pack with specific clinical objectives for newly qualified healthcare professionals (NQHP). Nominated practice supervisors may be tentatively allocated to each student prior to the start of the placement. Nonetheless, both practice supervisors and the student have cer-tain hopes and expectations of each other for the span of the practice placement. So, what does the student anticipate encountering at the start of the placement?

━━━━━━━━ ACTION **POINT 5.1** ━━━━━━━━

Student expectations from the placement

Your work base clearly has a wide range of specific knowledge and competence to offer students during practice placements. From your experience of having students on place-ment, make some notes on what you feel are the expectations that students might have on starting a placement in your practice setting.

On exploring students' expectations of practice-based learning, a study by Foster et al. (2015) concluded that students value targeted teaching, explaining, support and encouragement as some of the key features of a successful practice placement. In addition to students' expectations, the staff in the practice setting naturally also have certain expectations of students. They hope that the student will be punctual, make every effort to integrate with the team and be open-minded about the ways in which care is delivered in the particular practice setting. Practice supervisors usually expect students to seek out learning experiences and opportunities, and ask questions about aspects that they do not understand. The box below lists some of the personal qualities of 'good' learners that have been identified by registrants on previous mentor courses.

Attributes of Effective Practice-based Healthcare Learners

- Is keen, enthusiastic and motivated to learn
- Is open-minded
- Identifies own learning needs
- Is open to feedback and constructive comments
- Is punctual
- Reflects on experiences
- Knows own limitations
- Is able to adapt to different practice settings
- Does not have negative thoughts prior to start of placement
- Utilises learning opportunities
- Communicates effectively
- Wants to self-improve
- Reads round the subject area.

Placement-related factors that impinge on successful or unsatisfactory practice placement experience are summarised in Figure 5.1.

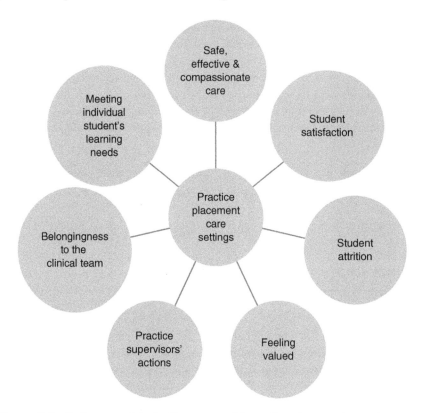

Figure 5.1   Factors associated with a successful practice placement experience

Advanced preparation of learners

Universities strongly advise students to contact practice placement settings prior to the placement start dates, mainly to introduce themselves, but also to enquire about practicalities such as what time shifts start, a room for changing into uniforms, possibly travel or car-parking facilities, as well as any other information that can be given (e.g. contact names). Initiating contact can be pivotal for a smooth and successful placement as, according to Webb and Shakespeare's (2008) research for example, good learning support depends to a great extent on students themselves initiating and building a relationship with those who are supervising their learning.

However, students find it useful if, prior to the practice placement, they receive a welcome letter from the practice setting, which may even invite the student to come over for an informal pre-placement visit. It is useful if the student can also be advised of any recommended preparatory reading related to the clinical specialism.

This action is in line with Ausubel et al.'s (1978) concept of 'advanced organiser', which suggests that learning is likely to be more effective if new experiences are linked to prior acquired knowledge.

The value of communication prior to the beginning of the placement is that the student begins to become familiar with the practice setting, gets to know more about the clinical specialism and meets one or more practice supervisors, and staff get to know the student as well. The aim of this would be to ensure that the clinical experiences that students will encounter meet their learning needs and enable the achievement of their practice objectives.

Creating and Maintaining a Learning Culture in the Practice Setting

Healthcare students acquire knowledge and competence at universities that are seen as well-established, natural learning environments. This is because they create and maintain environments that are conducive to learning through ensuring a relaxed and pleasant atmosphere in and outside campus buildings, encourage peer-learning and small-group learning by providing spaces where students can share knowledge and discuss their course-related issues in pairs or very small groups; and they provide cafés and refreshment areas, and departments that help students with course-related special issues. However, to what extent are practice settings learning environments?

━━━━━━━━━━ **ACTION POINT 5.2** ━━━━━━━━━━

A learning ethos in the practice setting

Using your current and past experience of factors that are significant in creating an effective learning experience for students during practice placements, make notes on the following:

- Who are the key people who are role models for learners (undergraduate and post-graduate, other) in practice settings?
- What are the factors that are important for the creation of a positive learning environment (including research-based factors) for everyone within any particular practice setting?

Being a role model for anyone can be a sobering prospect for most people. In response to who the role models in practice settings are, you would have identified a range of qualified health and care professionals, including:

- everyone who is a practice supervisor
- ward sisters/charge nurses

- team leaders
- specialist nurses (e.g. pain specialists)
- PEFs
- other registrants on pay bands 5 to 8
- allied healthcare professionals (e.g. physiotherapists, occupational therapists)
- lecturer-practitioners
- other students
- senior doctors, mainly consultants
- outreach workers
- clinical managers.

Role-modelling constitutes health and care professionals being practitioners of best practice in service-user care, and this is explored further in Chapter 6. However, poor care and neglect of patients were reported in the recent Francis (2013) report at one English NHS Trust. A number of the report's recommendations were subsequently implemented nationwide, which included:

- enhancement of patient safety
- staffing levels, 'to ensure the right people, with the right skills, are in the right place at the right time' (NHS England National Quality Board [NQB], 2014: 1)
- more openness and transparency, by providing information and acquiring feedback from healthcare service users and their family or friends.

These standards have to be met by the service provider to qualify as a suitable practice placement for health and care profession students. Similar recommendations were made in the Willis Commission Report (RCN, 2012), as noted in Chapter 2.

Practice settings as learning environments

In response to Action Point 5.2, that is, identifying the factors that are important for the creation of a positive learning ethos, you might have noted friendly and knowledgeable staff, positive attitude towards learning in clinical settings, and allocated time for teaching. Good communication is of course essential, as is the learner feeling that they are part of the team and valued. Team members with up-to-date knowledge of the latest research in their specialism generally make a positive impression. The availability and accessibility of research literature in the working environment, a well-stocked learning resources section or in a resource room, also create a positive image.

Furthermore, you might have noted that staff showing fair awareness of students' likely learning needs and their stage of knowledge and competence development, also create positive impressions. The enthusiasm of team members with responsibility for teaching in practice settings, and the input of PEFs/CHEFs, generate the impetus for learning. Constructive comments on performance of care interventions in an appropriate environment are usually appreciated by learners. A culture in which clinical staff are open to new ideas and share new learning from courses also presents healthy perspectives, as does good staff morale.

So, practice settings have to reflect learning environments. However, the concepts learning climate, learning culture and learning organisation all surface in relation to supporting learning in clinical settings. The difference between these concepts is that the setting can either have a learning climate, which can imply valuing learning but sporadically; or have a learning environment which signifies the longer-lasting value of learning. It can, however, have a learning culture which signifies a much more enduring outlook. 'Learning organisation' tends to refer to a more permanent and even more ingrained stance towards learning (see the progression illustrated in Figure 5.2).

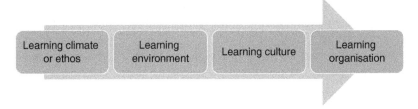

Figure 5.2 Progression from having a learning climate to being a learning organisation

Numerous research studies have been conducted on the effectiveness of practice settings as learning environments over the years, and new research in this area continues as the dynamics in practice settings evolve. Adverse research findings include Eick et al's. (2012) conclusion that one of the reasons for placement-related student attrition is non-acceptance of the student by the practice setting's staff, and thus also a perceived lack of support from them.

Lack of acceptance of the student leads to the student feeling that they do not belong to the clinical team, and research by Panda et al. (2021) on challenges faced by student nurses and midwives during practice placement, found that the attitude of clinical staff, instructors and significant others can negatively affect students' clinical learning, especially when they lack a sense of belongingness to the clinical team.

Furthermore, from their study of nursing homes as learning environments, Carlson and Idvall (2014) report with conviction that the 'supervisory relationship' (that is, the relationship between practice supervisor and student) has the greatest impact on student nurses' learning, and recommend that the work of supervisors of learning in the independent sector should be better recognised and that they should be supported through further collaborative activities (e.g. university-led workshops, practice supervisor updates).

More than three decades ago, Fretwell (1980) coined the term 'clinical learning environment' (CLE) as she concluded from her research that key components of an 'ideal' learning environment include 'anti-hierarchy', effective communication and teamwork between all those involved in the specific practice setting, and the availability of trained nurses to enable learners to meet their learning needs. Fast-forward to today, when the acronym CLE is extended to CLES+T (the S signifying supervision, and the T signifying additional teaching input from academics and practice-based teachers) and to CLEI (I signifies inventory), as will be discussed shortly.

ACTION POINT 5.3

Creating a learning culture in the practice setting

1. Based on the perspectives and ideas discussed above on practice settings being CLEs, make a list of your own of the factors in the health or care practice setting that you consider make it a good and effective learning environment.
2. How far does your own practice setting meet with the recommendations and factors that you have identified? Perform a SWOT analysis of your workplace as an effective clinical learning environment.
3. Then, consider what actions can be taken to enhance or improve your workplace as a CLE, focusing mainly but not exclusively on its weaknesses and threats.

The findings of studies on CLE also tend to reveal factors that promote learning in the practice setting and those that could hinder, a number of which are identified in Table 5.1.

Table 5.1   Factors that promote learning in practice settings and those that hinder

Factors that promote learning	Factors that hinder learning
• Registrants' level of knowledge of their clinical specialism	• Interruptions
• Adequate time to teach	• Over-busy ward area
• Practical demonstration of skills	• Lack of time
• Students feeling that they can take their time to practise the skills	• Staff, patients' and learners' attitudes
• A learning ethos	• Standards of equipment
• Teaching on a one-to-one basis	• Not enough information communicated
• Adequate staffing levels	• Learner–staff ratio too high
• Adequate planning and preparation	• Inadequate staffing levels
• Supporting learning resources and information	• Student uninterested
• Approachable staff	• Disorganised programme of teaching
	• Poor leadership

Due to a dearth of literature identifying ways in which non-hospital areas are learning environments, Gopee et al.'s (2004) analysis concluded with certain specific recommendations for enhancing primary care settings as learning environments, including:

- matching practice supervisor and student in accordance with the student's particular learning needs, for example by checking whether carrying out dressings is actually available in, say, placement with school nurses
- appropriate timing of practice placements, for example students are not allocated to a school nursing placement during school holidays
- management support to ensure designated time is identified for enabling learning, and ongoing professional development for all staff
- access to clinical supervision for all qualified staff.

Adequate staffing levels to safeguard patients and provide effective patient care are yet other features of a learning environment, and this was highlighted by the CNO for England (NHS England National Quality Board, 2014: 45), for example, who indicated that all 'nursing, midwifery and care staffing levels, and key quality and outcome measures should be discussed at Trust Board level in a public meeting'. For this to happen, the Board has to receive a monthly report of 'actual staff available on a shift-by-shift basis versus planned staffing levels' (2014: 45). Additionally, NICE (e.g. 2014) also publishes guidelines on staff capacity and capability, with its own perspectives on the issue.

Clearly, staffing levels have been a cause for concern for some years, and without sufficient and capable staff to provide safe and effective care, time might not be available to supervise students' learning. Additionally, the CNO has continually emphasised the need to ensure that a culture of compassionate care prevails, with concomitant staff education in this area (e.g. NHS England, 2016) (discussed in Chapter 6).

Furthermore, according to Campbell and Evans' (2016) qualitative research, managers' beliefs, attitude and role related to the effective facilitation of learning in their workplace have a major influence on the workplace also being a place for learning. Continuing and supported staff education and training, together with learning from service users and their families' experiences, comments and feedback are all components of an effective organisational learning culture.

Organisational learning culture

An organisational culture is defined as 'The collection of traditional values, policies, beliefs and attitudes that constitute a pervasive context for everything we do and think in an organisation' (Mullins, 2019: 686). Mannion and Davies (2018: 2) indicate that healthcare organisational culture refers to 'some of the softer, less visible, aspects of health service organisations and how these become manifest in patterns of care'.

These definitions refer to the values, beliefs, etc of staff, which is partly because the culture of groups of people generally comprises of the beliefs, values, norms, behaviour, social habits, etc of the individuals and groups that essentially are the resources that the organisation requires to support itself and enables it to function and achieve its mission and objectives. The organisation in the context of this chapter refers to all health and care practice settings that provide practice place-ments for students, in the NHS and the independent sector.

Organisation culture is variously explained by different writers, which include Schein (2017) and Mannion and Davies (2018), who both indicate that local cul-tures can be categorised as being at three levels, which, in the context of healthcare, flows from shallowest level to deepest (see Figure 5.3).

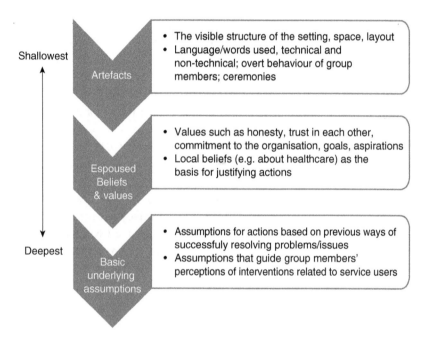

Figure 5.3   Levels of organisational culture

These artefacts, values and beliefs, and the underlying assumptions, are compo-nents of local culture that students encounter during the early days of the clinical placement in the practice setting. Beyond levels of organisational culture, organisa-tions also have different types of culture that newcomers to the setting encounter, which, according to Handy (2007), are: power culture, role culture, task culture or person culture. Briefly, in relation to care settings, they imply:

Power culture – depending on how much power is endowed in individual managers, power culture can be explicitly authoritarian or based on an individual's credentials, expertise and merit.

Role culture – based on the position individuals hold in the organisation and their knowledge and competence.

Task culture – can be too focused on tasks that need completing during the shift, rather than a more person-centred holistic view.

Person culture – where each individual member of staff is valued and their job aspirations are considered.

The extent and type of learning for individuals who work in the organisation can be influenced by all four types of culture, and, expanding on the person culture, Grealish and Henderson (2016) recognise the 'organisational learning culture', which, from their pre- and post-test study of nursing students' experience of learning in aged care settings, identifies four areas in which improvements were made which can be sustained when 'staff capacity to support learning is developed'. These four areas are:

- recognition of healthcare students and learning in the organisation
- accomplishment – staff's acquisition of new knowledge and skills
- affiliation – feeling part of the team in the practice setting, and of the organisation
- influence – feeling safe to express opinions and suggest ideas.

Thus, the culture that prevails in healthcare organisations and individual care settings can substantially influence how students get to perceive the practice placement area, and, for some time now, organisational learning culture in nursing and midwifery, in particular, has been referred to as a clinical learning environment. A wide range of research studies has been conducted over the years on what contemporarily constitutes an effective CLE, especially as the character of practice settings evolves with the times, for example with the continuing digitalisation of services.

Research on CLE by Henderson et al. (2012: 299), for example, revealed that students tend to value 'task accomplishment' highly, but, although the practice settings value safe practice, they were 'not readily open to innovation and challenges to routine practices'. More positive findings are also reported, such as students' working relationship with their supervisor of learning being seen as particularly significant in their achievement of practice objectives.

Based on the above accounts of the subject area, a clinical learning environment can be defined as a practice setting that manifests a psychosocial ethos and culture, with related supportive resources, that fosters mutual learning among all healthcare professionals, learners and clientele, and where care and treatment are founded on the best available evidence. The recommendations from earlier and recent studies regarding aspects that constitute good and effective learning environments form the key components of regular educational audit documents.

Further research on the continuing enhancement of practice settings as CLEs includes identifying what makes practice settings effective CLEs, such as Shivers et al.'s (2017) research on the Clinical Learning Environment Inventory (CLEI) and Manninen et al.'s (2022) research on the Clinical Learning Environment, Supervision and Nurse Teacher (CLES + T) scale.

Furthermore, from research on 'student satisfaction' with their practice placements in primary care centres, Cervera-Gasch et al. (2022) concluded that both student perception of the primary care setting as learning environment, and their overall level of satisfaction with the placement, were high.

Educational audit of practice placement settings

Several recent studies on CLEs have focused directly on exploring the factors that can be identified as the necessary criteria in educational audits that are used for identifying and monitoring the continuing suitability of each practice setting for student placement. Under 'Educational governance and quality', the NMC (2018d: 8) indicates that all learning environments are regularly reviewed to ensure that they are safe and effective, and therefore suitable for student placement. The HCPC (2017) also stipulates the requirement for the approval and quality monitoring of practice placement clinical areas.

These NMC and HCPC standards essentially signify the requirement for regular educational audits of every practice setting where students are placed for learning clinical skills and associated knowledge, and undertaken at least once every two years for each practice setting, while some require annual educational audits.

The criteria for suitability include a statement of the practice setting's philosophy of care, and a systematic approach to person-centred practice. Previously, Orton et al. (1993) had focused specifically on the criteria for educational auditing, review and approval of practice settings for students' practice placements under the following headings: (1) orientation to the placement, (2) theory and practice integration, (3) supernumerary status, (4) staff attitudes and behaviour, (5) mentors, and (6) progressive assessment. Currently, the strongly advocated Clinical Learning Environment Inventory (CLEI) is being applied for educational audits. The inventory comprises 42 criteria grouped under the sections: (1) personalisation, (2) student involvement, (3) task orientation, (4) innovation, and (5) satisfaction and individualisation. Research on CLEI, for example by Shivers et al. (2017), found that, overall, students are actually satisfied with practice settings that meet all the criteria in CLEI.

Another popular prevailing educational audit tool that measures the practice setting as a learning environment from the students' viewpoint is CLES+T, which stands for clinical learning environment, supervision and nurse teacher, consisting of a total of 34 criteria under five sections which are: (1) pedagogical atmosphere on the ward; (2) leadership style of the ward manager; (3) premises of nursing; (4) supervisory relationships; and (5) the role of nurse teachers (e.g. Manninen et al., 2022).

Furthermore, Anderson, A. et al. (2014) report on the implementation of an Inter-professional Clinical Placement Learning Environment Inventory (ICPLEI), from which they report that the tool is reliable and easy to complete, and that pre-registration healthcare students felt the items in the inventory were appropriate for CLE audit tools. Based on such continuing research on CLE, universities and local healthcare trusts jointly devise their own research-informed educational audit tools. These audit tools contain a range of criteria for determining whether the practice setting is suitable for the practice placement of healthcare profession students. Evidence needs to be available to auditors to demonstrate how each criterion is achieved.

═══════════ ACTION **POINT** 5.4 ═══════════

Strengths and weaknesses of your workbase as a learning environment

Locate a copy of the current completed educational audit document for your workplace, a copy of which is usually lodged in the practice setting electronically or maybe as a paper copy. If you cannot find the form, ask the ward manager or the PEF where the form can be found.

Then peruse each item or criterion in the document to decide for yourself whether the item are being fully achieved in your practice setting, or otherwise. This exercise will be your own professional judgement of areas of strengths and areas where improvements or enhancements can be made to your practice setting as a learning environment. Discuss your impressions with a peer if you have the opportunity.

Can you do anything about the weaker points? In fact, can you devise a SMART (specific, measurable, achievable, realistic and time-limited) action plan to make tangible improvements to the weaker areas/audit criteria?

Alternatively, view the CLES+T scale in Mikkonen et al. (2017: Table 3) or from another source of your choice. The scale is designed and worded in such a way that it endeavours to measure students' perception of the practice setting as a learning environment. Yet another alternative is to use the ICPLEI in Anderson, A. et al. (2014: Appendix). Using either of these two articles, peruse each item in the same way as indicated above for the educational audit document. (Full details of the articles are given in the References list at the end of this book).

Further research on the CLEI and CLES+T evaluation scales continues. For example, research conducted by Manninen et al. (2022) to explore the effectiveness of CLES+T from students' viewpoint, indicates that, overall, healthcare students are satisfied that the instrument is a valid tool for assessing the effectiveness of practice settings as CLEs.

In a previous multinational European study of the factors in the CLES+T scale that enhance students' learning experience during practice placement, Warne et al. (2010) found that student learning 'requires both significant time being spent working with patients and a supportive supervisory relationship' (2010: 809).

The educational audit document usually includes a section for recording the qualifications of each member of staff, of particular significance being which part of the profession's regulatory body's register they are on, and also whether they hold a practice assessor or similar qualification and have been attending updates related to practice supervision and assessment. Other post-registration qualifications are also recorded. Template 5.1 shows the content of the section at the front of the audit document that contains key information about the particular practice setting.

Template 5.1   Placement details page of educational audit document

Multi-professional Practice Environment Profile

Placement Details

1) Name and Address of Healthcare Provider/Organisation:
2) Name of Placement Area (Ward/Department/Unit/Team):
3) Placement Area Telephone No.:
4) Name of Manager of the Placement Area:
5) Manager's Email address:
6) Name and Contact Details of Person overseeing Quality of Learning Environment and students' learning:
7) Type of Service Provision/Speciality:
8) Work/Shift Patterns:
9) Date of last CQC visit:
10) Is the area compliant with CQC standards? Yes/No
11) Names of Reviewers:
12) Name of Academic Link Lecturer:
13) Names of Practice Education Facilitators:
14) What is the maximum number of students that your practice setting normally support at any one time?
15) Please identify the type of students regularly allocated to the placement area (child branch, adult branch, midwifery, work experience, ...)
16) What factors influence the number of students you can accept?
17) Name(s) of Academic Institutions Placing Students (University/College of Further Education/Other, e.g. for work experience):
18) Date of Previous Review:
19) Date of Review:

Naturally, each item in this section of the audit document is important. In addition to the placement details on the first two or three pages of the audit document, it identifies a number of criteria or 'standards' that have to be met for the practice setting to be approved as suitable for the practice placement of healthcare students. These standards are often based on research and national guidelines and can include, for example, the following:

- Care planning documentation reflects appropriate NHS England/NICE guidelines and DH directives.
- Confidentiality is in place to protect patients, staff and students.
- Training records demonstrate that all staff have attended mandatory training sessions.

The document also tends to have a section for clinical staff to identify and list all the formal and informal teaching and learning opportunities, that are, or can be, available in the particular practice setting.

━━━━━━━ ACTION **POINT 5.5** ━━━━━━━

Formal and informal learning opportunities

Identify and make two lists, one of all the formal learning opportunities that are available in your own practice setting, and one for the informal ones, which can include structured and unstructured, incidental or opportunistic learning. You might find it useful to make the lists in discussion with a colleague in the same practice setting.

For formal learning, you might have mentioned teaching sessions given by the clinical nurse specialist, for instance; and for **informal learning** opportunities, you might have mentioned an instance where you explain to the student why the doctor has changed a patient's medication. There are likely to be various teaching and learning opportunities in your work-based setting. Maybe one of the consultant medical officers holds regular formal teaching sessions for junior doctors, which all healthcare professionals in the particular area are welcome to attend. Maybe pharmaceutical or medical devices company representatives give talks and demonstrations/updates on their products in the practice setting. Further examples of formal and informal teaching and learning opportunities that tend to be identified when completing educational audit forms, are presented in Table 5.2.

Table 5.2 Formal and informal learning opportunities

Formal teaching	Informal learning opportunities
<ul><li>Lectures by senior doctors</li><li>Patient assessment-related teaching</li><li>Student progress reviews - initial, mid-placement and final</li><li>Teaching while carrying out patient care, i.e. work-based learning</li><li>Setting learning tasks to students</li><li>Practice development nurse's guidance</li><li>Teaching by PEFs or by 'cascade trainers'</li><li>In-service/postgraduate training</li><li>Observing RNs, physiotherapists and other AHPs, or doctors performing clinical interventions</li></ul>	<ul><li>Learning about or from a patient with a new condition</li><li>Change in patient's condition discussed at handover</li><li>Asking questions informally</li><li>Reflection-in-action and reflection-on-action</li><li>Informal chat in the staff room during coffee break</li><li>Updating procedures and clinical guidelines' folders and learning resources</li><li>Access to computer databases and internet</li></ul>

If preferred, the resources for learning available in the practice setting can be grouped as human and non-human resources. Formal learning opportunities, such as teaching sessions and skill demonstrations, require human resources and include inter-professional learning. Non-human resources include printed instructions on how to use equipment, learning about medication, ventilator monitors or a 'care programme approach'. Many of the resources needed to deliver patient care can also be used for learning and for achieving clinical and managerial objectives. Other learning resources include a room that can be used for teaching and learning, with internet-enabled computers, whiteboard or flipcharts, for instance. The learning resource files containing project or research reports compiled by individuals in the team, research articles, etc, are also usually available for consultation and learning.

Inter-professional learning

As for inter-professional learning (IPL) in practice settings, the concept is promoted in various authoritative documents (e.g. NMC, 2018d: 5, 9). Successful education programmes and projects (e.g. Goldsmith et al., 2009) are documented and presented at conferences. The Centre for the Advancement of Inter-professional Education's (2017: 14) *CAIPE Inter-professional Education Guidelines* indicate that inter-professional education (IPE) 'occurs when students from various professions learn from and about each other to improve collaboration and the quality of care'. It indicates that IPE includes work-based learning as well as that in academic settings, before and after qualifying, and it also provides guidelines on a variety of aspects of the implementation and evaluation of IPE.

Another similar definition of IPE is provided by Buring et al. (2009: 59) as follows: 'Inter-professional education involves educators and learners from two or more health professions and their foundational disciplines who jointly create and foster a collaborative learning environment.' They indicate that IPE results in improved health service-user outcomes and satisfaction, better teamwork, and lower error rates.

The basis for IPL is inter-professional working, in that to resolve an individual health service-user's health problem (or to avert it), a group of different healthcare professionals such as nurses, doctors, dieticians, physiotherapists, input their own areas of professional expertise as appropriate. Multi-professional or multidisciplinary working, on the other hand, is a different concept, in that it tends to entail different healthcare professionals attending to the patient, delivering their clinical input and withdrawing with minimal collaborative communication with other healthcare professionals. Such an approach reflects a fragmented service that is also inadequately coordinated and recorded.

Inter-professional working, however, does imply collaboration, and better coordinated patient care with fuller communication, verbal and written. Inter-professional learning extends the concept to the exchange of knowledge, of understanding and clinical skills, and signifies collaborative problem-solving and the identification of patient goals.

Inter-professional learning also comprises informal and formal learning. Informally, for instance, the nurse explains to the occupational therapist the plan of care for a particular service user and the rationale for each action. In turn, the occupational therapist designs a plan of action and explains the rationales from their perspective. Informal IPL refers to all modes of unstructured, incidental or opportunistic teaching and learning between different professional groups, while IPE is more in-depth and tends to refer to university-designed courses that result in students being awarded a diploma or degree.

Formal IPL involves attending structured short courses with substantial hands-on elements that are designed for specified healthcare professionals. These courses entail shared learning by, say, nursing and medical students (e.g. Lockeman et al., 2017), and can include modules on such activities as 'advanced life support', communication skills in complex circumstances, case-based learning, problem-based learning, patient safety, and mental health first aid.

The Academy of Medical Royal Colleges (2017), which is an organisation that represents the majority of healthcare professions in the UK, supports multi-professional team working, indicating that it delivers better outcomes for patients and more effective and satisfying work for clinicians. It adds that multi-professional work requires flexibility in attitude and behaviour and for professionals to value and respect the distinct contribution each profession makes.

─Reflection point 5.1─

IPL in your work setting

To what extent does IPL occur in your work setting, both informally and formally?

Research on AHPs' identity, conducted by Hean et al. (2006), concluded that different AHP student groups tend to see themselves as distinct from other professional groups, which is healthy as it enables healthcare professionals to be cognisant of their unique professional expertise. However, when asked which characteristics made them different, physiotherapy students, for example, indicated that being 'team players' made them different, despite teamworking not being unique to any healthcare profession group. This suggests that many of the characteristics of AHP groups are largely similar (e.g. teamworking, person-centred practice), despite their different areas of expertise.

Research on inter-professional education suggests that it tends to enhance inter-professional practice and increase understanding of the roles of different professions (e.g. Lockeman et al., 2017). However, from their review of research on inter-professional communication in healthcare, Foronda et al. (2016) found that doctors and nurses have different communication styles which are based on their pre-qualifying education. They identify structural hierarchies, lack of confidence, for example, as issues that hinder effective communication and relationships. They recommend that education pro-gramme planners should adjust the content of their teaching so that they include common elements on patient-related communication across the pre-qualifying education of healthcare professions, such as wider use of such constructs as inter-professional handover, and so forth.

Research conducted by McLeod et al. (2018) to test physiotherapy and adult nursing students' attitude towards IPL using a Readiness for Inter-professional Learning Scale questionnaire, found that the majority of students have a very pos-itive attitude towards IPL, in addition to greater understanding of other healthcare professionals' roles and skills.

On the other hand, on exploring ways of assessing three essential competen-cies of all health professionals, namely communication, team working and ethical practice, at five HEIs and in 16 professional groups, Holt et al. (2010: 264) report that multi-professional assessment 'accurately and fairly measure' students' capa-bilities. The researchers took into account professional statutory and regulatory bodies' requirements as well as the perceptions of practice-based and academic staff, and those of service users and carers on assessment of those competencies. Furthermore, healthcare students benefit from the care and treatment of healthcare service users being planned and delivered inter-professionally through integrated care pathways, which in turn can form the basis for constituting learning pathways for students.

Students' learning pathways

Students' placement learning in many care settings tends to benefit from being based on patient journeys and patient care pathways (e.g. McCarthy et al., 2016). The terms care pathway, patient pathway, collaborative care pathway, care map, multidisciplinary pathway of care, clinical pathway, and other ones, are often used interchangeably, and once the care pathway for a particular patient has been for-mulated, it can also form the basis for a student's learning pathway, whereby the student can track the patient's journey from the point of first contact with health-care through to recovery, and thereby gain knowledge of the interventions under-taken and the underpinning rationales for them. The student's learning can then be supplemented by self-directed study and by pre-arranged lectures and work-shops held at the university or within healthcare trusts.

A patient pathway (or care pathway) is the route that a patient might take from their first contact with an NHS member of staff (usually their general practitioner [GP]), through referral, to the completion of their treatment. The Centre for Policy on Ageing (2014) indicates that care pathways are designed to provide the best-known standard of care to patients with specific conditions, but they are also con-trary to the concept of person-centred care, unless 'variances' to care pathways allow for changes based on the service-user's specific health needs.

Furthermore, generic care pathways specifically designed for particular illnesses are well documented in the healthcare literature, such as van Wijngaarden et al.'s (2006) pathway on thrombolysis in acute ischaemic stroke. Several care pathways are also available on the internet, for example from the National Institute for Health and Care Excellence (NICE) (2022) website.

Research on care pathways tends to suggest that there are various benefits to the utilisation of care pathways, such as increased patient satisfaction and enabling staff to focus more on the clinical care they are providing. For example, an evaluative study of patient journeys conducted by Baron (2009) found various benefits of care pathways, including greater patient involvement in their recovery from illness and more effective inter-professional working.

A student on practice placement could encounter a patient whose relatively straightforward journey through healthcare takes them along the pathway identified in Figure 5.4.

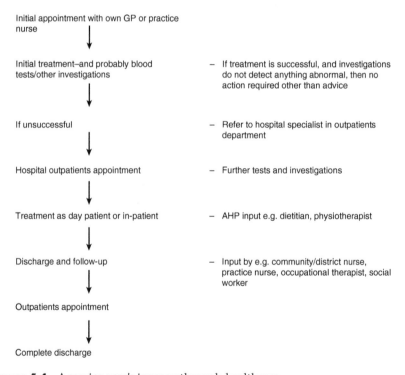

Figure 5.4 A service user's journey through healthcare

The student can follow a service user's care pathway through the healthcare system closely to gain knowledge and understanding of the care and treatment required for specific illnesses. The student's learning pathway through the practice placement would involve exposure to, and engagement with, selected care pathways, supplemented in various ways, for example, by practice-based teaching by the PEF, practice supervisor and other healthcare professionals.

Higher Education Institutes work in collaboration with local Trust clinicians to develop and implement learning pathway programmes in healthcare course curricula based on patient journeys, with web-based or simulated scenarios, for example, for students to explore and learn from. As for defining learning pathways related to healthcare students' learning, it essentially constitutes an individualised plan of learning that is based on care interventions that are received by specified patients as they progress on their journey through healthcare to resolve their current health problem. Furthermore, as care pathways incorporate the involvement of an appropriate combination of nursing or midwifery, medical, social work and AHP professionals, learning pathways are increasingly referred to as 'inter-professional learning pathways'.

The learning pathway for a student on an Emergency Department placement could include the student starting with a day with the ambulance services, following a healthcare service user with a suspected fracture through the Emergency Department to the X-ray department, witnessing the doctor's decisions, spending time working with plaster technicians, and so on. Furthermore, if the same patient or service user also suffers from, say, Type 1 diabetes or displays aggressive behaviour, then these themselves present instances for further learning for the student, the management of which can be explored up to maximum patient recovery.

The effectiveness of learning pathways in making learning more comprehensive was explored by Anderson (2009: 835), for instance, who found that the use of learning pathways enabled students to develop 'a greater awareness and understanding of the delivery of healthcare in primary care settings and ... expanded their nursing knowledge and skills'. However, Anderson also notes that some students felt that learning pathways fragmented their learning in the base placement area.

The downside of the fragmentation of learning needs to be heeded as the subjects of Anderson's study were final placement student nurses who felt that their priority in this placement was to consolidate their clinical skills. This can clearly also impact on the achievement of all required standards of proficiency by students during the final practice placement to be able to register their qualification with the NMC.

It is useful to note, however, that the notion of learning pathways is found in other contexts, one of which is the arena of general adult education in which individuals who have missed education opportunities during the compulsory education years are enabled to learn through NVQ and other routes (e.g. McGivney, 2003).

The student learning pathway during practice placement is widely favoured, with some useful developments that can counteract the weaknesses of learning pathways identified by Anderson (2009). The model is referred to as the 'hub and spokes' model. The hub is the base placement setting to which the student has been allocated and at which their main practice supervisors are based, and from there the student can accompany the health service user to whichever department of healthcare or social care professional they have been referred (the spoke).

The 'hub and spokes' medium for practice learning pathways is widely applied, except a spoke visit by a student on practice placement cannot be downplayed as 'you might find it interesting', for instance. In fact, to optimise learning from the spoke experience, the student should articulate in writing, usually on the relevant pages of the practice assessment document (PAD), one or more aims for the spoke visit against the name of the spoke to be visited (see Template 5.2).

Template 5.2 Record of learning from 'spoke' experience

Date of visit to spoke area	Name of spoke	Aim(s) of visiting spoke area	Summary of learning from spoke	Nominated practice supervisor's comments

The spoke-based practice supervisor may be required to sign the relevant section of the student's PAD to confirm the student did attend and engage. After the visit, the student needs to write down the specific learning acquired from the spoke visit. A number of studies have already been conducted on the hub and spokes model, which include Roxburgh et al.'s (2012) research that, in conclusion, identified the beneficial effects of using this model of placement learning as a mechanism that promotes deep and meaningful person-centred learning.

The results of an evaluative study by Thomas and Westwood (2016) of students' experiences of the 'hub and spoke' model of placement allocation, identified that the model enhances students' understanding of the whole patient journey which in turn offers students a breadth of experience and transferable skills such as communication and adaptability, and also increases a sense of belonging to the hub area. However, when the aims of the spoke experience weren't clearly identified, the experience was problematic.

Yet another study on hub and spokes as a student learning pathway during practice placement conducted by Millar et al. (2017) revealed similar beneficial findings to the above-mentioned study, but also other potential issues such as some spoke areas being in high demand and possibly becoming 'resistant' to students, as well as benefits such as being able to appreciate the patient/service user as an individual, their lifestyle's effect on their health, and thereby also enhancing person-centred practice.

In conclusion, recognising the components of patients' journeys or pathways through healthcare can provide healthcare students with fuller insights into the beginnings of individual service users' ill health and the stage-by-stage events that they undergo in the endeavour to resolve their health problems. Under the guidance of their practice supervisors, students can personally witness some of the clinical interventions that occur away from the practice placement setting, which should enrich their learning.

Becoming a learning organisation

Going beyond the concept of practice settings being effective learning environments is the exhortation that whole healthcare organisations should establish a culture of learning with a view to becoming learning organisations (see also Figure 5.1). The development of a learning culture needs to be a dominant theme in the strategic plans of healthcare organisations, and to incorporate a drive to improve the quality of practice by creating the means of integrating learning with practice. Some of the initiatives that support such a change include CPD, reflective practice, clinical supervision and WBL.

A learning organisation is therefore one that facilitates learning for all team members. This concept is part of a trio of notions that include lifelong learning and learning society. It evolved with the development of various non-healthcare organisations such as banks, supermarkets, and industries as learning organisations, on the basis that they all learn from customer feedback and actively engage in ongoing staff training. As for a learning society, this refers to everyone in a community having the opportunity to be educated to the level of achievement that they aspire to and of which they are capable.

Formal and informal learning occurs in various forms in the workplace, and, based on the increasing value derived from inter-professional learning in practice settings, Holland and Lauder (2012) suggest that practice learning should be part of the wider concept of 'communities of (learning in) practice', while healthcare providers become 'learning organisations'. The concept of 'communities of practice' has prevailed for some time, and Wenger (2000), for example, explains that they constitute groups of people who share a common passion for something, about which they extend their learning together, some of which may also be incidental, i.e. unintentional.

As for the whole of the healthcare provider, for example an acute NHS Trust, becoming a learning organisation, this can only be healthy in that all its practice settings as well as all departments that are not practice settings have learning and open-mindedness structured within their culture. This ethos is usually well established in UK hospices and university-linked healthcare providers, except that, at times, senior healthcare managers have previously linked learning organisations only with 'learning from mistakes or incidents' (e.g. Dixon-Woods et al., 2014). Alternatively, as found by Campbell and Evans (2016) and others, when supervisors and line managers are themselves effective facilitators of learning, this tends to encourage the team to support formal and informal learning more enthusiastically, which in turn leads to improved team performance.

The concept of a learning organisation is consistently becoming a feature of healthcare settings, which is mostly related to evidence-based practice and new medical devices, and partly because healthcare providers are required to learn from 'near misses' and any mistakes that have occurred. These dimensions therefore form the impetus for keeping up to date and for career-long learning. A learning organisation constitutes of five core strategic building blocks, namely: shared vision, mind-set and perceptions, personal mastery, team learning and interrelationships between the organisation's systems, according to Choi et al.'s (2016) research. Alternatively, the key features of a learning organisation, according to Wilkinson et al.'s (2004) analysis, include:

- an absence of complacency, and always seeking improvement
- a tolerance of mistakes and failures, and learning from them
- a belief in the human potential for creativity and innovation
- an openness and sharing of knowledge, and learning across teams
- trusting staff to work towards corporate goals, without close monitoring
- being outward looking at competing organisations, and potentially learning from them
- celebration throughout the organisation of the success of individuals and teams.

Additionally, the general literature indicates that successful healthcare learning organisations also have:

- a coherent, well-resourced, organisation-led learning strategy that is explicitly linked to the roles and skills needed to deliver local service improvements for patients, and to the learning needs of staff
- staff development that is based on a system of appraisal and professional and personal development planning for all staff, which is linked to organisational and individual development needs, and is regularly reviewed
- an education and training strategy that includes a learning infrastructure such as access to library resources
- regular publication and evaluation of in-house and external learning activities.

Most healthcare settings in both public and independent sectors now partly or fully portray the above-mentioned attributes. You might wish to check for yourself how far your employing organisation demonstrates the above-mentioned features of a learning organisation, and maybe you will be nicely surprised. See Akhnif et al. (2017), under Further Optional Reading at the end of this chapter, for more ways in which the learning organisation idea applies to health services.

Shared responsibilities for effective practice placements

Various stakeholders have responsibility for ensuring effective learning occurs during students' practice placements, according to the RCN (2017), which includes HEIs, service providers, course directors, students themselves, and PEFs. The responsibilities of the student encompass those before, during and after the placement. The student's responsibilities before the placement include:

- perusing the practice competencies that must be achieved by the end of the placement, and comprehending them
- recognising the purpose of the practice placement experience, that is, to develop specific competencies related to the specialism
- contacting the placement setting
- acting professionally with regard to punctuality and attitude, and dressing according to the local uniform policy.

During the placement, the student's responsibilities include being proactive in seeking out learning experiences. After the placement, the student has a responsibility to take stock of their achievements, ensure that all practice placement documentation is completed by due dates, complete the placement evaluation form, and reflect on the experience after completing the placement.

The RCN publication also states that a successful practice placement depends on well-planned learning opportunities and the provision of support and coaching for students. It lists and explains several actions that supervisors of practice-based learning should take to fulfil their responsibility, which include:

- contributing to a supportive learning environment and quality learning outcomes for students
- being approachable, supportive and aware of how students learn best
- having knowledge and information of the student's programme of study and practice assessment tools.

Complementarily, the NMC (2018d: 9–10) provides further substantial guidance on effective practice placements, and under 'Student empowerment' provides details of ways in which students must be supported and protected during placements, which includes having access to a wide range of opportunities and healthcare professions, and receiving 'constructive feedback'.

Consequently, a dynamic and proactive approach to the organisation, provision and assessment of practice experience is a requirement. Higher Education Institutes and service providers strive to think creatively about a range of ways in which to provide practice placements that meet the needs of the NHS and the wider healthcare sector, as also acknowledged by Knight et al. (2021). Planning and provision both have to take into account and value the ideas and suggestions of students and draw on the experience and knowledge of other stakeholders. Additionally, for effective student practice placements, the practice learning environment also needs to have:

- a stated philosophy of care that is reflected in practice and in the aims of students' curricula
- care provision that is founded on relevant research and evidence-based findings, where available
- students endeavouring to gain, whenever possible, experience as part of a multi-professional team
- a learning resources area with relevant learning materials and equipment that are easily accessible
- student feedback, which is actively sought.

Issues Related to Practice Placements

As can be expected, issues related to pre-registration students' practice placements do surface now and again. One potential issue is students' supernumerary status (which was discussed in Chapter 3), which could well be because some students do not engage fully because have a family to support, while others might be holding down a part-time job, which can result in their learning being compromised to some extent. Immaterial of the cause of the issue, the student could well need extra structured support during a practice placement which academic link lecturers and others can provide, and without necessarily being physically present.

On evaluating the use of short message service (SMS) texting by university staff to students as an additional means of support for healthcare students (including nursing, radiography and occupational therapy students) during practice placements, for example, Young et al. (2010) found that texting does enable students to access additional support when needed during practice placements.

One of the reasons for various guidelines on practice placements being issued by the RCN, the QAA and the DH at the turn of the century is the publication of research (e.g. Phillips et al., 2000) identifying various weaknesses in the prevailing practice-based teaching and learning. Another reason is the increase in the number of students in the endeavour to rectify the shortage of qualified healthcare professionals. This meant that more students could be allocated to fewer RNs. This also coincided with other research findings that some students were being given a pass for practice competencies, with scant evidence of their competence (discussed in Chapter 8), and that some newly qualified RNs were not 'fit for practice', that is, not clinically competent.

Furthermore, the Care Quality Commission (CQC) – which is an organisation that was set up by the government to regularly monitor the quality of care and treatment being provided to healthcare service users by each service provider in England – can also decide whether a practice setting is suitable as a learning environment for students. If deemed unsuitable, it has the authority to stop the particular practice setting from having students on placement with them until the identified weakness is rectified.

The CQC's (2022) fundamental standards are for service providers such as hospitals, care homes, GP services, dentists, and mental health services, and can be accessed on the CQC's website. Currently, there are 13 fundamental standards, which the CQC asserts are those below which care must never fall. These standards are detailed under the following headings:

- Person-centred
- Dignity and respect
- Consent
- Safety
- Safeguarding from abuse
- Food and drink
- Premises and equipment
- Complaints
- Good governance
- Staffing
- Fit and proper staff
- Duty of candour
- Display of ratings.

Examples of further details for three of the standards are provided in the box below. In essence, if the practice setting's standards do fall below those specified by the CQC, then the setting is deemed unsuitable for student placement.

Examples of Details of Some of the CQC's Fundamental Standards

Dignity and respect: You must be treated with dignity and respect at all times while you're receiving care and treatment. This includes making sure:

- You have privacy when you need and want it.
- Everybody is treated as equals.
- You're given any support you need to help you remain independent and involved in your local community.

Consent: You (or anybody legally acting on your behalf) must give your consent before any care or treatment is given to you.

Staffing: The provider of your care must have enough suitably qualified, competent and experienced staff to make sure they can meet these standards. Their staff must be given the support, training and supervision they need to help them do their job.

Furthermore, the heightened awareness of evidence-based practice means that students are often more inquisitive about the reasons for each step of clinical interventions. Nevertheless, for various day-to-day reasons, some procedures are not performed exactly as the procedures' manual states and consequently the so-called theory and practice gap at times surfaces. From qualified healthcare professionals' and their managers' viewpoint, these still constitute competent practice because procedures are adapted in accordance with resource availability and patient circumstances.

For instance, if the moving and handling procedure or guidelines state that a hoist should be used to help a patient above a certain weight, but a hoist is not immediately available, then the RN could use alternative measures. The reason for this might not be immediately obvious to the student, and, at times, students refuse to participate in procedures that are not being performed precisely according to the guidelines. They should be exploring different and maybe creative ways of applying theories to practice instead.

However, because a number of healthcare profession lecturers are often not active clinicians, unlike medical academics who are also practising doctors, this tends to create a theory–practice gap that practice-based supervisors of learning have to redress during student practice placements, argue Lakasing and Francis (2005). The authors indicate that practice-based supervisors of learning should therefore be provided with protected time and extra remuneration to enable them to fulfil this demanding role more effectively. Where extra funding is made available for this, the money can be utilised to employ additional pro rata staff to create protected (or supported) time for a more effective practice-based facilitation of learning.

The likely issues related to the effectiveness of clinical settings as learning environments can be prevented or resolved in several ways however, as concluded by Pienaar et al. (2022) from their integrative review of supportive CLEs. Pienaar et al. identified eight prominent models of students learning supervision during practice placements, and then grouped ways of facilitating students learning under three components:

(1) Student supporters – practice learning supervisors, academic staff, peers but with appropriate qualities and interest in enabling learning, and who in turn are appropriately prepared and supported

(2) The relationship between the students and student supporters – whereupon students feel accepted, valued and belong to the clinical team

(3) Effective partnership between the students and student supporters.

Chapter Summary

As with other components in this book, creating and maintaining an effective clinical learning environment is also identified as a key dimension of facilitating students learning during practice placements. This chapter has focused on the different ways in which practice settings can be effective learning environments, and has therefore explored:

- Students' perspectives on practice placements such as their hopes and expectations; a ward orientation or an induction programme; the advanced preparation of learners; and ensuring that course practice competencies are achieved.
- Organisational learning culture and research on clinical learning environments, which underpin development of the tool for regular educational audits of practice placement areas; learning resources (human and material), including inter-professional learning and learning pathways; and role models for learners in the practice setting.
- The part played by national guidelines, standards and current policy documents on practice placements.
- What work-based learning is and how it applies to health and care profession students' learning; and how healthcare providers can become true learning organisations.
- Some of the main issues related to practice placements for students.

Further Optional Reading

1. For a number of ways in which learning organisation as an idea applies to health services, see:
   - Akhnif, E., Macq, J. and Meessen, B. (2017) 'Scoping literature review on the Learning Organisation concept as applied to the health system', *Health Research Policy and Systems, 15*(16): 1–12.
2. For the QAA's stance on effective WBL, see:
   - Quality Assurance Agency for Higher Education (2018) *UK Quality Code for Higher Education Advice and Guidance: Work-based Learning.* Available at: www.qaa.ac.uk/quality-code/advice-and-guidance/work-based-learning# (accessed 6 March 2022).
3. For practical measures that can be adopted to create a welcoming practice environment for students, see:
   - Tremayne, P. and Hunt, L. (2019) 'Has anyone seen the student? Creating a welcoming practice environment for students', *British Journal of Nursing, 28*(6): 369–373.

6

PRACTICE LEARNING SUPERVISORS' AND ASSESSORS' LEADERSHIP

Introduction

One of the preconditions of healthcare registrants undertaking practice learning supervisor duties is that they have to be proficient in care interventions to the highest contemporary standard. For nurses, the components of duties in which they have to be proficient are grouped by the NMC (2018c) under seven platforms; for midwives, they are grouped under six domains (NMC, 2019a); and for AHPs, they are grouped under 15 generic statements which apply to all AHPs regulated by the HCPC (e.g. 2014); and numerous SOP are identified under those sections.

Moreover, the duties and responsibilities of registrants have also often been grouped under four headings, which has, at times, also been referred to as 'the four pillars' of advanced clinical practice for health and social care professionals. These four pillars are: (i) person-centred clinical practice, (ii) leadership and management, (iii) educating others, and (iv) research (HEE, NHS Improvement and NHSE, 2017: 8; NHS Employers, 2019). On the other hand, in the NHS Knowledge and Skills Framework (NHS KSF) (CIPD, 2021b), all healthcare professionals' duties have been identified under six 'core dimensions', namely: (1) communication, (2) personal and people development, (3) health, safety and security, (4) service improvement, (5) quality, and (6) equality and diversity. Leadership was later added as an optional dimension following requests from NHS leaders.

Clearly, all these categorisations acknowledge registrants' duties to provide thorough and high-quality care, as well as enabling students and colleagues to further develop their care intervention skills. As the NMC (2018b: 25) asserts, providing leadership entails identifying priorities, managing time, staff and resources effectively, and dealing with risk to make sure that the quality of care or service being delivered is maintained and improved. Consequently, practice supervisors have to embody leadership in the above-mentioned groups or dimensions of their duties, in the course of their practice, continually ascertaining the evidence base of all care interventions, and of the various factors that affect the provision of effective care delivery to health or care service users.

This chapter therefore addresses ways in which practice learning supervisors' duties incorporate leadership in the supervision of students' learning and assessment, which includes components that apply to student midwives. Simultaneously, practice supervisors have to be role models of person-centred, evidence-informed clinical practice (as noted in Chapter 1), for leading practice that is safe, sensitive and effective, as well as for educating those who need to learn to do so in clinical settings.

Chapter objectives

1. Appraise ways in which forward planning and prioritising work comprise important components of practice learning supervisors' and assessors' leadership, with an extra focus on midwifery students as an example.
2. Critically evaluate ways in which practice supervisors fulfil their leadership duties effectively in the facilitation of students' practice-based learning and student assessment.
3. Explain how healthcare professionals engage in high-quality and effective, evidence-informed person-centred care, and therefore also feature as role models for learners.
4. Understand how to influence and implement changes in practice as essential components of the registrant's responsibilities, and overcome any incidental barriers or obstacles in doing so.

The Practice Learning Supervisor's Leadership

Healthcare policy documents are awash with recommendations, commendations as well as rhetoric on healthcare leadership. The ways in which practice supervisors forward-plan and supervise a range of learning experiences for students on placement, and oversee them accessing pertinent learning opportunities, are reflections of the leadership characteristics that were alluded to in Chapters 1 and 4 to some degree. Prioritising work to ensure time is allocated for supervising and supporting students' learning is another key feature of the practice supervisor's leadership, which includes designating time for establishing effective supervisory relationships with students and with other professionals whom students will encounter during the placement.

Leadership therefore also applies to facilitating students' learning so that they can achieve their placement competencies in good time, and also to acting proactively to pre-empt and avert the likely problems of assessments (explored in Chapter 8 of this book), as well as dealing with those that do occur.

Registrants' leadership related to learning for all staff in their practice settings, including for pre-registration and post-qualifying education students, has been identified by research for some time (e.g. O'Driscoll et al., 2010; Adelman-Mullally et al., 2013). According to O'Driscoll and colleagues' research, personnel whose leadership is more immediately apparent include clinical nurse specialists, modern matrons, nurse consultants, nurse practitioners, nurse managers and others of similar seniority, but their role in student teaching during practice placements is less well defined. They also found, however, that the ward manager's leadership is crucial in creating and supporting a learning culture in the practice setting, and also that it is healthcare professionals who regularly teach learners who are those who exercise leadership in the facilitation of learning more effectively.

Several definitions of leadership prevail in the healthcare literature, most of which emphasise the leader's ability to *influence* the activities, behaviour or actions of their 'followers' towards goal achievement. In the context of healthcare, Gopee (2022: 69) indicates that 'leadership is a two-way process based on a leader–follower type relationship (whereby healthcare professionals) involve, inspire and energise team members towards the achievement of the organisation's or the care setting's goals'. These influential processes also apply to effective practice supervision. For a thorough analysis of leadership as a concept that applies to most areas of society, the reader is referred to Kouzes and Posner's (2017) *The Leadership Challenge*, and Chapter 3 of Gopee's (2022) *Leading and Managing Healthcare*, which, as the book title suggests, applies to leadership in healthcare.

In all above-mentioned instances, leadership entails being a role model for juniors, for learners, as well as for colleagues, which is leadership, in effective person-centred, compassionate care, in evidence-based practice, in the organisation of care, and in teaching and assessing learners, as also indicated above (see also Figure 6.1).

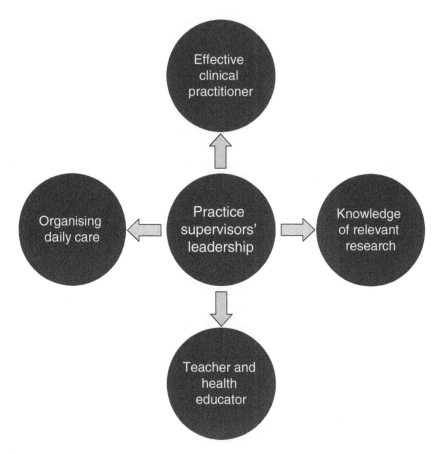

Figure 6.1 Areas of practice supervisors' leadership

The practice supervisor as the role model

From their research on student nurses' satisfaction with practice placements, Suliman and Warshawski (2022) deduced that placement-based learning supervisors feature as significant professional role models for their students, while also enhancing students' resilience and student satisfaction, which leads to higher retention of students. In their study of leadership in the facilitation of practice learning, Adelman-Mullally et al. (2013) also identify various ways in which learning supervisors and assessors exemplify leadership through role modelling and providing vision to students.

Consequently, practice supervisors and assessors are embodiments of exemplary professional practice that is evidence-based and person-centred, and thereby are role models of best practice. Their leadership in relation to their duties and responsibilities thus also makes them amenable to change and improvement in practice that enhance service user care. Various other research studies also indicate that practice-based learning supervisors represent role models for their students in their clinical specialism, as well as being a role model of teaching (e.g. in patient health education) (e.g. Darling, 1984; Jack et al., 2017).

Being a healthcare professional thus also signifies being a role model for colleagues, and, for juniors and learners, which of necessity incorporates being highly proficient in one's practice as well as having the associated knowledge and manifesting the appropriate behaviour.

─Reflection point 6.1─

Practice supervisors as role models

Consider the terms 'model' and 'modelling'. Next, consider what a role model is. Consider also why healthcare professionals need to be role models, who else for, and what it is about a person that makes them a role model.

In response to Reflection Point 6.1, you might have felt that healthcare professionals who are role models are those who perform clinical interventions to the highest standard, and who provide person-centred, safe and effective evidence-informed care. They should, furthermore, also be role models of organisation and management of care, and in leadership, albeit within the parameters of their post.

As with many tentative concepts, a concept analysis or a STEP (social, technological, economic and political) analysis can enable further clarification of role-modelling, and a systematic understanding of various facets and components of the concept. Alternatively, a SWOT (strengths, weaknesses, opportunities and threats) analysis can be undertaken. Such an analysis can help the individual decide whether any problem-solving, avoidance or developmental actions need to be taken.

ACTION POINT 6.1

STEP analysis of role models

Using the headings 'social', 'technological', 'economic' and 'political', conduct a STEP analysis of 'the practice supervisor as a role model'.

Being a role model is a feature of Bandura's (1996) social learning theory, which stipulates that substantial learning occurs as a result of observation of appropriate professionals, which is appropriate for healthcare students as they learn substantial clinical intervention skills working with qualified professionals in healthcare settings, which is also consistent with 'work-based learning', which was discussed in Chapter 5. Bandura indicates that individuals learn behaviour through observing experts or proficient professionals, the mental retention of the process and procedure applied, reproducing the behaviour usually under supervision, and reinforcement of the newly learnt behaviour.

Being amenable to adopting changes in modes of clinical intervention, of new medical devices, diagnostic techniques, and medicines that benefit or enhance the patient's health is a characteristic of a role model that those who are open to learning can emulate and adopt. There are, however, instances of poor practice that get reported to the NMC or hit the national news, which suggest that certain individual healthcare professionals may not be role models for others.

A role model is 'a person regarded by others as a good example to follow' (Brookes and O'Neill, 2017: 810), that is, someone whose practice standards, attitudes and beliefs can be emulated by the observer. Individuals choose their role models, such as someone who is good at time management, at self-organisation or at how they interact with service users.

On evaluating the perceptions of undergraduate students on role modelling within the clinical learning environment, Donaldson and Carter (2005) found that students valued highly the availability of good role models whose competence they could observe and replicate when required. Constructive feedback was needed on their practice from their role models to develop their competence and build up their confidence, and to convert observed behaviour into their own behaviour and skill set.

Consequently, role models are those whom we look up to, emulate and admire as professionals, as well as those in society in general, and subsequently people base their character identity, values and lifestyle on selected celebrities or characters in television programmes. All teachers in the practice setting (e.g. practice supervisors) should therefore be aware of their impact as role models on students' learning of skills and professional attitudes. However, there are mixed views on nurses being role models of healthy habits when off duty. An appropriate level of self-awareness and self-discipline related to one's public behaviour should nevertheless be observed by healthcare professionals.

Having explored the general nature of practice supervisors' leadership, the next section explores practice learning supervisors' leadership with regards to effective, person-centred, evidence-informed practice, and practice development; and later, the chapter examines leadership in the supervision and assessment of students and in management of change.

Leadership in Effective, Evidence-Informed, Person-Centred Practice

The HCPC (2014), the NMC (2018b, 2018c), and other healthcare regulators clearly indicate that registrants must continually question the evidence base and effectiveness of the care they deliver. They must also recognise that standards of practice involve being open-minded with regard to novel methods of clinical interventions, of research findings and of developments in one's own specialist field of practice.

Evidence-based practice (EBP) is one of the essential components of effective practice and quality assurance in healthcare. It is a concept and practice that has been gradually adopted in all areas of healthcare. 'Safe and effective care' is a phrase that is often mentioned by the NMC in its standards publications (e.g. 2018b: 9) and by the HCPC. Safety of healthcare service users in practice settings is therefore also a strand of healthcare professionals' codes of conduct (e.g. HCPC, 2016: 8), and is therefore obligatory. So what does the term 'effective practice' mean?

Effective practice

'Effective clinical practice' is a concept that is closely related to quality of care and treatment, and is also related to such concepts as clinical governance and audits. The word *effective* is an adjective, which, according to the dictionary (e.g. Brookes and O'Neill, 2017: 286), means 'producing an intended or desired result'. It can be used interchangeably with 'efficacious' and 'productive'. Effective practice therefore means that the clinical interventions that healthcare professionals perform as part of the patient's care pathway (or care plan) do achieve the goals of the care interventions. For example, if certain actions are taken to reduce a patient's body temperature, and after a specified number of minutes the temperature does go down, then the actions were 'effective'.

Ways of achieving effective practice signify ensuring that practice is evidence-based, and is therefore adjusted based on new evidence. Effective clinical interventions are therefore closely associated with EBP and also with practice development, which will be discussed shortly. It is also juxtaposed with the concept of patient outcomes, but there is a lack of consensus with regard to how patient outcomes are gauged, and it therefore remains in the background as a notion warranting further research and refinement.

Related to the practice supervisor leadership, the word 'effective' therefore signifies that as proficient healthcare professionals, practice supervisors accomplish the goals in their patients' plans of care and treatment, as intended in their individual care pathways. Effective care and practice development are terms that are integral to service improvement as also advocated by NHS England's (2022: 1) Improvement Capability Building and Delivery Team, whose purpose is 'to build improvement capability in teams, organisations and systems to help them improve services to enhance patient care'.

Person-centred practice

As advocated by several researchers, person-centred practice refers to holistic approaches to care whereupon service users are treated with respect and dignity, are informed of their care and treatment, and their preferences are listened to. Person-centred care 'is about focusing care on the needs of the individual (and) ensuring that people's preferences, needs and values guide clinical decisions, and providing care that is respectful of and responsive to them', according to HEE (2022c: 1).

Furthermore, 'person-centredness' is:

> an approach to practice established through the formation and fostering of healthful relationships between all care providers, service users and others significant to them in their lives. It is underpinned by values of respect for persons (personhood), individual right to self-determination, mutual respect and understanding. It is enabled by cultures of empowerment that foster continuous approaches to practice development (McCormack and McCanse, 2017: 4).

Every single concept in these assertions is an important component of person-centred practice, and applies to all service users across clinical specialisms, across age spans, and to people of all ethnic groups. Principles and frameworks of person-centred practice have been advocated and tested by research, but will continue to evolve with new generations of people and socio-political influences. For example, McCormack and McCanse's (2017) framework for person-centred practice comprise of the following person-centred processes:

- providing holistic care
- working with the person's beliefs and values
- engaging authentically
- sharing decision-making
- being sympathetically present.

Also being vociferously advocated presently as a component of person-centred practice is compassionate care, which was identified as lacking in healthcare provision in the Francis Report (2013), a report that was the result of a thorough investigation into suspected malpractice in terms of patients being 'neglected', and concluded with approximately 300 recommendations, one of which refers to strengthening compassionate care in healthcare organisations.

As also noted in Chapter 2, compassionate care is one of the competencies that student nurses have to gain a pass in during their pre-registration programme (NMC, 2018c: 16), and the Department of Health and Social Care's (2021) NHS Constitution for England states that healthcare professionals' responsibilities include treating every individual with compassion, dignity and respect. Furthermore, compassionate care is a feature in England's CNO guidance entitled *Leading Change, Adding Value: A Framework for Nursing, Midwifery and Care Staff* (NHS England, 2016).

ACTION **POINT 6.2**

Exactly how are person-centred and compassionate care practised?

Either in your own words, or in discussion with a colleague/peer whom you trust, consider ways in which your practice is person-centred and compassionate in your day-to-day care delivery; and then articulate these in writing.

As a practice supervisor, your ways of providing compassionate care are the ways that your student is likely to adopt for their future practice because, as a registrant, you are the role model for them. So, you are likely to incorporate acting with warmth and empathy, actively listening, being sensitive and accessible, respecting dignity and privacy, as components of compassionate care when interacting with service users, which are characteristics also found by Bray et al. (2014) in their study of healthcare professionals' understanding of compassionate care. It can therefore be learnt through experiential learning and reflection.

However, on exploring students' process of professional socialisation, Curtis et al. (2012) found that healthcare profession students' socialisation tends to elicit doubts about whether they will have time to practise compassionate care on qualification and as a registrant. Nevertheless, compassionate care does not always depend on time, because it is an inherent component of most clinical interventions and interactions with patients, and is therefore another instance where the role modelling of practice supervisors is so crucial for the student's learning.

Leadership as an evidence-informed practitioner

As indicated at the beginning of the chapter, evidence-based practice (EBP) is one of the essential areas of proficiency of practice supervisors, and it is also usually a component of healthcare professionals' codes of practice, such as the NMC (2018b: 9) and the General Medical Council (2013: 8 [clause 16] – updated 2019). EBP, practice development and leadership apply to all registrants, and therefore, especially, to practice supervisor roles, as well as to practice assessors.

Codes of professional practice in healthcare often include the requirement that registrants' care interventions have to be based on the 'best available evidence' (e.g. NMC, 2018b: 9), and updated as new evidence warrants making changes or adjustments to practice. Furthermore, the NMC (2018c: 32–37) emphasises the 'use of evidence-based best practice approaches' in all aspects of care interventions.

Evidence-based practice (also referred to as 'evidence-informed practice') is closely associated with evidence-based medicine (EBM), for which Archie Cochrane is renowned for being one of its principal initiators (Smith and Rennie, 2014). Strauss et al. (2019) indicate that EBM requires the integration of the best research evidence with our clinical expertise and our patient's unique values and circumstances, emphasising that the patient's values and preferences must be taken into account in addition to research evidence.

Evidence-based practice is defined by Polit and Beck (2021: 384) as 'a practice that involves making clinical decisions based on clinical judgement, patient preferences, and on the best available evidence, usually evidence from disciplined research'. The key reason for the adoption of EBP in healthcare is the endeavour to ensure that each action taken by the healthcare professional is a 'well-informed' action, that is, it is based on evidence of its effectiveness, as well as patient preferences, and so on, as noted in Polit and Beck's definition above. It thereby constitutes a shift from previous traditional or routine procedures to more objective scientific working.

Other terms related to EBP are 'evidence-based healthcare' (EBHC), evidence-based nursing, evidence-based management, and so forth. EBHC refers to evidence-based decision-making about groups of patients, or populations, which can manifest itself as evidence-based management of their care. Although the two terms overlap substantially, EBHC can be distinguished from EBP in that the former tends to refer to groups of patients, while the latter can refer to single clinical interventions.

Reflection point 6.2

Best evidence

EBP therefore refers to the use of 'best evidence' and is based on national and international standards. How do we know that every clinical intervention that we perform in our workplace is based on the 'best evidence' currently available?

Research evidence is available from national computer databases (e.g. Cochrane Collaboration, 2022). There are several likely sources of best evidence for good practice, including:

- clinical guidelines (e.g. from NICE)
- specialist research conferences
- professional journal articles
- assertions and suggestions from patients with a long-term health problem/ their family
- colleagues and peer contact – uni- or inter-disciplinary professionals.

Because all registrants (obviously including practice supervisors) have to be role models of good practice for their learners (e.g. NMC, 2018a), this signifies that they should always be reflecting on whether their clinical interventions are of the highest standard known and based on the best available evidence, with a view to making changes to enhance practice further. There are various ways in which EBP can be achieved. Healthcare professionals can search for evidence of the effect of particular clinical interventions and best evidence on electronic databases such as MEDLINE or Cumulative Index to Nursing and Allied Health Literature (CINAHL), on the internet, or they can do a manual search of targeted literature.

Identifying existing research on particular components of clinical practice has gradually become increasingly easier, as various organisations have evolved that store and provide systematically reviewed, meta-analysed or critically appraised research on different healthcare topics. The wide availability of electronic databases includes the Cochrane Collaboration (2022) which stores research evidence that has been appraised or systematically reviewed. It indicates that a systematic review summarises the results of available carefully designed healthcare studies (controlled trials) and provides a high level of evidence on the effectiveness of specific healthcare interventions.

Whether it is the findings of the healthcare colleague's own research or those of studies encountered at conferences or on courses, the ultimate stages of research studies entail critically appraising the study or studies, before deciding on whether to implement their findings and recommendation, and then later disseminating them. Other organisations that store critically appraised research on healthcare topics include:

- NHS Evidence
- Joanna Briggs Institute
- York University NHS Centre for Reviews and Dissemination
- the quarterly journal *Evidence-Based Nursing*
- Health Technology Assessment.

The Health Technology Assessment programme, which is funded by the National Institute for Health and Care Research (NIHR) (2022), supports the search for evidence that is immediately useful to patients, to clinical practice and to policy or decision-makers. It also conducts research on health technology to establish its effectiveness and compares the technology to current devices for NHS interventions to see which works best. It also examines the costs and effectiveness of health technology, and results are made available on its website.

The strengths of the assembled research literature can be classified as a hierarchy of levels or grades of evidence, in order of validity and significance. Polit and Beck (2021), for instance, classify the hierarchy of evidence at eight levels, from the highest level of evidence being that from systematic reviews/meta-analyses of RCTs to the lowest level being expert opinion, as is shown in Figure 6.2.

Hierarchy of evidence	
• *Highest level evidence*	I: Systematic review/meta-analysis of RCTs
	II: Randomised Controlled Trial (RCT)
	III: Non-Randomised Trial (quasi-experiment)
	IV: Systematic review of non-experimental (observational) studies
	V: Non-experimental/observational study
	VI: Systematic review/metasynthesis of qualitative studies
	VII: Qualitative study/descriptive study
• *Lowest level evidence*	VIII: Non-research source (e.g. Expert Opinion, internal evidence)

Figure 6.2   Hierarchy of evidence

You would have already encountered some of the terminologies in Figure 6.2, but if not, their meanings are easily found on the internet. Other organisations categorise evidence differently, but they are essentially similar.

Although RCTs have long been considered the gold standard of medical research, some express reservations with regards to this notion – for example, as Jones and

Podolsky (2015: 1503) note, gold standard suggests 'that there is (only) one best way to do something', and methodological shortcomings could be present. On the other hand, when the evidence comes from just one research study, maybe along with a small sample size, and is funded by industry, then extra care is required before accepting its findings as evidence. Consequently, evidence should be a combination of research evidence and patient values and preferences. Use of healthcare professionals' personal experience and intuition have also been advised.

Several benefits or advantages of EBP in healthcare have been documented over the years, such as: a higher quality of care and improved patient outcomes; increased safety of healthcare service users; increased healthcare professionals' confidence in the care they provide; and more efficient and effective use of available resources. Without EBP, otherwise, practice risks rapidly becoming out of date, to the detriment of patients.

The difference between research-based practice and EBP is that research-based practice of clinical interventions usually only allows for consideration of findings of quantitative research, while EBP also considers descriptive or qualitative studies, professional experience, intuition and tacit knowledge (when we know more than we can evidence or tell) (Benner, 2001). For a critical appraisal of research, several frameworks are widely published such as CASP (Critical Appraisal Skills Programme) (CASP UK, 2022) which comprise of approximately 11 questions in relation to the validity and value of the research. It is in the interest of the implementer of a particular component of EBP to examine closely and carefully the appraisal or systematic review already conducted by established organisations, who, in fact, are also likely to have accessed and appraised the original study report.

There can, however, be obstacles to the implementation of EBP and research findings, which are examined later in this chapter.

Practice development

The core concepts 'effective practice', 'EBP' and person-centred practice all potentially imply that there is scope for making improvements to practice, for the benefit of service users. Such changes are, at times, referred to as 'practice development' (or clinical practice development), which is about improving and enhancing hands-on clinical interventions.

Practice development is defined as 'a continuous process of improvement towards increased effectiveness in patient centred care, which is brought about by enabling healthcare teams to develop their knowledge and skills, and to transform the culture and context of care' (McCormack et al. 2013: 4). Thus, practice development is a systematic approach that enables healthcare teams to look critically at their practice and identify how it can be improved, and the improvement sustained within their systems. It therefore also refers to a broad range of innovations that are initiated to improve practice and healthcare services.

The term *innovation* differs from practice development in certain respects, especially in that the former refers to implementing something new and unprecedented.

According to the dictionary (e.g. Brookes and O'Neill, 2017: 464), to 'innovate' means 'to introduce new ideas or methods', implying that a new product, practice or method is being introduced for the first time. An innovation refers to implementing a relatively radical new practice, which is developed necessarily in response to patient care needs. 'Development', however, refers to a gradual progressive change and advancement. Change as a concept, however, can mean substituting something with something new, a development, or reverting to an older (but effective) practice.

Clinical practice development is often triggered by a need for new actions to resolve a health problem. For example, falls among older people have presented as an issue for some time, and one of the actions taken to prevent or manage falls is the use of sensor alarms that alert nurses when an 'at risk' patient gets out of bed unaided, for example. Moreover, in most instances practice is not developed or improved by individuals (e.g. practice supervisors) acting on their own, as it often takes a team approach to change to a new practice. The team may be a small group of colleagues based at a specialist centre (e.g. a day surgery unit, a nursing home, an intensive care unit), a hospital-level team, when a change is introduced at organisational level, or at national or supra-organisational level (as in the development of person-centred practice).

Practice development thus continually aims to enhance the quality of patient-centred care, and to mobilise this Heyns et al. (2017) advocate the appointment of practice development facilitators, whereby facilitation involves enabling practitioners to adjust their culture of practice so that changes in practice are sustainable and positive. These facilitators therefore also have to be role models as well as change agents.

Naturally, implementing a new way of practice (changing how a clinical intervention is performed) might require new resources in terms of new equipment, medical devices or disposable materials, and a step-by-step procedure for performing the new practice, along with staff training. We also have to be completely clear about the 'purposes' and 'consequences' of the novel practice, and ensure that it is systematically evaluated by, for example, applying the Donabedian (1988) 'structure–process–outcome' model of evaluation of change.

The Donabedian model is a very practical framework for implementing and monitoring or formatively evaluating (see Chapter 9) the progress and effect of a new or an existing form of practice, as also asserted by Moore et al. (2015). The framework can be introduced or utilised by individual practitioners, at team level, at organisational level (e.g. in a hospital), at supra-organisational level (across organisations), or nationally. Thinking, for example, in relation to evaluating the effectiveness of patient-controlled analgesia (PCA), the 'structure–process–outcome' model comprises of the following:

- Structure: the material items required for implementing the new practice, such as new devices (e.g. PCA devices) and attachments, easy to follow information for the service user, and premises.

- Process: the step-by-step procedure for healthcare professionals to apply, and for teaching the patient how to use it, and when to call for help, etc.
- Outcome: identifying clearly the effectiveness of PCAs – for example, pain relief in x seconds, saving staff time, quicker patient relief from pain.

The practice development framework suggested by Donabedian should enable you to take these developments further systematically if you so wish, maybe within the context of management of change (discussed later in this chapter).

Nursing posts for practice development include neonatal practice development nurse, lead nurse for practice development, and practice development facilitator. The resources that can help healthcare professionals include the journal *Practice Development in Healthcare*, and national conferences specifically on effective and safe innovative practice. Several NHS Trusts employ practice development nurses or facilitators, or have practice development incorporated in existing senior clinical posts.

Leadership in Practice-Based Supervision of Learning

Nurses', midwives' and AHPs' teaching roles start soon after registering their qualification with the NMC/HCPC and being employed by healthcare organisations that have students on placement with them, which is another reason for ensuring that their practice is safe and effective, up-to-date, evidence-informed and person-centred. Practice is also firmly inter-disciplinary, and inter-professional education fully supported. Furthermore, learning from or between healthcare professionals is reinforced by Amy's (2008: 212) research conclusion that learning can be 'institutionalised' in organisations (e.g. healthcare trusts) through facilitative leadership.

Practice learning supervisors' leadership

Applied to midwifery as an example, practice supervisors' and practice assessors' duties include participation in the educational preparation of student midwives to enable them to develop their knowledge and competence in midwifery practice. Their leadership entails ensuring that students' development and education prepare them appropriately for safe and competent practice, and for registration with the NMC, the professional body that governs midwifery.

The NMC's (2019a) standards of proficiency (SOP) for midwifery identify the knowledge and competence that newly registered midwives must be proficient in at the start of their career. The revision of the pre-2019 standards was required to meet the needs of the everchanging midwifery practice as well as an acknowledgement of additional healthcare needs of both mother and baby. The SOP were developed by midwifery experts and relevant stakeholders, alongside service users, and they communicate the midwife's role using the Framework for Maternal and Newborn Care (Quality Maternal and Newborn Care, 2022), with evidence from The Lancet Series on Midwifery (Renfrew et al., 2014).

Some of the key changes to midwifery education incorporated in the new standards include a shift in language, moving away from terms such as 'low risk and high risk' to 'universal care and additional care', the requirement for all student midwives to be trained in proficiency of examination of the newborn and preparing for the future in relation to taking on prescribing qualifications.

Accordingly, practise-based midwifery learning supervisors' leadership also involves having a partnership approach with midwifery lecturers from the associated HEI in order to meet students' learning needs and to ensure that the practice setting is an effective learning environment. Furthermore, the current support that is available for student midwives in the practice setting in conjunction with the HEI, tends to include (in addition to practice supervisors, of course): nominated practice assessors, academic link, personal tutors, academic assessors, and the midwifery placements co-ordinator. The duties of most of these different support positions were explained in Chapter 1 of this book.

Practice supervisors' leadership in midwifery is also applied through systematic approaches to supporting students' learning in practice settings, one of which is by the application of the Collaborative Learning in Practice (CLiP) coaching model for facilitating students' practice-based learning, which is also supported by Health Education England (e.g. James Paget University Hospitals NHS Foundation Trust, 2017) and the RCN (2022a). The CLiP model involves students being encouraged to take the lead in their learning needs through identified daily learning outcomes. Thus, students are coached by their practice supervisor with support from more senior student midwives. This mechanism allows for students to learn from one another, develop their skills in taking the lead in care provision as well as take responsibility for their own learning needs (see illustration in Figure 6.3).

The CLiP coaching model has been successfully implemented in many NHS Trust areas in both nursing and midwifery, and research suggests that consequently students feel better prepared for registration, feel more confident and enjoy teaching each other (e.g. Hill et al., 2020). The model also supports practice settings to increase the number of student midwives they can accommodate for practice placements, as the model requires a number of students to be allocated per shift for its success. This has also resolved some issues with placement capacity, for example those documented by Knight et al. (2021), except that the nature of the model is not suitable in all areas of care. For example, it is not effective on the labour ward where women require one-to-one care, and therefore the CLiP model is not advantageous to that environment.

Assessors' leadership in managing assessments

Leadership is essential for ensuring the timely assessment of students' practice competencies. Practice settings are generally informed of the students allocated to them well before their practice placement starts, to which practice supervisors respond by structuring tentative plans of learning experiences for the students for the duration of the placement. However, as will be seen in Chapter 8 of this book,

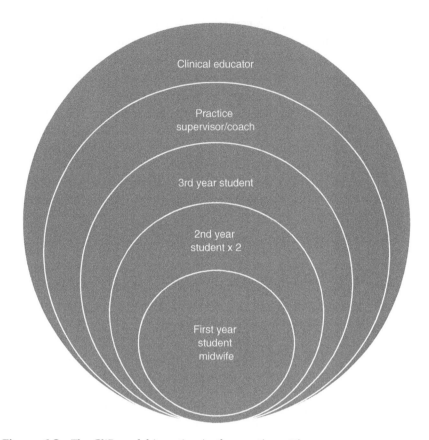

Figure 6.3   The CliP model in action in the practice setting

research (e.g. Gingerich et al., 2020; Hughes et al., 2021) highlights various alarming issues that could undermine the assessment of students' competencies during placements.

That assessments are conducted 'on the hoof' by registrants that the student 'bumps into' and as part of 'multiple roles', were issues highlighted two decades ago by Phillips et al. (2000). Then, 'failure to fail' is a problem that has been highlighted for more than two decades (e.g. Hughes et al., 2021) when sometimes students are awarded a pass without sufficient evidence of their competence in specific clinical skills. Furthermore, on occasion, students have reacted in very unfriendly ways when given a fail on specific competencies by assessors, as found by Hunt et al.'s (2016) for example.

Similarly, O'Driscoll et al. (2010) identify such issues as registrants' workload interfering with the facilitation of students' learning during practice placements, and registrants feeling pressurised to take on practice learning supervisor-type roles for their career development. The variety of potential problems associated with student assessments make early and careful planning of assessment imperative. Consequently, the purpose of proactive planning is to endeavour to prevent issues such as those mentioned above from arising.

Such problems can also be averted by practice supervisors' and assessors' leadership through accepting the role as a serious responsibility, and early, careful forward planning of their own workload and the student's practice learning. Practice assessors' leadership in relation to the assessment of students' practice competencies is also noted in Chapter 8 of this book in the appropriate sections.

Leadership in assessing pre-registration student midwives and grading clinical competencies

The practice setting in midwifery practice is where students learn under direct supervision and become competent through engaging in hands-on care of women and their families through the pregnancy and parenting journey, and later in their learning stage through indirect supervision. It is also where student assessment takes place to ascertain their clinical intervention skills, and therefore the NMC's competencies in which the student midwife will be deemed competent or otherwise.

Academic institutes, in collaboration with their healthcare provider partners who offer midwifery courses in England, have adopted the Midwifery Ongoing Record of Achievement (MORA) document to record evidence of the achievement of competencies, and to monitor students' learning and progress in line with the NMC's (2018a) SSSA. The MORA was developed by the Midwifery Practice Assessment Collaboration (King's College London, 2020), and is designed in a way in which competencies are not stated for each academic year, but instead it offers a flexible approach, taking into consideration that practice learning varies in relation to clinical opportunities and the placement programme structures.

The MORA also supports the grading of practice using a holistic assessment approach, which it does in two stages. First, practice supervisors provide regular feedback and grade the student during their placement using the grading criteria. Second, at the end of the placement, practice assessors decide on the final holistic grade using the set marking criteria, and this is the grade which contributes to the course. Different descriptors are used for the varying levels of study. An example of Level 5 descriptors for a second-year student midwife to achieve a pass at 'Excellent' grade (extracted from MORA) are:

- their behaviour meets the professional conduct criteria and they contribute to care provision in a safe, sensitive and woman-focused way
- has an excellent level of knowledge and understanding of the evidence and policies that relate to their practice at this level
- is developing a critical approach to reasoning and reflection and always shows insightful integration of theory and practice
- identifies problems and applies their knowledge and skills to problem-solve in straightforward and some complex scenarios
- is always self-directed in identifying their learning needs, seeking out new learning opportunities

- is self-aware and always seeks feedback and responds positively
- proactively contributes to effective team working.

Alternative grades for practice competencies at other levels are 'Outstanding', 'Very good', 'Good', 'Satisfactory' and 'Unsatisfactory'. Grading of practice for midwifery students has been implemented since around 2009, and as a positive, it bestows equal importance to students' achievements in practice learning as to their academic grade achievements. Clinicians have also reported the benefit of grading practice, and their contribution towards the student's overall course grade enables them to feel recognised as 'gate keepers to the profession' (Way et al., 2019: 252). The recent introduction of MORA has also helped to alleviate some previous concerns about differences in the way that HEI grade their midwifery students in the clinical area.

MORA contains all the competencies that students need to achieve, and spans the woman's pregnancy journey and therefore includes competencies in antenatal, intrapartum, postnatal and neonatal care. Competencies are divided into universal care and additional care, ensuring that students are skilled in caring for women who require enhanced care.

Consequently, student midwives must also become competent in a full systematic examination of the newborn in line with local and national evidence-based protocols. In England, this is referred to as the Newborn Infant Physical Examination, which comprises of four key components of examination: the eyes, heart, hips and male testes (Public Health England, 2021). Other examples of midwifery competencies include proficiencies in medicine management, recognising signs of labour, the ability to communicate effectively and work within a multi-professional team, and providing support to breastfeeding women.

However, there can be challenges to practice supervision and assessment in the practice setting, and practice supervisors' and assessors' leadership is also reflected in pre-empting and managing issues related to students' practice-based learning and achievement of agreed competencies, which can become apparent during the placement or at post-placement evaluation, as illustrated in Case Study 6.1.

At the end of each practice placement, students are encouraged to evaluate their experiences and provide feedback to their HEI, and to the NHS placement area. The results are shared anonymously and discussion can take place between the HEI and placement area for the results to inform future planning, and to ensure an adequate learning environment which meets student needs. Post-placement evaluations tend to show that students value practice supervisors and assessors who invest in their learning, and that they benefit from the support they receive and from being valued as a team member, although these things can be affected by issues such as staff shortages and high workload.

Students' experiences in the clinical area are highly impacted by the relationship they have with their supervisors and assessors, and by the culture to which they are exposed, which in turn can affect student retention (e.g. Panda et al., 2021). Both organisational learning culture and student retention were examined in detail in

Chapter 5 of this book. On some occasions, a formal approach is required when concerns have been raised in relation to a student's progress or performance to ensure that issues are addressed as soon as possible. Subsequently, a progression plan can be initiated to support the student with SMART (specific, measurable, achievable, realistic and time-bound) objectives that can enable students to achieve the objectives in the plan.

─Case study 6.1─

Addressing students' clinical skills and progress

Karolina is a third-year student midwife on a labour ward rotation. Practice supervisors have provided mostly positive daily feedback with some feed-forward comments. However, when Karolina worked her intermediate shift with her practice assessor, the assessor was concerned that Karolina was not meeting the required standard of practice and showing the knowledge expected of a third-year student midwife. The concerns were documented in the student's MORA and the assessor informed the student's academic assessor of this. A tripartite meeting was arranged between the student, the practice assessor and the academic assessor to discuss this further and initiate a progression plan. It was explained that the student had not been able to demonstrate the application of aseptic technique when performing female urinary catheterisation on a couple of occasions, and the student was deemed to inaccurately commence CTGs (cardiotocograph) a number of times. The student did not agree with the concerns and challenged the assessor's observation, and felt that because her supervisor comments were positive, then the issue related to her and the practice assessor having a personality clash. She reported that her practice assessor often thinks she is being difficult and that she is unable to take on board constructive criticism.

Progression plan templates are included in MORA and encourage objectives to be written using SMART principles. Examples of SMART objectives for Karolina are as follows:

Specific objectives - noting the competencies where concerns have arisen and any other general performance concerns:

1. Apply the correct aseptic technique when performing female catheterisation.
2. Accurately assess foetal well-being by ensuring that a pinard is used prior to commencement of the CTG.
3. Develop a positive working relationship between practice assessor and Karolina.

Measurable objectives - referring to the expectations of the student at this level in her education programme and ensuring they are **achievable** and **realistic** goals:

1. Competently complete the skill of catheterisation without support, including the procedure to maintain aseptic technique. This can be done in any setting, e.g. a labour ward, theatre or a postnatal ward. Karolina to revise the theory in relation to catheterisation and attend a supported session with her academic assessor on the performance of this skill in a simulated scenario. Karolina can

(Continued)

achieve the skill in the clinical area by ensuring that practice supervisors and assessors supply the clinical opportunities for catheterisation.

2. Ensure that a Pinard stethoscope is used prior to the commencement of a CTG. This is to be documented in the clinical records.

3. Be cognisant of the feedback provided: Karolina to keep a daily diary of her own performance on the shift which she can then map against the practice assessor feedback, and then any differences can be discussed between Karolina and her practice assessor and used to inform feed-forward comments and actions.

Time-bound aspect of objectives – consideration of when the progression plan will be revisited:

1. Karolina and the practice assessor to meet at the end of each shift to discuss and provide comments on the above and discuss the daily diary.

2. Overall performance and achievement to be discussed in two weeks' time, with regular ongoing feedback during that time frame. The academic assessor is to organise further tripartite discussion in one week's time.

In this instance, there will also be opportunities for Karolina to practise clinical skills in a simulation setting, which is a safe space to allow for open discussion, questions and practice without consequences to the health of the woman. This should help develop competence and confidence prior to commencing the skill in the clinical area. Recommended prior reading should encourage Karolina to take responsibility for her own learning. The daily diary allows for an open and honest discussion to take place between the student and the practice assessor. It also serves as the foundation for a productive conversation starter, and the student may also decide on which sections within MORA to gain feedback on from the women and families for whom she is caring, which may further inform discussion with the assessor.

Support for further learning for registered midwives, and therefore also midwifery learning supervisors and assessors, is included in the Ockenden report (Gov.uk, 2022) which published the findings of an investigation at a NHS Trust in Shropshire, where there was a series of failings resulting in preventable maternal and neonatal deaths. The report identifies essential and immediate action for all maternity services in England, some of which will have a direct impact on support and learning upon qualification, including ensuring that all Trusts offer a supportive preceptorship programme. Accordingly, an interim £95.6 million of investment for maternity services was made available in 2021 to support newly qualified midwives as they start their career, as well as for employing an additional midwife in every maternity unit in England (NHSEI, 2021).

Leadership in Managing Change Using Frameworks of Change Management

All healthcare professionals will have encountered changes in the way care and treatment are organised and delivered in various practice settings, and it is almost inevitable that practice supervisors will have been involved as participants in change, and may have also initiated change. It should therefore prove useful for practice supervisors to have good insights into how to manage change. It is important to distinguish between the concepts of 'managing' change and 'introducing' or 'imposing' change; the latter can be effected at short notice, but managing the change implies longer-term, planned and systematic activities.

Other than EBP and practice development, there are various other reasons for change in clinical practice, which are identified in Table 6.1.

Table 6.1 Reasons for change in healthcare

Reasons for changes	Brief details
1. Change in medical technology	• New medical devices and equipment; use of computer networks and easier access to information
2. New knowledge	• Research and audit findings; expert guidelines
3. Safer and more effective products	• Consumable materials; hardware being superseded by more efficient or effective ones
4. The nature of the workforce	• Workers of different age groups and with domestic responsibilities; changes in qualified:unqualified staff ratio, e.g. registered nurse associates with different skills
5. Revised policies and strategies	• Use of strategies and equipment to prevent injury to staff, or to avoid 'hospital acquired infections'
6. Quality-conscious consumers	• Patient satisfaction surveys, with suggestions for changes that should be made
7. Funding and budgets	• Availability and allocation of required resources

At times, change occurs in reaction to dictats from government departments, or because of poor CQC audit results, or based on the publication of new clinical guidelines, or as service efficiency measures. For the effective and systematic management of change, a range of proformas and frameworks for managing change has been published, such as NHS England's (2017b: 1) Change Model, which is a framework for achieving 'transformational, sustainable change' and comprises of eight elements that should be considered when leading change. These eight elements need to be applied to each individual change being implemented, and they are:

- our shared purpose
- leadership by all
- spread and adoption
- improvement tools
- project and performance management
- measurement
- system drivers
- motivation and mobilisation.

A relatively more straightforward but comprehensive framework for managing change was constituted by Gopee and Galloway (2017) and is composed of seven essential and interrelated factors for managing change successfully, which are: Recognition, Analysis, Preparation, Strategies, Implementation, Evaluation, Sustaining (RAPSIES). The RAPSIES framework therefore entails (in sequence):

1. **Recognition** of the need for change to solve a problem, for instance, or to improve an element of practice.
2. **Analysis** of the available options related to the contemplated change, the environment or setting where change will be implemented, and the users of the change.
3. **Preparation** for the change, such as identifying a change agent to lead the implementation of the change, education, defining the intended outcomes and involving all relevant colleagues.
4. **Strategies** for planned implementation of the change.
5. **Implementation** of the change, which may be preceded by piloting the change; timing of implementation.
6. **Evaluation** of the impact of the change against the intended outcomes, continuing evaluation and at pre-determined times.
7. **Sustaining** the change, i.e. how to ensure the change endures and is mainstreamed.

The change might succeed or fail, depending on the effectiveness of each of the seven steps in the framework. For example, when managing change to flexible-hour rostering, each of the seven steps needs to be managed effectively. A simpler model of change management is Lewin's three-stage change process which entails unfreezing the situation, implementing the change, and then refreezing it, which corresponds with Analysis, Implementation and Sustaining of the change, respectively, in the RAPSIES model. The implementation of the change is referred to as 'movement', and 'refreezing' refers to sustaining the change. This is obviously an extremely simplistic explanation of activities that warrant careful consideration of all related factors and careful planning and implementation.

To provide more details of step 4 of the RAPSIES model, for instance – the concept 'Strategies' for implementing the change, which is similar to 'Unfreezing' – there are several strategies that can be considered before deciding on the relevant ones, which includes a SWOT analysis, a PESTLE analysis and a **forcefield analysis** – see, for example, a SWOT analysis of changing to family-witnessed resuscitation in the emergency department of acute hospitals (Figure 6.4).

Following analysis by the team, the change agent takes action to manage any weaknesses and threats, build on the strengths, agree on the success criteria of the change, and implement any staff training required. Some of these actions can be executed by using a format like the one presented in Template 6.1, which can contribute to designing and implementing a local protocol for this intervention.

Strengths	Weaknesses
• Comfort for the family that all that could be done was done • Psychologically beneficial to the family • Facilitate grieving • Family members as support for each other, and enhance bonding between them • Enable closure and facilitate acceptance of death • Is more holistic and family-centred practice	• Is a stressful event for healthcare professionals • Deficient healthcare professionals' education of the topic • Lack of self-confidence in technical abilities and what to communicate to the family • Lack of experience, • Fear of emotional/physical reactions of family • Lack of time to provide comfort to the family during the dying process • Can be traumatic to family seeing invasive procedures being carried out • Family members might not understand what is happening • Too many people and therefore lack of physical space in small area / room • Family member can become very distressed, and need staff time to support them • Family might not want to observe resuscitation.
Opportunities	Threats
• Forming a working relationship with the family • Education for juniors to learn about CPR and FWR, especially seeing cardiac arrest team in action • Further develop expertise in FWR • Develop / adapt a protocol for FWR locally • Role expansion • Specialist role • Enhanced family-centred patient care.	• Delay in waiting for family members to be present • Family member could try to help with procedure • Family might feel CPR was stopped too early, and risk of litigation • Family not leaving their loved one's side, which implies more staff time required • Family members could physically get in the way or ask questions at inappropriate times • Patient information overload.

Figure 6.4 SWOT analysis of changing to family-witnessed resuscitation in emergency department

Template 6.1 can be used for actions to take in relation to the likely weaknesses prior to beginning implementation of the change; the same can apply to threats, and also strengths and opportunities.

Template 6.1 Subsequent actions following SWOT analysis of proposed family-witnessed resuscitation in the emergency department

SWOT analysis - *Weaknesses*	Probable actions
• Is a stressful event for healthcare professionals • Deficient healthcare professionals' education of the topic • Lack of self-confidence in technical abilities and what to communicate to the family • Lack of experience, • Fear of emotional/physical reactions of family • etc • etc	• Teamwork is essential, as it also provides mutual support • Beneficial to all healthcare professionals because this suggests further education is required • Opportunities for learning by observation of senior healthcare professionals • ...

The weaknesses and threats that surface in SWOT analyses can be further compounded by general obstacles to the implementation of research findings, and can include:

- deficient critical appraisal and research skills
- not having ready access to the right resources
- an organisational and managerial ethos and culture that expect change to be implemented very quickly
- lack of power and financial control to implement change
- lack of valid research on the topic, or of user-friendly reviews and guidelines
- organisational factors such as funding, staffing and education
- accessibility to research and databases.

The management of change, however, requires a systematic approach and takes time. Full details of the management of change is available in relevant textbooks, including Gopee's (2022) *Leading and Managing Healthcare*, Chapter 9.

Reflection point 6.3

Barriers to implementing research evidence

As a practice supervisor, consider or discuss with an appropriate colleague whether any of the above-mentioned obstacles to the implementation of research findings still prevail in your workplace. Which of the likely obstacles have been largely resolved?

As for access to research at the workplace, most NHS Trusts now have a postgraduate department or library, which tends to provide access to electronic databases and have subscriptions for specialism-specific journals. Nonetheless, in an extensive review of literature to ascertain the barriers to the implementation of EBP, Williams et al. (2015) identified the five most commonly occurring barriers as:

- workload
- other staff/management not supportive of research
- lack of resources
- lack of authority to change practice
- workplace/professional culture being resistant to change.

Because of the issues related to the implementation of EBP, education curricula for healthcare professionals have, over the years, endeavoured to rectify these problems by the inclusion of research modules in their health profession courses at both pre- and post-registration levels. Of course, undergraduate healthcare education curricula have been required (e.g. by the NMC, 2018c, 2019b) to incorporate research appraisal and application of research knowledge and skills to care delivery regularly for more than a decade, and therefore some of the issues discussed by Williams et al. (2015) may also have gradually been resolved.

Some of the other ways in which barriers to research implementation can be managed include a mechanism for providing research advice and support to the care team; enabling healthcare professionals to develop negotiation and management of change skills; and support to establish self-belief in one's research appraisal skills.

Managerial and organisational input and support tend to be as important as individual skills in the implementation of research findings, except that such implementation needs to be 'managed'. Research-based practice is an inherent component of practice supervisors' clinical practice, and the healthcare trust's clinical procedure and guidelines almost always include the evidence base for practice.

Eventually, when the change has been implemented and embedded in the practice setting successfully, it can be disseminated to others within the healthcare organisation and maybe externally as well. However, there can be barriers to dissemination, the main ones being lack of knowledge of where and how to disseminate and lack of time.

Furthermore, instances of more novel and more effective practice tend to be published and thereby disseminated as news items in healthcare journals, presented at conferences, and sometimes as stories in newspapers and on television. Dissemination of research findings should, however, aim to ensure that key messages are conveyed to specific groups of staff; it should be executed by utilising a wide range of methods to generate a strong reaction, preferably implementation, and wth greater impact. The range of methods of effective dissemination of research findings include:

- journal articles or short reports
- journal clubs
- seminars, study days
- conference presentations
- poster presentations
- publishing the findings as books or book chapters
- inclusion in curricula
- newsletters.

Chapter Summary

This chapter has focused on registrants' and practice supervisors' leadership, which comprise of leadership in facilitation of learners' learning, of evidence-based person-centred practice and practice development, as well as on the management of change and student assessment, and has therefore examined:

- Practice supervisors' and assessors' leadership in careful forward planning and managing students' practice-based learning and assessment during practice placement, and prioritising daily work to accommodate support for learners.
- Why and how practice supervisors' leadership is underpinned by high-quality person-centred, evidence-informed practice that is also safe and effective, and comprises being role models to all in the practice setting.

- How practice supervisors influence and implement changes in practice as essential components of the registrant's responsibilities, and through application of frameworks for managing change; and overcome any incidental barriers or obstacles in doing so.
- Ways in which evidence-informed practice is achieved, and the practice supervisor's role in identifying, appraising, applying and disseminating changes.

Further Optional Reading

1. For a more detailed account and analysis of leadership in healthcare and on systematic management of change using a framework, see Chapters 3 and 9 respectively of:

    - Gopee, N. (2022) *Leading and Managing Healthcare*. London: Sage.

2. An excellent resource for the best ways of critically appraising research papers is:

    - Greenhalgh, T. (2019) *How to Read a Paper: The Basics of Evidence-Based Medicine and Healthcare*, 6th edn. Oxford: Wiley-Blackwell.

3. Various detailed examples of service improvement and innovations (case studies) in healthcare are available on NICE's website, e.g.:

    - National Institute for Health and Care Excellence (2021) *Transforming the Care of Children and Young People in London with Asthma*. Available at: www.nice.org.uk/sharedlearning/transforming-care-cyp-london-with-asthma (accessed 22 June 2022).

7

ASSESSING STUDENT KNOWLEDGE AND COMPETENCE

Introduction

The primary function of the practice assessor is to assess students' healthcare intervention skills and associated knowledge. This chapter explores student assessment from the perspectives of what assessments are, a number of reasons for performing them, at which specific points in their programmes students are assessed, who other than the practice assessor assesses students (e.g. peer assessment), as well as the range of methods of assessment that are available to select from. The specified procedures that have to be followed for conducting assessments, along with the validity and reliability of assessments, are other inherent components which are also addressed in this chapter. These points essentially constitute the principles and processes of assessments. The concepts that are inherent within the principles of assessment are therefore essential, and the practical considerations as well as the theoretical base are addressed in both this chapter and Chapter 8. Potential problematic facets of assessments, as well as past and present issues related to assessments and how they can be averted or resolved, are also essential components addressed in Chapter 8.

Chapter objectives

1. Identify what assessments are, and the elements of healthcare courses on which students are assessed.
2. Enunciate several reasons for the assessment of clinical skills and the knowledge base of students on healthcare profession courses.
3. Cite instances of various staff members who are involved in assessment, including the roles of self- and peer assessment.
4. Explain a range of methods of assessment that practice assessors can apply to conduct student assessments, and the various fundamental principles of assessments that they need to abide by to fulfil this function.
5. Explain the requirements that practice assessors have to meet to ascertain students' achievement of proficiency, and the significance of the 'ongoing achievement record'.
6. Explain the ways in which student assessments can meet validity and reliability criteria of assessments.

Assessing Practice

Assessment is an integral part of all credit-awarding healthcare courses, and one of the principal purposes of practice assessor preparation is to equip registrants with the ability to conduct student assessment that meets the validity, reliability and fairness criteria of assessment of identified practice competencies during practice placements (e.g. HCPC, 2017). Other components of assessor preparation, according to the NMC (2018a), are:

- ensuring competence in interpersonal communication skills, relevant to student learning and assessment, and the ability to provide constructive feedback
- the ability to conduct objective, evidence-based assessments of students.

The NMC (2018a) indicates that the assessment of nursing and midwifery students is conducted by practice assessors and academic assessors, with input from practice supervisors. At the end of each assessment by direct observation, the assessor has to make a decision regarding whether the student is competent to perform the assessed skill independently, unsupervised, safely and effectively, and signs the appropriate section of the student's competency document as pass or fail.

There are a number of factors that assessors have to consider to fulfil their assessment duties effectively. Specifically, for nursing and midwifery students, in the *Standards Framework for Nursing and Midwifery Education* (NMC, 2018d: 12) document, under 'Curricula and assessment', the NMC stipulates a range of considerations related to student assessment, including that assessment must occur throughout the programme and across practice settings to determine student progression, and that practice assessments are 'evidenced by (direct) observations and other appropriate methods'.

Additionally, the NMC's (2018a: 9) SSSA identifies a number of facets of the 'practice assessor' role, such as 'practice assessors conduct assessment to confirm student achievement of proficiencies and programme outcomes for practice learning'. Such statements identify requirements such as the need for educational preparation (attending a course) for the practice assessor role, and ways in which the assessment of students is to be conducted to ensure the evidence base and effectiveness of the assessment process. Furthermore, the NMC (2018a: 7) also details the practice supervisor's role in student assessment and progression through four clauses reproduced in the box below.

Practice Supervisors' Contribution to Assessment and Progression

Practice supervisors

4.1 contribute to the student's record of achievement by periodically recording relevant observations on the conduct, proficiency and achievement of the students they are supervising

4.2 contribute to student assessments to inform decisions for progression

4.3 have sufficient opportunities to engage with practice assessors and academic assessors to share relevant observations on the conduct, proficiency and achievement of the students they are supervising

4.4 are expected to appropriately raise and respond to student conduct and competence concerns and are supported in doing so.

So, clearly, practice supervisors have a fundamental and crucial role to play in monitoring the development and achievement of the student's healthcare skills, knowledge and attitude. Technically, practice supervisors thus conduct formative assessments (discussed later in this chapter), and their duties include recording the student's achievements and taking action if they have concerns that the student is under-performing and under-achieving. Practice supervisors therefore provide relevant information to practice assessors about the student's achievement and progress during practice placement.

The practice assessor role in nursing and midwifery is complemented by the 'academic' assessor's role, the latter normally being a university-based lecturer, who, in collaboration with the practice assessor, determines whether the student has met all NMC's pre-registration education requirements to be able to become a registrant with the NMC.

What are assessments?

To begin to examine the principles and processes of assessment, it is useful to establish first what you, as the healthcare professional, already know about assessment of competencies.

━━━━━━━━━━━━ ACTION **POINT 7.1** ━━━━━━━━━━━━

What you already know about assessments

1. Think of the courses that you have already attended, and any one(s) you might currently be on. Think also of your contact with other learners and students on various programmes of study. What are the various methods of assessment that are used to assess learners' knowledge and skills? Jot down as many methods as you can think of.
2. Consider what else you already know about assessments, which aspects of assessments you are unclear about, and what else you feel you need to know about assessments. Make written notes of your responses.

So, what do you already know about assessments? In response to Activity 7.1, you may have thought that the assessment of practice-based competencies are best carried out by direct observation of the learner's performance, while other practice objectives can be assessed by asking the learner specific questions, or by their reflective write-ups. Essays and written examinations are used for the assessment of theory (also referred to as knowledge base). Most of these will be examined in this chapter under 'How to assess'. In addition to assessment of practice-based competencies by direct observation, other examples of methods of assessment of practice and theory in healthcare education programmes are:

*   OSCE (i.e. Objective Structured Clinical Examination)
*   assessment of practical skills in skills laboratories by simulation, using assessment stations
*   written examination
*   portfolio, with reflective accounts
*   care studies/case studies

- objective tests or multiple-choice questions
- short-answer questions
- structured essays
- seminars/poster designs and presentations – individually or in 2s or 3s
- numeracy test/medication calculation test
- end-point assessment (for apprentices and nursing associates)
- audio- or video-recording on an agreed topic, with PowerPoint slides
- individual student negotiated project (e.g. in a dissertation)
- viva voce (to defend or justify the outcomes of a project).

Other assessment methods that usually contribute to the summative assessment of students include the testimony, rating or comments of service users and carers, peer assessment and student self-assessment. The HEE (2017: 25) adds storyboards and 'professional conversations' to the methods of assessing nursing associates. Video recordings by healthcare students on digital video discs or other means that can be utilised instead of direct observation, with the permission of any service user involved of course, for the assessment of students' competencies, according to Tweed et al. (2010).

Furthermore, assessments have to be appropriate for the component of knowledge and competence being assessed. For example, the knowledge of medication calculation is assessed by unseen invigilated written examination, incidents or innovations encountered during practice placements are assessed by reflective account in PAD, evidence-informed decision-making by appraisal of research, and vaguer topics such as leadership by small group presentations. With regard to the last bullet point in the above list, a viva voce is a face-to-face question-and-answer examination between the student and the examiner. This is standard practice for PhD student assessments, and in apprenticeship and other academic programmes.

Your response to what else you feel you need to know about assessments obviously depends very much on your experience, existing knowledge and understanding of the concept, and it varies between individuals. You might have felt, for instance, that you could do with knowing more about formative, summative, continuous, peer/self-assessment or about practice competencies.

Furthermore, you might need to know about student assessment in programmes for more recent nursing titles such as apprentices, and nursing associates. For nursing associates, the training and assessment of competencies are based on the current Skills for Health (2022) Care Certificate Standards which are designed mainly for non-regulated vocations. For apprenticeship undergraduate programmes, the end-point assessment method can include a 'professional discussion' on the achievement of nationally published KSBs (knowledge, skills and behaviours) (IATE, 2022c).

━━━━━━━━━━ ACTION **POINT 7.2** ━━━━━━━━━━

Assessments that I've passed

To explore this area further, first look back to a course that you attended, preferably recently, and make notes on the following:

- A list of assessments that you had to pass in order to complete the course successfully.
- When exactly during the course were you assessed, and on which components of the course?
- Specifically, what was assessed?

What do we mean by assessments?

A number of assessment methods such as written examinations, practical assessments and projects have been identified above; and if you were assessed by continuous assessment, then you would have been exposed to a range of assessment components on different occasions, during both practice placements and in university skill laboratories and classrooms.

Definitions of assessment

The dictionary (Brookes and O'Neill, 2017: 48) states that the word 'assess' originates from the Latin word *assidere*, which means to sit by or beside, which implies a close relationship and the sharing of an experience. The word also means 'estimate the value or worth of someone or something' and 'to judge the worth or importance of'. Based on general current understanding of the term, assessment therefore tends to imply observing the student closely while they perform a specific clinical intervention, with a view to stating at the end of the performance whether the intervention was performed competently. It also seems to imply being supportive and identifying subsequent learning needs.

Taking a step back, however, it is important to note that an assessment is not an activity that only appointed assessors perform in order to fulfil our work role. We assess life situations all the time before we take any action, whether it is to do with assessing whether to wear a coat when going out based on the perceived weather and temperature outside, whether it is safe to overtake when driving, or whether we can treat ourselves to a delicious cake while bearing in mind the day's calorie intake. Such assessments do not result in someone awarding us a pass or fail but they still involve assessing stimuli or data, and then making a decision.

Assessment is also reflected in health assessment of the health service user, which entails collecting information and identifying any actual and potential patient problems from the data, from which decisions are made regarding the action to be taken. Student assessment, however, is related to collecting information as evidence of the student's ability to perform specified clinical interventions as competencies, and their critical thinking skills. Some of the core skills necessary for assessing patients' needs and problems are also relevant for assessing learners. These are observing, measuring, questioning and making decisions. So, these skills also apply to the assessment of students' knowledge and skills.

With regards to assessing health profession students' clinical competencies and related knowledge, assessment can be defined as the process of systematically appraising the student's knowledge and competence to ascertain the extent to which they have achieved the specified outcomes for the particular stage of their programme of study. Curzon and Tummons (2013) suggest that assessments involve collecting, measuring and interpreting information related to students' responses to the process of instruction.

Assessment is also a measurement of the quantity of learning, as well as the quality. While quantity of learning implies the number of skills or part-skills that the learner has already learnt, quality of learning refers to how fully the skills (or knowledge) have been learnt (see also reliability of assessments discussed later in this chapter). The two elements also provide a measure of progress, and thereby also form the basis for identifying areas of further learning.

What do we assess?

As noted in Chapter 2, acquiring professional competencies involves learning in all three inherent components, or domains – cognitive, psychomotor and affective. That means learning the professional knowledge base required to perform our healthcare duties, the skills required for performing care interventions, and also having the appropriate attitude. Attitude in this context is also referred to as values and behaviours.

The NMC's (2018c) standards of proficiency (SOP) for nurses identifies the exact learning outcomes that pre-registration students need to achieve to gain registered nurse status on the NMC's professional register. These standards are detailed under seven 'platforms', as noted at the beginning of Chapter 2, and also under 'Communication and relationship management skills' (Annexe A of NMC, 2018c) and 'Nursing procedures' (Annexe B). The same standards apply to all four fields of nursing (adult, child, learning disability and mental health), and students have to be competent in all of them at the point of registration.

More details of the NMC's (2018c) SOP are documented as specific practice placement objectives in students' Practice Assessment Document (PAD) or MORA, on which students are assessed, but they are discussed between practice supervisors and assessors before the student arrives to start the particular placement. For NMC-based pre-registration programmes, practice assessors assess student achievement on all competencies stated in the student's PAD or similar document, and make decisions about the student's level of achievement.

For apprenticeship programmes leading to Registered Nurse qualification, the Institute for Apprenticeships & Technical Education (IATE) (2022a) has published full details of the content and modes of delivery of the programme, which includes the NMC's (2018c) SOP as well as additional knowledge, skills and behaviours. The methods of student assessment are detailed in the publication *End-Point Assessment Plan for Registered Nurse Fully Integrated Degree Apprenticeship Standard* (IATE, 2022b).

Similarly, the HCPC publishes specific areas of knowledge and competence for different pre-qualifying AHP courses. These standards and competencies are reflected in the course's and modules' aims and learning outcomes, in theory components as well as in practice elements. There are also specific SOP for SCPHNs (NMC, 2018d) and 'competencies' for advanced nurse practitioners that have to be met (e.g. RCN, 2018).

As we shall see later, it is absolutely vital for the practice assessor to establish very early on during the practice placement exactly which specific competencies the student on the particular practice placement is to be assessed on. Otherwise, the assessment may not meet the curriculum's requirements. In the notes that you made in response to Activity 7.2, you may have mentioned that the NMC or the associated university has already laid down the components that practice assessors need to assess in the form of competencies, but more specific guidance can usually be accessed from PEFs and associated academics such as the academic assessors and course directors.

All assessments of the pre-registration curriculum are mandatory, and those in the first year of the programme are set at academic level 4 (higher education certificate level); those for the second year are set at level 5 (higher education diplomas and foundation degrees); those for the third year are set at level 6 (Bachelor's degrees with or without Honours); and those set at level 7 are for Master's degrees, postgraduate diplomas and postgraduate certificates (QAA, 2014). Various other ways of differentiating between academic levels have also already been developed (e.g. Steinaker and Bell, 1979; Anderson, L. W. et al., 2014).

The competencies PAD that students bring with them to the practice placement contains other useful information such as the process of assessment, the roles and responsibilities of the practice supervisor and the practice assessor, those of the student, and the university support available to them. Furthermore, at a number of university–trust partnerships, an electronic version of the PAD and assessment record is utilised, referred to as the Practice Assessment Record and Evaluation (PARE) (HEE, 2022d), for instance. PARE can be accessed by practice supervisors, practice assessors, students, lecturers and other appropriate personnel such as PEFs.

In addition to constituting a record of practice assessment for each student in their electronic PAD, advantages of PARE include the ease of access to these records from anywhere via computers, which saves time, markedly reduces paperwork, is potentially more accurate and reduces the risk of cross-infection through paper-based PAD being handled several times and across practice placement areas. It also facilitates student evaluation of placements and the resulting appropriate action taken.

The NMC's SOP documents are usually available in a 'learning resources' folder for students in practice settings, but it might prove useful to obtain a copy of this for yourself for revisiting if required.

━━━━━━━━━━ **ACTION POINT 7.3** ━━━━━━━━━━

Pre-registration student assessment

Find out from your partner university all the assessments that the pre-registration student needs to pass for the specific field in which you practice. You could access this information via the named academic link for your practice setting, or the PEF.

In addition to the placement competencies set by the university, students are encouraged to achieve as many other competencies as the placement can offer and thereby maximise learning. A number of clinical areas have their own clearly identified competencies or learning objectives that can be achieved during placement. A number of them are optional for pre-registration students but compulsory for newly appointed registrants on induction or preceptee programmes.

In addition to the regulatory bodies' SOP, professional bodies (or colleges/societies) such as the Chartered Society of Physiotherapy (CSP) publish further specific standards, such as those in the publications *Physiotherapy Framework* (CSP, 2011 – updated 2020) and *Learning and Development Principles* (CSP, 2020). The *Physiotherapy Framework* comprises knowledge and skills under four elements, which are:

1. Professional values
2. Physiotherapy knowledge
3. Physiotherapy practice skills
4. Generic behaviours, knowledge and skills.

Extensive details of knowledge, skills and behaviour are provided in the framework document for each the four elements, which are referred to as 'Domain descriptors' for different levels of practice from 'Novice' level to 'Expert' level. These elements also incorporate inherent physiotherapy activities such as leadership, research, and education. The *Learning and Development Principles* publication (CSP, 2020) indicates a further nine principles that contemporary pre-registration physiotherapy programmes should incorporate, such as inter-professional education.

In addition to the assessment of healthcare students' competencies, practice supervisors and assessors also assess each student's professional values in practice (this was referred to as the student's character in the past). Professional values tend to be judged against ethical and legal frameworks, such as the sections and clauses in the NMC (2018b) code of practice; and they are assessed continuously and documented in the student's PAD under such areas as:

- maintaining confidentiality
- maintaining every service user's privacy and dignity
- seeking consent prior to care interventions
- being non-judgemental towards service users
- exercising candour.

Furthermore, the practice assessor may also be required to assess non-regulated care workers, such as healthcare support workers (HSW). In terms of what to assess, the information will be provided by educators responsible for the HSW's learning programme, which leads to a 'Care Certificate' being awarded. National standards for Care Certificate programmes are identified by Skills for Health (2022). As for nursing associates, the required standards are identified in HEE's (2017) Nursing Associate Curriculum Framework.

Why do we Assess our Students?

We have already referred to some of the aims of assessments. Most individuals have mixed feelings about being assessed as, on the one hand, it creates anxiety but, on the other hand it is rewarding because on passing the assessment, the learner can be given permission to practise the particular clinical skill with less supervision. To begin our discussion on why we need to assess, consider for yourself what the range of purposes of assessments is, in addition to the NMC's (2018a) requirement for practice assessors to assess students.

ACTION POINT 7.4

Purposes of assessments

Think of all the methods of assessment that you noted during Activity 7.1, and of the reasons for assessing students and other learners. Make notes of these reasons for assessment. What did each assessment test?

According to the NMC (2018a: 9), the nominated practice assessor in partnership with the nominated academic assessor must indicate whether the student has achieved the NMC (2018c) standards for pre-registration nurse education, and therefore whether they are safe and effective in practice, and thus the practice competencies are designed to test the student's ability to perform service-user care interventions safely. Structured essays test the student's knowledge and understanding of concepts in nursing, but practice assessors are not involved in marking essays as this is the remit of the HEI (including the academic assessor).

In addition to knowledge and clinical skills, assessments also ascertain learning in the affective domain (Bloom, 1956; discussed in Chapter 3), that is, values and attitudes. Several purposes of assessments are identified by different researchers. In summary, we assess learners in order to:

- establish and then authorise learners as developing health professionals to practise specific clinical intervention with fair autonomy
- provide a mark or grade that informs the student of their level of performance at that point in time
- determine the student's progress with the learning programme
- ascertain the learner's overall competence and fitness for practice
- motivate the learner towards new components of learning
- judge the level of professional learning in the psychomotor (dexterity with clinical skills), affective (attitude) and cognitive (knowledge and thinking) components
- identify further learning needs based on self-assessment and assessor feedback
- provide potential employers with details of knowledge and competence achieved by the individual, and therefore their fitness to practise.

Assessments therefore constitute an opportunity for identifying learning needs, which suggests that learning is an integral component of the assessment process, and not simply a means of measuring attainment. Students are encouraged to undertake self-assessment and to reflect on their learning. It could be argued that all learner assessments are learning situations, in that the assessment provides scope for improvement or enhancement of the way the intervention was performed or adjusted when managing different categories of service users. This notion also suggests that even if the student performs the skill competently, there is still scope for progressing from 'competent' to 'proficient' levels, as identified in Benner's (2001) skill acquisition continuum. Additionally, if the learner makes an error, then they are likely to be aware of it, or the assessor will point it out to them and identify relevant learning needs.

From the teacher's perspective, assessment also provides a measure of teaching effectiveness. It provides some feedback on the teams' effectiveness at teaching specific healthcare interventions during practice placements. Normally, the student will have had some teaching related to those competencies at the university beforehand. Assessments of theory also provide nurse lecturers with a fair measure of the effectiveness of their university-based teaching.

In addition to the aims of assessments already mentioned, another function of assessments is to fulfil one of society's needs directly, in that they identify which healthcare professionals have acquired the necessary repertoire of knowledge and competencies for safe and competent practice, and therefore given license to practice as a registered practitioner initially, and probably as a specialist later.

Who Assesses Learners?

Having explored what are assessments, and why they are conducted, the following section briefly examines who are the different personnel who conduct them. An obvious answer to the question of who assesses learners is qualified healthcare professionals who have completed the relevant assessor preparation programme, and therefore have been given 'a licence' to assess students' competencies. However, it is pertinent to consider the broader question of who else are the relevant professionals who assess student competencies.

—Reflection point 7.1—

Who assesses?

Think about assessments that you and your colleagues have been involved in recently, either while on a course or in the work setting. Spend a few minutes thinking about who conducted the assessments, why, on what, on whom and how. Is it only the practice assessor who assesses the student's competencies, or are other individuals also afforded this responsibility?

Perhaps an immediate response to Reflection Point 7.1 is that it is the practice assessor who assesses students in the practice setting. In fact, you might have concluded that all qualified healthcare professionals, including doctors, are involved in assessments, albeit often informally or indirectly. So, the answer to the question 'Who assesses?' could be broader, and include students' self-assessment, peer assessment and assessment by care service users. However, as in the role of practice supervisors, the majority of these personnel 'contribute' to the assessment process, with final decisions being the remit of practice assessors and academic assessors.

However, there are likely to be student-related, practice assessor-related or placement-related issues that the academic assessor has to explore and address before deciding that the proficiencies have definitely been achieved, as also noted by Drayton and Edmonds (2020). A student-related issue may be sub-optimal performance or progress by the student. Reliability and sufficiency of evidence presented by assessors and the appropriacy of the placement for adequate opportunities for the student to learn the competencies, are other possible issues.

Student self-assessment and peer assessment

Self-assessment is one of the most valuable forms of assessment for students. It is almost always formative and therefore a learning exercise. As implied, the student uses a set of criteria or a checklist, written or mental, to self-assess their knowledge of a sub-topic area or of a specific competency. It also enables them to own the learning and to control the learning that meets their needs. Self-assessment may be performed informally or more formally by the use of profiling documents or reflective diaries.

Much informal or subconscious self-assessment carried out by learners is based on their own individual aspirations, values and beliefs. These could be influenced by their views on patient care, based on their own personal and professional experience.

Self-assessment is often applied deliberately by practice supervisors and assessors whenever students are asked how effectively they performed specific clinical interventions; and they occur at review meetings with the assessor.

━━━━━━━━ **ACTION POINT 7.5** ━━━━━━━━

Self-assessment

Take a critical look at the idea of self-assessment by students, and of the strengths and weaknesses of self-assessments, and identify as many of these as you can think of.

Self-assessment is characterised by the involvement of students in identifying standards and/or criteria to apply to their work, and making judgements about the extent to which they have met them, according to Boud (2016). A number of areas of strengths as well as weaknesses of self-assessment can be identified, of which strengths include:

- inspires a conscious effort to be honest with themselves
- has an opportunity to 'take stock' and identify limitations of their knowledge, and their learning needs
- identifies where more practice/knowledge gain is required
- is less traumatic than traditional methods of assessment such as written or practical examinations
- promotes reflection-on-action and critical thinking.

As for the weaknesses of self-assessment, it is possible that some students are too self-critical while others can be too lenient in their judgement of their own performance. Some, however, may not be capable of gauging the effectiveness of their own performance sufficiently objectively and accurately, and thus self-assessment could worsen a student's poor self-image. Based on the diversity of each individual student's values, motivations, interests and aspirations, it seems advisable to implement self-assessment gradually and cautiously within education programmes.

For peer assessment, the value and impact of peers' and colleagues' impressions of our competence in various aspects of our roles cannot be underestimated. This is often an informal exercise, with colleagues, friends and even family members having different perceptions of our capability and performance, based perhaps on their different professional experiences. More structured peer assessment is generally incorporated within pre-registration programmes whereupon peers assess how well a student conducts a seminar, a short teaching session in the practice setting or in a classroom, or certain non-invasive clinical intervention in simulated situations.

In distance and e-learning modes of education delivery, facilitators often encourage students to form their own 'learning sets' for the purposes of learning together, for discussions and questioning each other. In this case, peer assessment is not formal in that other students or colleagues do not usually award a summative 'pass' or 'fail' to the peer-assessed. They do, however, provide valuable thoughts, impressions and feedback on the individual's knowledge, which can be formally incorporated into a profile or a record of reflective learning. In this way, peer assessment usually presents an opportunity to verbalise uncertainties and reservations about one's learning without having to deal with the anxiety of academia-based assessments and therefore pass or fail situations.

Because of its value to students, peer assessment has increasingly become accepted as an educationally sound activity and been built into assessment processes (e.g. Ashenafi, 2017). Many of us may find assessing our peers uncomfortable. We usually aim to provide constructive comment, but do not wish to seem over-critical and therefore tend not to assess or voice our views fully – or we may feel that as we have such a good rapport with our peers, we could damage their self-confidence with our 'criticisms'. It is also important to recognise that being assessed by our peer group can be more daunting than being assessed by a qualified assessor. If it is done badly, peer assessment can quickly destroy students' confidence or make them feel unable to face their peers again, and therefore it is an activity that needs to be supervised or facilitated, and with certain ground rules.

Following a systematic review of peer assessment and closely related concepts, Wong and Shorey (2022) identify both its benefits and potential issues. The benefits include enhanced engagement with learning as well as skill development in teamwork and leadership skills. However, students also find peer assessment an uncomfortable learning experience, especially when confronting disagreements between peers. Furthermore, for an effective assessment, peers who are doing the assessing, as well as the person being assessed, can be helped by the expertise of a facilitator in recognising the parameters of their role. When one group of post-registration students were asked to list the advantages and disadvantages of peer assessment, they felt the advantages included the following (Gopee, 2001):

- It can confirm previously held belief in skills or the lack of them.
- It is a chance to share colleagues' perception of the performance.
- It is an opportunity to identify one's weaknesses, which can later be worked on, to improve.
- The feedback from colleagues/students of equal status has impact.
- It is usually formative, so will not result in a pass or a fail for the course.

However, as with self-assessment, there can well be problematic areas related to peer assessment in that some students can find it hard to take any criticism at all from equals; someone could be unknowingly or deliberately over-critical and destructive; the individual might not accept their peers' views; it could destroy self-confidence and lead to deserting the course altogether; and there could be complete disagreement between peers.

Service-user involvement in the assessment of student competencies

One of the judges of how competently a healthcare profession learner performs a clinical intervention could be the healthcare service user, especially in relation to so-called softer skills such as compassion and empathy. User involvement in learner assessment and the provision of feedback on how competently the learner functioned in particular care interventions is increasingly built into pre-registration courses (e.g. NMC, 2018d, 2022b).

So, what are the specific ways in which supervisors and practice assessors incorporate service-user involvement in student assessments? Usually, the practice supervisor or assessor gauges how content the care service user is with the care that they receive, by observation and even by casually asking them. The service user can provide feedback to the practice supervisor or assessor about the learner's communication skills, or use of aseptic techniques when undertaking wound care, for example, which are competencies under the NMC's (2018c) 'Annexe A: Communication and relationship management skills' and 'Annexe B: Nursing procedures', respectively, and the relevant platforms. However, one or two negative comments being made by the service user or their carer should not, by itself, constitute a 'Fail' on a communication competency.

User involvement in the assessment of competencies related to professional values and attitude can be achieved by the practice supervisor or assessor asking the patient or service user if they felt that their consent had been obtained by the student prior to the clinical intervention, if they felt that they were treated with dignity and whether confidentiality was maintained in the presence of others, for example. These actions are also consistent with the current definitions of person-centred care.

Service-user feedback or testimony is recorded in the student's PAD by the practice supervisor, and to make the feedback even more useful, the student is advised to write a short reflection on this, which includes stating why they think what they did were the correct actions with reference to any relevant publication, and the learning actions that they are going to engage in subsequently.

Evidence of effective service-user involvement in students' learning and assessment is readily available (e.g. Haycock-Stuart et al., 2016), although it is acknowledged that it is a time-intensive activity that also requires additional infrastructure.

How are Assessments Conducted?

Broadly, pre-registration healthcare students' knowledge base (cognitive learning) is assessed at the university, and professional skills and attitude are assessed in the practice setting during practice placements. This involves an initial supervisor–student interview and a practice assessor–student meeting when the competencies to be achieved are ascertained, and often a learning contract (also referred to as a learning and development need) is constituted.

Approximately halfway through the placement, a mid-placement review takes place so as to ascertain the student's progress with the contracted competencies. Learners deemed competent in performing a particular clinical skill can move on to learn other skills identified in their PAD. During the last week of the placement, a final interview is conducted, and the nominated practice assessor makes a final decision on whether all clinical competencies have been achieved, and if so, they are signed and dated accordingly.

Assessing paramedic students' practice competence

For paramedic students, for instance, practice educators can assess the competence of students on each of the paramedic standards during practice placement in a number of different ways, using some of the different methods of practice assessment identified earlier in this chapter. However, for standard 14.4 ('know how to position or immobilise patients correctly for safe and effective interventions'), for example, the practice educator requires the student to demonstrate their ability to do so, and the practice educator observes the student performing this intervention directly (i.e. by direct observation of clinical performance).

A number of paramedic standards can be assessed by continuous assessment, but many of them logically lend themselves to assessment by direct observation. The PAD or practice competencies document usually requires the practice educator to assess students on each competency by two or three different assessment methods. The PAD identifies the specific competencies that comprise service-user clinical interventions that must be assessed by direct observation, whereby the learner performs the clinical intervention while being closely monitored by the practice educator.

For assessment by direct observation, there can be several practicalities that need to be considered and instituted for episodic and end-point formal assessment to be conducted effectively. The practicalities for assessing student nurses are detailed in the first box in Chapter 8 of this book.

━━━━━━━━━━ ACTION **POINT 7.6** ━━━━━━━━━━

Paramedic students' practice assessment document

If you are a student practice educator, try and gain access to an up-to-date PAD as it contains competencies that students in your allied health profession must achieve by the end of a specific practice placement, either for year one, two or three of the course.

To become a practice educator, paramedics initially need to have consolidated their learning from their pre-registration education (e.g. by shadowing or being supervised) and acquired the responsibilities and further competence related to the responsibilities that they have in the practice area where they are employed.

Following preparation for the practice educator role, they will be able to facilitate students' learning and teach them. Learning occurs in a variety of clinical settings, such as in the patient's home, the ambulance hub, at the roadside, in a vehicle and at the ambulance station or while on a standby position, and includes planned and opportunistic learning. However, teaching and learning for students need to be planned in advance, and with creativity, and where possible every opportunity used wisely to enable students to learn more widely and effectively, and be assessed for competence to practise. Student practice educators as relatively new registrants gradually assimilate further new roles and responsibilities and also adopt various teaching and learning methods.

What this generally means then is that some assessments are typically carried out during placement hours, 'shadowing' a student during usual working hours, and some assessments occur in the university setting, viz:

- Example of placement assessment 'Communication Skills' – communication skills can be assessed during placement hours. This is because an assessor can view the actual interaction with a patient.
- Example of university assessment 'Advanced Life Support' – more invasive skills are typically assessed in a simulated environment within the university.

Next, in this major section on how to assess, further principles of assessment are addressed, and comprise:

- ensuring the learner has learned the clinical skill
- the assessor's essential interpersonal skills
- dimensions of assessment
- assessing different levels of competence
- fairness of assessment
- assessment criteria and pass or fail decisions
- accurate ongoing recording of the process and outcomes of assessment.

Additionally, the process of assessment of competencies has to be managed, decisions made and feedback given to the learner. These latter points, along with how the practice assessor averts and resolves problems of assessment, are examined in Chapter 8.

Ensuring that the learner has learned the clinical skill

An important prerequisite of the assessment of a learner is to ensure that they have been taught the clinical skill systematically and given the necessary practice opportunities over time and under supervision prior to the point of assessment. Which care intervention skills and competencies students are required to learn was discussed in Chapter 2, and how they acquire the required competencies, including stages and levels of skill acquisition (e.g. Steinaker and Bell, 1979; Benner, 2001), in Chapter 3. But, crucially and logically, before the student is asked to demonstrate that they are competent in any care intervention, they naturally need to learn to perform the skill according to approved procedures, and under the guidance of registrants. The learning also has to be in the context of eventualities in the practice setting and of changing patients' health conditions.

The assessor's essential communication and interpersonal skills

Assessment is a role that has to be executed responsibly by the practice assessor, and, to do so effectively, certain specific personal and interpersonal skills are essential to enable the student to feel at ease when they are being assessed performing clinical interventions. These skills and techniques form part of effective supervisory relationships, and are some of the most important tools the practitioner undertaking the practice supervisor or assessor role has in their armoury. The healthcare professional should already be a skilled communicator in healthcare settings through their pre-registration education, and therefore it is useful to establish which other communication techniques they need to develop in order to extend their skill base for more effective teaching and assessing.

Various generic modes of communication can be applied by practice supervisors and assessors, including:

- written, e.g. handwritten, printed, emailed, as a text message
- oral (spoken), e.g. face to face, one to one, in groups, by telephone, by video link
- non-verbal, e.g. body posture, eye contact, tone of voice.

Oral (spoken) communication is always accompanied by non-verbal messages, vocal and non-vocal. In fact, non-verbal hues (or cues) are more powerful than verbal messages. Furthermore, Argyle (1994) suggests that non-verbal signals of a friendly attitude (as opposed to an unfriendly one) are:

- proximity: moving closer, leaning forward if seated
- orientation: more direct, but side to side for some situations
- gaze: more gaze for each other, and mutual gaze
- facial expression: more smiling
- gestures: head nods, lively movements
- posture: open arms stretched towards each other rather than arms on hips or folded
- touch: more touch in an appropriate manner
- tone of voice: higher pitch, upward contour, pure tone
- verbal contents: more self-disclosure.

After reflecting on the SOLER (which stands for: 'Sit squarely'; 'Open posture'; 'Lean towards the other'; 'Eye contact'; 'Relax') framework for non-verbal communication, Stickley (2011) suggests that the framework (or model) can be enhanced by using the acronym SURETY (which stands for 'Sit at an angle'; 'Uncross legs and arms'; 'Relax'; 'Eye contact'; 'Touch'; 'Your intuition'). This latter model incorporates the function of touch as a means of non-verbal communication, and intuition. Normal communication processes, however, are often presented as information processing theory in the context of cognitive learning theory, which is discussed in Chapter 2.

═══════ ACTION **POINT** 7.7 ═══════

Interpersonal skills in assessing a student

Make a list of what you consider to be the general communication skills required in all assessment situations, and then a list of the more specific communication skills required by the assessor for conducting assessments effectively.

Several communication skill items emerge when exploring in detail what and how practice assessors communicate with students. Table 7.1 lists many of the essential interpersonal skills required during assessments that were identified by just one group of registrants on a previous mentor course.

Table 7.1 Communication and interpersonal factors related to student assessment

Generic communication skills	Specific interpersonal skills
• Non-verbal communication – e.g. eye contact, facial expression • Body language – posture, body orientation, proximity, attitude, behaviour, space • Being non-judgemental – warmth, empathy, respect • Always remaining calm • Openness • Questioning – open or closed questions • Reflecting • Active listening • Verbal communication – pace, volume, tone, clarity • Diplomacy • Considering environmental factors • Being enthusiastic, interested • Making time, using silence • Constructive comments/advice • Approachable and friendly, non-intimidatory	• Putting the learner at ease • Enabling learner to relax if anxious so that they can perform the skill to their full potential • Building confidence by positive feedback if necessary • Giving clear directions • Continuous feedback • Being non-judgemental by not criticising verbally or non-verbally • Giving prompts/clues if student's mind goes blank • Allowing enough time for the student to perform the care intervention fully, including appropriate documentation • Making time to listen, and to maintain rapport • Preventing observer bias and observer effect • Ascertaining level of understanding of terminologies/jargon • Confidence – in the student/in self • Reinforcing what has been discussed

Dimensions of assessment

There are a number of other essential facets of assessment that we need to consider to gain a more comprehensive picture of how to assess. Hughes and Quinn (2013: 245) and others identify what are generally known as 'dimensions of assessments'. Particularly relevant is whether assessments are:

1.   continuous or episodic
2.   formative or summative
3.   criterion-referenced or norm-referenced
4.   authentic or traditional.

Continuous or episodic assessments

Until the latter half of the 1980s, the assessment of pre-registration students used to take place at predetermined points during their course. The student on the general nursing course was assessed on their ability to administer medications in Year 1 of the course, and to use aseptic techniques when redressing a wound, and organise the total care of an individual or a group of healthcare service users on specific subsequent occasions. They also had to pass written examinations at the end of the course. These were episodic summative assessments, and implicitly progression points on the programme. However, these snapshot assessments were not seen as representing the wide range of skills acquired during placements, nor were they seen as a genuine representation of how students usually deliver care, and they therefore fell into disfavour, and were replaced by continuous assessment involving assessment of practice and theory on numerous occasions throughout the course.

Students have to learn all care intervention skills that are identified in their PAD, and signed as appropriate because they are necessary for them to perform their duties as registered healthcare professionals when they qualify. For current healthcare apprentices and trainee nursing associates, the assessment of competencies is undertaken by continuous assessment as well as a form of episodic assessment referred to as 'end point' assessment (HEE, 2017: 25; IATE, 2022b) (sometimes referred to as 'terminal assessment').

Episodic (or intermittent) assessments therefore involve testing the student at specific times or on particular occasions during an educational programme, such as at the end of a module, placement or year. Continuous assessment aims to increase the quality and quantity of evidence gathered in relation to the achievement of competencies by the student. It involves a continuing awareness by the practice supervisor of the student's level of competence and knowledge, and is thus a cumulative judgement about progress and achievement.

━━━━━━━━━━ **ACTION** POINT 7.8 ━━━━━━━━━━

Advantages and disadvantages of continuous and episodic assessments

Consider what you think might be the advantages and disadvantages of episodic and continuous assessments, and make some notes.

The principal reason for episodic assessments being discredited in nursing and midwifery in the past is that decisions about the student's competence were being made on the basis of one-off performances. These performances, be they excellent or otherwise, might be atypical. Another disadvantage is that several key skills remain untested if they do not present themselves during the identified assessment episode.

Subsequently, current pre-registration programmes include identified 'progression points', by when students will have been assessed and achieved a 'Pass' on several key competencies before progressing to the subsequent stage of their education programme (NMC, 2018d, 2019b). These assessments can also be examples of episodic assessment, and students are required to demonstrate that they are competent in those competencies to be able to register subsequently with the NMC as an RN or RM, or with the HCPC.

Formative or summative assessments

Another dimension of assessment is whether the assessment is formative or summative. Derived from the words 'form' and 'forming', 'formative' relates to the developmental and improvement stages of learning an activity (e.g. a clinical skill). Formative assessment of a professional practice skill is conducted with the aim of promoting learning, so that afterwards the learner can perform the skill safely and effectively, and knows the rationale for every step of the intervention. The student's clinical intervention skills thus develop under conditions in which they reflect-in-action, and, at the same time, think creatively without being too concerned about final pass or fail grades. The student also has the opportunity to take time to learn the skill thoroughly with the support of practice supervisors.

Formative assessments apply to the assessment of practical skills as well as to the required knowledge base and their application (i.e. theory). For the theory component of education programmes, the student thereby obtains feedback on the evidence they are presenting to the academic marker on how far they are demonstrating knowledge of the subject area, its application together with critical analysis, and coherence and general structure and presentation of their script. Formative assessments are therefore instituted to provide feedback to the student on their progress, and their aims are to:

- allow for individual development
- identify strengths and weaknesses
- inform the student of how they are progressing
- maximise learning.

As a concept and an activity, formative assessment has been advocated for decades, but implementation proves erratic even today, which could be due to it being yet another extra requirement to create time for in busy day-to-day professional activities in both the practice setting and HEIs. Thus, it has resource and efficiency implications. It is, however, an educationally sound concept and students tend to be grateful for the feedback that they receive from it.

After providing students with free access to formative web-based quizzes as a form of formative self-assessment, Bijol et al. (2015) found that those who did participate in the quizzes performed much better (statistically significantly better) at final examinations than those who didn't engage with the quizzes. The researchers therefore argue that the formative quizzes promote learning and improve the student experience.

'Summative' relates to a point in time during a unit of learning, for example a practice placement, when the practice assessor makes a decision about whether to declare the learner as competent or otherwise on specified components of learning. Summative assessments are conducted to determine whether the learner is now competent to work without direct supervision and, if so, then this is recorded in their competencies' assessment document.

Summative assessments also constitute a periodic record of the student's achievement of the aims and outcomes of a module or course. The grade awarded for these assessments, along with those for coursework and examinations, contributes to the final classification of the student's university award.

It might prove useful to ask your student, or to look back yourself on any long course that you have been on in recent years, to identify the range of formative assessments related to summative assignments incorporated in the programme. As to assessment in the practice setting, the student learning part-skills (e.g. some of the sub-skills required for administering an intramuscular injection) itself constitutes a formative assessment. The 'professional discussion' at the end of apprenticeship programmes (IATE, 2022c), and dissertations for university degrees are summative assessments.

On healthcare courses, summative assessments are concerned with healthcare service-user safety and standards of practice. They are also concerned with justice for the student and the credibility of the university's awards. They must therefore meet the highest standards of validity (accuracy) and reliability (consistency by assessors) (e.g. IATE, 2022b; NMC, 2022b), which are discussed in some detail later in this chapter.

Criterion-referenced or norm-referenced assessments

The third dimension of assessment we consider is norm referencing and criterion referencing. In norm-referenced assessment, the student's score, marks or grades are determined to an extent by those achieved by other students in a given group or cohort. Programme Assessment Boards (also known as Award Boards) have the discretion to raise or lower the marks required by a particular cohort to achieve a particular grade if unusual circumstances have prevailed. Criterion-referenced assessments are more straightforward in that the score or mark given to a particular student for a particular piece of coursework is decided entirely on the basis of a predetermined set of marking criteria. Students will have been informed of these criteria long before the assessment date.

─Reflection point 7.2─

Norm-referenced or criterion-referenced assessments

Think about some of the assessments that you have mentioned for Action Point 7.1 and decide whether they are norm-referenced or criterion-referenced assessments.

Occasionally, a criterion-referenced assessment can be marked on a norm-referenced basis at the discretion of the appropriate Programme Assessment Board. The approved detailed procedure or clinical guidelines used in healthcare trusts to perform clinical care safely and effectively also constitute criterion-referenced student assessment for the specific clinical intervention.

Authentic assessment or traditional assessment

For some years now, discussions have taken place about the relevance of student assessments at their time in education and the relevance of those assessments and the qualifications gained to the knowledge and skills required for work when the student starts employment after gaining their qualification. Therefore, the value of assessment is judged also by whether they test knowledge and competence that will be required during employment, and if they do, then they are considered to be authentic assessments.

Authentic assessment is applied through assessment components that students have to pass during the course as well as in their final project or dissertation when they are asked to apply their knowledge and understanding to 'real-world contexts'. On comparing authentic versus traditional assessment in the fields of health and of education, whereupon the latter refers to assessments that test knowledge and memorisation, Saher et al. (2022) found that the best models of assessment comprise of a combination of both types or dimensions of assessment, based partly on the qualification the student is aiming for. Student assessment on health profession courses is of necessity often authentic as it tests students' ability to apply their knowledge to real-life healthcare situations, and which they will use on gaining employment.

Assessing different levels of competence

Healthcare profession students tend to be taught and assessed at different academic levels during Year 1, Year 2 and Year 3. The NMC's (2018c) SOP for nurses, for example, are configured at different academic levels in the PADs that students take to practice placements. Healthcare apprentices, nursing associate students, and healthcare support workers studying for diplomas, degrees or national vocational qualifications are also assessed at different levels as learners progress to subsequent years of their preparation programme.

To teach and assess competencies at different levels of learning, a number of current nurse education curricula tend to apply Steinaker and Bell's (1979) model (or taxonomy) of experiential learning. This taxonomy consists of exposure level, participation, identification, internalisation and dissemination. A broad guide to how the experiential taxonomy levels equate with the QAA's (2014) academic levels is:

- Certificate level/academic level 4 – exposure, participation (Year 1)
- Diploma level/academic level 5 – participation, identification and internalisation (Year 2)
- Degree level/academic level 6 – identification, internalisation and dissemination (Year 3).

This is a very simple classification and just a general guide that underpins the specific wording of competencies to reflect the different levels. Alternatively, some programmes use Benner's (2001) stages of skill acquisition model, which was discussed in Chapter 2. Others use Bondy's (1983) five levels of competency that learners can achieve, namely dependent level, marginal, assisted, supervised and independent level, usually in post-registration courses. Alternatively, the skills are acquired at an increasing level of complexity, i.e. more complex clinical intervention skills, in the latter years of the programme.

The assessment of theory at different levels in healthcare professions, however, is usually based on Bloom's (1956) taxonomy of cognitive learning or Anderson, L.W. et al.'s (2014) taxonomy, which were discussed in Chapter 3. You may wish to look back at the appropriate section to remind yourself of the details of Bloom's model, which comprises knowledge, comprehension, application, analysis, synthesis and evaluation; or of Anderson et al.'s model, which constitutes: remember, understand, apply, analyse, evaluate and create. In all taxonomies, the first points – that is, exposure, knowledge and remember – represent lower-level learning and the last points represent the higher levels.

Fairness of assessments

Because in practice assessments, we are measuring the performance of the individual student on particular patient-related competencies, wouldn't you agree that assessments have to be as objective as possible and must be fair and unbiased for every student? The NMC (2018d: 11 and clause 5.8), the QAA (2018: 4), the HCPC (2017: 9) and the IATE (2022c: 7) all state that assessments must be objective, fair, reliable and valid to enable students to demonstrate that they have achieved the proficiencies for their programme. So, what does fairness of assessment mean?

━━━━━━━━━ ACTION **POINT 7.9** ━━━━━━━━━

Barriers to 'fairness'

Think about your own experiences of assessment (either assessing or being assessed) and consider instances where students' practice assessments might, or could, have been deemed 'unfair', and how we could have ensured that they were 'fair'. Identify all factors that you feel can interfere with the fairness of the assessment, using the three headings: (a) student factors; (b) assessor factors (practice supervisor or assessor); and (c) environmental (the practice setting) factors. If you can't remember being assessed, then make some notes of your own ideas of aspects that we should be aware of during an assessment to ensure that it is being conducted fairly.

It is conceivable that, on occasion, the demands being made on a student during assessment or the questions being asked may seem beyond the boundaries of what would generally be expected. Fairness of assessment refers to being aware of external or internal circumstances that could adversely affect the student's performance of the clinical skill. There are several factors that could hamper the fairness of assessments. An unfair assessment could also mean that it might not be a valid assessment. Student factors that can make an assessment unfair include:

- expecting an unjustifiably higher level of knowledge
- not enough opportunities to practise the competencies
- last-minute delays or changes
- undeclared physical illness or fatigue
- a theory–practice disjunction/gap.

You should be able to think of other student factors, including personal circumstances. Assessor factors include practice supervisors' motivation to supervise learning, having a bias towards or against the student, not having had adequate educational preparation to become a practice assessor, having an overpowering attitude and a lack of knowledge of the student's course. Some of the factors in the clinical environment that might unfairly affect assessments are interruptions, a lack of resources in the practice setting (e.g. equipment), the suitability of placement and low staffing levels.

Assessment criteria and pass or fail decisions

Following a fairly conducted episodic assessment, for example, the practice assessor has to decide whether it's a pass or a fail for the student for the particular competency.

This decision may well depend entirely on whether the student closely followed the Trust's approved procedure to perform the clinical skill, or the written (or unwritten) protocol. The items in the procedure are the actual 'assessment criteria'.

The term *assessment criteria* refers to the predetermined set of components that are used for deciding whether the learner performed the clinical intervention competently. They can therefore constitute a checklist of the step-by-step actions that should be taken by the learner when performing the care intervention. These step-by-step actions are normally the Trust's approved procedure or clinical guidelines for that intervention and are set down in two columns as 'actions' and 'rationales', and are usually supported by references to make them evidence-informed. They are normally kept in the practice setting's 'Policies and Procedures' section for use and for reference purposes. There is likely to be a separate folder for clinical guidelines or protocols that refer to more specialist or advanced care interventions.

─Reflection point 7.3─

What am I looking for during student assessment?

Consider two examples of assessment of competence that you have been involved in. This could be a pre-registration or a post-registration course competency:

- How did the practice assessor determine what criteria to use to decide on a pass or a fail for the learner?
- What influenced them to choose these particular criteria?
- Furthermore, for student paramedic assessment related to invasive interventions, for example, why do you think more invasive procedures are more likely to be carried out in a simulated environment rather than on an actual patient? What do you think are the ethical implications? What do you think are the moral implications?

In response to the above reflection point, you may have thought that anyone who hasn't yet demonstrated and proved their competence at an invasive procedure, should not perform the procedure on an actual service user as they can potentially, maybe unknowingly, harm the service user, i.e. it is unethical, and also in breach of the HCPC (2016) Standards of Conduct, Performance and Ethics.

So, the student paramedic will be assessed through a mixture of assessment episodes and instances, to ensure not only competency but also consistency, for example on one or multiple occasions. As for the pass/fail assessment criteria, there are generic ambulance service 'clinical practice guidelines' in the UK published by the Joint Royal Colleges Ambulance Liaison Committee (JRCALC) & the Association of Ambulance Chief Executives (2021). The aim of these guidelines is to ensure effective clinical risk management and 'uniformity in the delivery of high quality patient care' (p. 1), and therefore they also underpin the pre-registration paramedic programme. However, different ambulance services and organisations may still have different guidelines, drug protocols for different treatment and care pathways, which is because paramedic teams in the UK work within the scope of practice specified by their employer.

Conversely, it is noteworthy that for nursing the PAD is widely standardised, such as the cross-London PAD, which essentially means that the translation of NMC's SOP for nurses is identically implemented by all London healthcare settings where students have practice placements (e.g. Baillie and Fish, 2021). Additionally, for the majority of healthcare professions, there are clinical guidelines published by other UK authoritative organisations such as the National Institute for Health and Care Excellence ('NICE'), Resuscitation Council UK, and so on, which are also relevant to paramedic practice.

─Reflection point 7.4─

Protocols/guidelines for paramedic interventions

Why do you think there are differences in scope of practice between different ambulance organisations? What could be the advantages of all paramedics working to exactly the same protocol, and what could be the disadvantages?

As noted earlier in this chapter, paramedicine is a relatively new health profession, and good practice for various service-user interventions is still emerging. However, you are likely to agree that concerted effort must be made to establish communication between different paramedic services as this can create a medium for identifying more effective practices, and therefore benchmarking good practice.

The significance of having specified assessment criteria is also recognised by Helminen et al. (2017), for example, who indicate that it ensures a good quality process in practice assessments. However, for those healthcare activities for which there is no identified step-by-step approved procedure, the performance criteria can be established by asking the skilled practitioner to describe to someone in detail everything that they would do to perform the intervention competently. For instance, there might not be a procedure for assessing communication skills, for bed-making, for taking body temperature using tympanic thermometers or, say, for doing patient handovers. A set of performance criteria for patient handovers (or 'reporting on patients' progress') using the increasingly widely utilised SBAR (situation – background – assessment – recommendation) framework or technique (e.g. Stewart and Hand, 2017), is presented in Table 7.2.

Table 7.2   Performance criteria for patient handovers using SBAR

Assessment Criteria for Assessing Competency – Patient Handovers	Possible SBAR component
• Have the right documentation, e.g. care plan/pathway, to refer to	Situation
• Have a good understanding of the patient's/service user's health conditions	Assessment
• Observe confidentiality, especially for bedside handovers	Background
• State the interventions that have been performed, e.g. removal of drains, sutures	Background
• Keep the information concise and focused	Situation
• Use appropriate English and technical words	Assessment
• Pitch the amount of information imparted to the level of knowledge the handover recipients already have, e.g. more detailed information may need to be imparted if new staff or if students are present	Assessment
• Ensure that information that must be given, is given	Assessment
• Inform about individual service user's overall progress	Assessment
• Note any relevant communication from the service user's family or from members of the multidisciplinary team	Background
• State any investigation results received, and any subsequent action required	Recommendation
• State any changes in medication, and service user's reaction to them	Background / Recommendation
• State the plan of care for the rest of the day	Recommendation
• Include service user's awareness of own condition, e.g. in mental health	Situation

Thus, the assessment criteria for deciding on a pass or fail for a student on their ability to do patient handovers can be quite involved, despite those listed in the box being generic, and will need to be more specific, depending on where and when the handover is taking place. A more detailed analysis of handover can be found in Ballantyne's (2017) article, for example (full details of which can be found in the References section of this book).

For competencies for which there are no written assessment criteria in the practice setting as procedures or clinical guidelines, they might be found in, for instance, *The Royal Marsden Manual of Clinical Nursing Procedures* (Lister et al., 2021). They might also be available from NICE, the World Health Organisation, the Scottish Intercollegiate Guidelines Network and other reputable authoritative organisations via their websites.

Students' record of achievement

From one of its periodic reviews of pre-registration education curricula some years ago, it emerged that supervisors of practice-based learning and assessors of practice competencies would benefit from having access to their students' progress documentation of preceding practice placements as evidence of skills that they are already deemed competent in, prior to establishing the student's learning requirements and needs in their current placement.

This mechanism was implemented as an 'ongoing achievement record' (OAR), and is currently either incorporated in PAD, or used in conjunction with the PAD, or as MORA (explained earlier in this chapter and in Chapter 6) instead of PAD. With the information in OAR, a 'diagnostic assessment' of competencies is made at the initial meeting with the student at the beginning of the placement so as to establish the student's specific learning needs and objectives.

The student's learning needs are therefore established through a review of requirements in the OAR document, the student's practice competencies' document, any other relevant skill achievement document, and from certificates of attendance from additional study days/workshops already attended by the student. The practice competencies document tends to have a section where supported learning time is also recorded (see Template 7.1 for an example of this).

Accurate recording of supported learning time with the student has several advantages. When evidence of this NMC requirement is asked for, then the record will be proof of this provision. Recording supported learning time is also likely to act as a trigger to ensure that this contact time happens, which can also mean increased support for the student to achieve the necessary competencies. The contact must however be recorded straightaway, and not retrospectively.

Template 7.1   Recording supported learning time for supervision and practice placement

Week 1	Notes on learning during this week:	
	Signature of student:	Date:
	Signature of practice supervisor:	Date:
Week 2	Notes on learning during this week:	
	Signature of student:	Date:
	Signature of practice supervisor:	Date:
Week 3	etc. ...	

The reasons for the assessment of competence and ensuring proficiency during the final practice placement include ensuring competent, safe and effective practice, and must achieve the validity and reliability requirements of assessments, as well as fairness of assessments. Final documentation needs to be carried out by a practice assessor and the academic assessor who are on the same part or sub-part of the NMC's professional register as that which the student is aiming to enter.

Finally, the pre-registration student is assessed by the practice assessor and academic assessor whose roles essentially are to ascertain and vouch that the student has achieved all practice competencies and the NMC's (2018c) SOP, which they do by a combination of means, and sign and date the appropriate pages of relevant documents, or not. When all evidence has become available to indicate that the student has successfully completed all theory and practice requirements, then the HEI informs the NMC accordingly, leading to the student applying to have their name entered on the NMC register as an RN.

So, for assessment of practice, students' PADs clearly identify the specific requirements and the procedure for assessment of competencies. Case Study 7.1 is of a student for whom an action plan had to be constituted after the mid-placement review.

Case study 7.1

A successful action plan

Kayleigh is a 33-year-old third-year mental health student nurse who is a new mother, and whose return from maternity leave was delayed for medical reasons. On her return, she had two theory modules and the final practice module to pass in order to complete her pre-registration programme. For the practice module, Kayleigh was placed for 12 weeks at a 9-5 day services centre for adults with mental health problems and who have been referred to secondary mental health services for further therapy and rehabilitation.

Although an initial interview with the practice supervisor and practice assessor took place in the first week, and the required supported learning time was utilised to monitor progress with practice competencies, Kayleigh struggled to re-engage after the break from the course, and in subsequent weeks found it difficult to achieve the agreed competencies and was unable to express why this was so to her practice supervisor. Both practice supervisor and the day services manager were very accommodating and supportive. The student failed various objectives at the mid-placement review and an action plan was compiled in the presence of the student, practice assessor, academic link and day services nurse manager. The competencies that were identified in the action plan, which were related mainly to 'interpersonal skills', included:

- Be consistently on time for shifts and planned activities, and thereby demonstrate reliability, punctuality and good time management.
- Take responsibility for meeting professional codes of practice and organisational policies while prioritising the care of service users, and work with team members to promote health with high standards of practice, while acting with integrity.
- Take responsibilities that are appropriate for Year 3 students by demonstrating the ability to take the lead in reviews, admissions and group work.

The student felt disappointed but had anticipated being given fails during the mid-placement review and needing an action plan. The support that would enable Kayleigh to achieve the action plan objectives was identified as named practice supervisors and the manager; and resources included the NMC's guidelines and codes of practice, as well as the Trust's policies and procedures. The PEF would regularly contact the practice supervisor to check on progress and offer any further help and advice required, and made himself available during the subsequent weeks for further support.

The student composed herself and, with the above-mentioned support during subsequent weeks, put the required time and effort in, and went on to achieve the competencies in the action plan and the remainder of her practice competencies, and subsequently passed the practice placement.

If Kayleigh had not managed to achieve any of the objectives in the action plan, then she would have failed the practice module. However, students are usually allowed a second attempt at any fail component, which in this case could constitute extending the placement by four to six weeks or changing to another placement for a similar period of time.

Protected learning time, however, for supervisor and student to work together, has often proved difficult to achieve in a number of very busy practice settings, or during particularly busy periods, as was also found in research conducted by Hutchison and Cochrane (2014), for example. Moreover, if a student is awarded a fail on this final placement, then this can raise questions about the quality of practice supervision and assessment of the competence that the student has experienced over the preceding two-and-a-half years of their education programme. To resolve the 'challenges' of time, workload, responsibility related to the role and practicalities of the assessment of competence, more concerted proactive forward planning of the work roster is required to ensure that students and their supervisors and assessors work together on the same span of duty.

Assessing care support workers and other learners

Registrants periodically get allocated students for practice placement who are on other health or social care profession programmes than the one they are themselves qualified in. This is of course fully acceptable, especially in the current ethos of inter-professional learning, and endeavours towards a health and social care seamless service. This is also so that the underlying principles of supervising learning comprise core healthcare knowledge and skills that apply to all registerable professions. However, logically registrants might be required to undertake further information sessions or to attend relevant workshops, in particular to comprehend the technicalities of their role towards learners from other specific healthcare professions.

To assess support workers' competence on NVQ courses, for example, they would need to have successfully completed the Certificate in Assessing Vocational

Achievement (CAVA) programme (which replaced the A1/2 and D32/33 assessor qualifications) (CTC Training, 2022). If the nurse is facilitating practice learning for a medical student, then they have to acquaint themselves with the competencies that the medical student has to achieve by the end of the placement.

Validity and Reliability of Assessments

Having considered the principles of assessment that assessors need to adhere to for assessing students' clinical intervention skills correctly, the assessor has to pause before deciding on a pass or fail for the student, and to consider the validity and reliability as well as the discrimination and practicability (or usability) attributes of assessments. These four attributes are absolutely crucial in all assessments of competencies.

Validity

'Validity' is the most crucial aspect of an assessment in that it refers to the extent to which the assessment measured what it is aimed to measure. For an assessment to be valid, the assessor must have focused on the component that the assessment aimed to assess, and to have done so accurately. It should have assessed the competency or learning outcome(s) that it set out to assess and did not digress into formal assessment of other competencies that had not been agreed with the student beforehand. The five main types of validity, which are also recognised by Hughes and Quinn (2013), are: content validity, predictive validity, concurrent validity, construct validity and face validity, some of which apply more to the overall curriculum and assessment of theory, and not necessarily to the assessment of competencies in practice settings.

Content validity

'Content validity' refers to the extent to which the assessment adequately covers the content of the whole curriculum. Therefore, the assessment questions and assignment guidelines have to assess all the learning outcomes of the module, or of the whole course, as initially intended. Note that, for various reasons, not everything that the student learns during the course can be assessed. How far assessments address content validity depends primarily on the structure of the assessment components of the module or course, and is generally monitored by the course director or the programme manager for the course.

Predictive validity

The extent to which the result of assessments can predict the future performance of the student is referred to as 'predictive validity'. It is important for the assessor to determine if the student's performance during, say, a particular practical assessment, can predict how far they will perform to the same standard in future situations, and also whether the student can adjust the performance to different practice settings, for example from a ward setting to community care and to service users of different age groups (within the field of practice).

Concurrent validity

The extent to which the assessment results correlate with those of other assessments administered at the same time is referred to as 'concurrent validity'. In other words, if two different assessments are designed to measure the same learning outcomes, then the student should do equally well in both, for example asking a student to talk through how they would perform a skill, and actually to demonstrate it.

Construct validity

Validity that refers to the extent to which the results of the assessment are related to impressions or evidence gained from observations of the individual's behaviour with regard to their attitudes, values and developing character (which are also known as 'psychological constructs'), is referred to as 'construct validity'.

Face validity

'Face validity' involves stopping to consider the overall impression of how competently the clinical skill was performed, and whether the student actually demonstrated the complex array of observational, analytical, interpersonal and technical skills required for the competency.

—Reflection point 7.5—

Types of validity

A first-year student is being assessed on a surgical ward changing a patient's dressing using aseptic technique. The purpose of this particular episode of assessment is specifically to do with changing a dressing using aseptic technique skills. However, during the procedure, the patient makes some statements that clearly reflect marked disorientation, and the student is unable to respond therapeutically to disorientation. The aseptic technique is performed correctly. Should the assessor pass or fail the student? Which result is the 'valid' result?

Reliability

According to the QAA (2018: 2), 'Assessment ensures that qualifications are awarded only to those students who meet specified learning outcomes'. Furthermore, the QAA (2018: 4), the NMC (2018d), the HCPC (2017) and the IATE (2022c) all state that student achievement of learning outcomes must be measured accurately, transparently and reliably. Therefore, in addition to validity, another essential consideration of any assessment is its 'reliability', which is a term that is used to indicate the consistency with which an assessment measures the areas that it is designed to measure. This means that if the assessment is conducted again, the same level of performance should produce the same result, provided other variables remain similar.

To take this a step further, reliability has to do with consistency in the grade or result awarded for a particular piece of work:

- between different assessors
- between different occasions on which the work is done
- between different methods of assessment.

In all cases, the result or grade awarded should be almost, or preferably exactly, the same for the assessment to be deemed 'reliable'. Consistency in the assessment of student competencies in this way is referred to as inter-assessor reliability and is discussed in detail in Chapter 8.

Reflection point 7.6

Reliability of assessments

Think about any assessments that you or your colleagues have been involved in recently. Then spend a few minutes thinking about how reliable the assessment was. Decide why you think that the assessment was or was not reliable.

Generally, there are certain factors that might negatively affect reliability being achieved. These are practical issues, such as:

- individual biases
- the halo effect
- insufficient time being allocated for the assessment
- the ambiguity of questions being asked
- competence as an assessor
- whether more than one assessor was involved, as two assessors could mean more objectivity
- whether the assessment criteria had been agreed.

Discrimination

Discrimination in assessment refers to the ability of assessment to differentiate between the different levels of competence demonstrated by students, such as Year 1, Year 2 or Year 3 students. Steinaker and Bell's (1979) taxonomy of learning is generally used to differentiate between these levels of competencies. However, by and large, learners should be given the opportunity to demonstrate their true level of ability, regardless of the level that they are expected to reach at the particular stage of the course.

Discrimination also refers to the distinction between all learners. A healthcare assistant would be assessed against certain adjusted criteria for a particular care intervention from a medical student or from a student nurse, for instance, mainly because the level of theoretical knowledge expected of each is different.

Practicability (or usability)

The concept 'practicability' refers to whether the assessment can be conducted within the time, and with the resources, available. Practice assessors might encounter problems of practicability of assessment when practice placements are too short, or when, for some reason, the episodic assessments have been left until the last few days of the placement. However, despite effective assessments being complex and challenging, the validity and reliability attributes of assessments remain the benchmark of rigour in the assessment of healthcare competencies (e.g. Moniz et al., 2015).

Strategies for assessments

As for all their courses, each university identifies clearly in their healthcare course documents exactly which assessments students have to pass to be awarded the intended qualification on successful completion of the course. The assessments to be conducted in practice settings are documented in the practice assessment document (PAD), and for assessment of theory, assessment requirements are supported by the detailed assessment guidelines specified in module and course documents.

The course curriculum and specific assessment requirements, including the assessment of practice competencies, will have been planned well before students start on the course. These requirements will be under the scrutiny of the university's quality assurance guidelines and protocols for designing courses and modules, which will have gone through a rigorous approval process before being offered to students. They would have then been approved by an assembled panel of experts, which usually includes representations from the NMC, and/or the HCPC, other relevant authorities and subject specialists from other universities.

During the planning stages, the modules will have been fully discussed by the course or module curriculum planning teams. There are specific assessment strategies within each course and module. The pass marks for assessments may vary by a few points between different universities, as may the weightings between practical and theoretical assessments, or different assessment components. The number of assessments may vary, as may the number of formative assessments related to the summative ones. Students taking the course or module are assessed on their achievement of its learning outcomes and/or competencies.

Overall monitoring of module or course assessments are conducted by designated university committees and Boards, which do so by following the university's protocols and rules. Finally, each student's assessment results are scrutinised and ratified by the Examinations Board or Assessment Board.

To assess students' competence during practice placements, various assessment strategies are advocated, such as direct observation of skill performance, unobtrusive observation of the learner's behaviour and interaction with the service user they are caring for, writing reflective accounts and questions and answers. It is usually up to the practice assessor to decide which NMC competency area can be assessed by each strategy. For example, direct observation can be utilised for assessing care intervention, attitude, communication skill; and questions and answers for the rationale for each action taken, knowledge of the reasons (or indication) for specific medications and possible side-effects.

Variety in modes of assessment is also recommended by the QAA (2018: 5) and by Skills for Health (2022) for the achievement of care certificate standards, which should also achieve inclusivity and equitability of assessments, because thereby students with different cultural or educational backgrounds, and those with additional learning needs, can demonstrate their knowledge and competence through different assessment methods. For the assessment of theory components, students have to demonstrate critical analyses and the application of key concepts through their coursework, seminar presentations, projects, written examinations, and so forth. It is, however, well known that some assessment methods, for example written examinations, enable some students to demonstrate their capabilities more effectively, while other methods suit other students better.

Additionally, the NMC (2018d), under 'Student empowerment', indicates that students should be assessed utilising a range of different assessment methods. Furthermore, on exploring the feasibility and outcome of allowing students a choice of assessment methods, Garside et al. (2009) found that this is achievable, as some students chose to be assessed by seminar discussions, others by poster presentations, and others by essays, to good effect.

In addition to the principles and essential attributes of assessments explored throughout this chapter, especially under discussions of how assessments are conducted, the QAA (2018) identifies a number of generic broader principles of assessment that HEIs should follow. They include the following:

- assessment methods and criteria are aligned to learning outcomes and teaching activities
- assessment is reliable, consistent, fair and valid
- assessment design is approached holistically (with a variety of assessment methods used, as appropriate)
- assessment is explicit and transparent
- assessment and feedback are purposeful and support the learning process
- assessment is timely
- students are supported and prepared for assessment
- assessment is efficient and manageable.

Another set of principles of assessment, which incidentally overlap with those published by the QAA, has been published by the Joint Information Systems Committee (JISC) (2022), details of which are given in the Further Optional Reading section.

Chapter Summary

This chapter has focused on the assessment of learners' clinical knowledge and competencies, taking the approach of what assessments are, why we conduct them, who assesses, when and how, which encompassed:

- What the term 'assessment' means in the context of assessing professional knowledge and competence. This involved considering various definitions of assessment, and the exact competencies to be assessed.
- Why we need to assess our students and learners, that is, the exact purposes and aims of assessment, and at which particular points in students' programmes of study to assess them.
- Who assesses learners, including practice supervisors, student self-assessment and peer assessment, and service-user involvement in the assessment of competencies.
- How assessments are conducted, which includes ensuring that the learner has learned the clinical skill, the use of essential interpersonal skills, and the dimensions of assessment, namely continuous or episodic assessment, formative or summative, criterion-referenced or norm-referenced, and authentic or traditional assessment.
- Assessing different levels of competence, fairness of assessment and the use of performance criteria.
- Validity, reliability, discrimination and practicability as essential attributes of assessment; and the role of approved assessment policies, procedures and strategies.

Further Optional Reading

1. For detailed and well-argued guidelines on the assessment of students on apprenticeship programmes, see:

   • Institute for Apprenticeships & Technical Education (2022) *Developing an End-point Assessment Plan*. Available at: www.instituteforapprenticeships. org/developing-new-apprenticeships/developing-an-end-point-assessment-plan (accessed 5 April 2022).

2. For a recently published set of principles of assessment that HEIs are advised to follow, see:

   • Joint Information Systems Committee (JISC) (2022) *Principles of Good Assessment and Feedback*. Available at: www.jisc.ac.uk/guides/principles-of-good-assessment-and-feedback# (accessed 10 May 2022).

3. For very recent national guidelines and principles of student assessment, see:

   • Quality Assurance Agency for Higher Education (2018) *Assessment (UK Quality Code for Higher Education – Advice and Guidance)*. Available at: www.qaa.ac.uk/quality-code/advice-and-guidance/assessment# (accessed 9 April 2022).

8

MANAGING STUDENT ASSESSMENT, ASSOCIATED CHALLENGES AND ACCOUNTABILITY

Introduction

Having explored the nature and different facets of student assessment, as well as the principles of assessment, in Chapter 7, along with the validity and reliability of assessment as its essential attributes, this chapter focuses on the importance of careful planning and management of student assessment, on ways of managing the likely problematic areas related to the assessment of health and social care students, and on the assessor's accountability.

—Chapter objectives—

1. Explain specific ways in which forward planning and prioritising work are important components of the management of student assessments.
2. Identify the likely challenges or problems of assessment of student competencies, and the ways in which assessors avert or resolve them.
3. Present an analysis of the responsibilities and accountability of practice assessors in the assessment of practice competencies, along with related ethical and legal aspects of student assessment.
4. Cite the various ways in which practice assessors achieve and monitor intra- and inter-assessor reliability in the decisions that they make in relation to the assessments they conduct.
5. Establish the practice supervisor's role in supporting the struggling or underachieving student, and ways of harnessing the various lines of support that are available to them, including resources and guidelines.

Managing Student Assessment

Practice assessors have a professional duty to comply with the underlying principles of assessment (e.g. QAA, 2018) identified in Chapter 7 of this book. Forward planning of assessments also reflects the practice assessor's leadership in terms of prioritising their duties and supporting students. Forward planning involves identifying exactly which competencies the assessor will assess the student on, and on which dates, this being conditional on the appropriate service user being in the clinical setting and giving their consent to student assessment. Then, the day before the assessment, the assessor might contact the student to check that they are happy for the assessment to proceed on the following day.

The nominated practice assessor normally introduces themselves to students who they will assess very early on in the placement, preferably during the first week of placement soon after the student has had a structured orientation to the placement setting. The practice assessor and the student agree on a relatively firm plan for ways in which the student's practice competencies will be assessed, and these are documented on the appropriate pages of the PAD. The plan includes practice supervisors facilitating the student's learning, episodes of assessment carried out by the practice assessor via direct observation, a mid-placement review, and a summative final review of the achievement of competencies in the last week of the placement.

If the student is deemed to be underachieving, that is, not making substantial progress with the achievement of competencies, then at the mid-placement review (if not before), an action plan has to be constituted, and all associated parties informed, such as the PEF and academic assessor. Then, at the end of the placement and the final review or interview, the practice assessor has to inform the student of their levels of achievement, and of a decision to award the student a pass or a fail for those assessment components. It is in relation to the assessment of competence that the challenges of practice placements tend to surface.

Assessment of competencies, at times, involves one-off short episodes of direct observation of the learner performing clinical interventions, but mostly it is a continual process occurring throughout the practice placement. One danger associated with this is that if interruptions do occur during episodes of assessment, then the assessor could miss vital steps in the performance of the care intervention, incorrect or unsafe practice can also be missed, and a pass decision (or fail) could be made, wrongly, with incomplete information. Consequently, it is of paramount importance that all avoidable interruptions are managed during student assessments.

Managing the process of assessment in the practice setting

━━━━━━━━━ ACTION **POINT** 8.1 ━━━━━━━━━

Planning and managing the process of assessment of practice

This activity asks you to explore in detail how to manage an episode of assessment of students' practice competencies or clinical skills by direct observation. To do this, focus on the specified outcomes or competencies of a specific practice module of the pre-registration course for your healthcare profession, or the NMC's (2018c) competencies for, say, second-year students in your field of nursing, or the outcomes of a post-registration healthcare course. Practice competencies are normally found in the student's practice competencies or practice assessment document (PAD).

You might choose to work on this activity with a colleague or course peer who is in a similar specialism as you. Identify in detail everything that needs to be done, from arrangement to completion of the assessment of these competencies by direct observation, from the time that the student starts on the practice placement to when the student is signed off as competent for the particular competencies. Include everything, such as how you would ensure that the skills have been learnt, as well as the organisational aspects that have to be considered to ensure the assessment proceeds as planned.

From your response to Action Point 8.1, you would have verbalised the various preparations needed to ensure that the assessment of competencies is completed effectively and efficiently. Maybe the practice supervisors can compile a teaching and assessment schedule that identifies which competencies will have been learnt by the student by the end of week two and week three for example, and at which points the practice assessor will ascertain and acknowledge the achievement of those competencies. The learning and assessment schedule of course needs to be flexible enough to allow for opportunistic or incidental learning, otherwise it needs to be adhered to as planned, and can form part of a 'learning agreement' (as noted in Chapter 2) and an assessment plan.

For all assessments, there are usually certain curriculum regulations that need to be adhered to, such as submission dates for practice competencies' documents for post-registration students and the procedure to follow if the student fails a competency. A number of key points specifically related to managing practical assessments using the 'direct observation' method, are identified in the box below. They relate to any of the specific standards of proficiency under the seven 'platforms' in the NMC's (2018c: 14–15) document, two examples of which under platform 3 are:

> 3.5: demonstrate the ability to accurately process all information gathered during the assessment process to identify needs for individualised nursing care and develop person-centred evidence-based plans for nursing interventions with agreed goals.

> 3.12: interpret results from routine investigations, taking prompt action when required by implementing appropriate interventions, requesting additional investigations or escalating to others.

Table 8.1 Planning and managing assessment of an episode of care

Prior to the assessment (practice supervisor and assessor input)	• Student and assessor agree, during week 1 of placement, the objectives/competencies that need to be achieved and assessed.
	• Ensure that the learner has learnt the skill, designated practice supervisors facilitate learning of those clinical interventions in accordance with approved procedures or clinical guidelines. The skill is taught at the appropriate academic level. The learner is given sufficient practice opportunities and has been formatively assessed during the placement.
	• Agree assessment criteria.
	• Practice assessor feels: (a) up to date with interventions being assessed; (b) competent to assess/has attended practice assessor updates; (c) takes a supportive and positive approach.
	• On day of assessment – ensure that the student is aware of the time of the assessment, and feels ready for the assessment.
	• Consider 'practicability' and fairness of assessment issues.
	• Obtain consent of patient/service user involved.
	• Practice assessor checks with ward / shift manager if it is ok to proceed with the assessment; and of any change on the patient's circumstances that they should be aware of
	• Ensure student has PAD available for recording result of the assessment
	• Check student is punctual, and appropriately dressed
	• Colleagues are aware if and when they can interrupt (if necessary), assessor gives bleep/pager to another person.

During the assessment, assessor	• Uses appropriate communication skills (see Table 7.1 titled 'Communication and interpersonal factors related to assessments').
	• Creates a climate that enables the student to relax so that they can perform the clinical intervention correctly.
	• Indicates to the student to start the clinical intervention(s) when ready.
	• Safety issues – if the learner is about to make a mistake, or does so, consider the seriousness of the mistake, and intervene, ask questions about next step, or provide prompt/clues, as appropriate.
	• Responsive assessment – taking into account the patient's changing healthcare needs.
	• Situated assessments, i.e. in the context of available resources and circumstances in the setting.
	• Considers predictive validity of assessments, i.e. whether the learner can perform as well in future and in other patient care situations.
After the assessment	• Need to exercise professional judgement throughout.
	• Check that student has correctly documented the intervention in the service user's care pathway/plan.
	• Decide on whether to award a pass or fail for the competency assessed.
	• Give feedback according to established good practice (discussed shortly).
	• Ensure documentation is completed – for care interventions performed, student competency and of feedback given.
	• If the result is a fail, then the assessor needs to follow the university's procedure for subsequent actions to take, which normally includes informing the PEF, academic assessor, and others as per local protocol such as the personal tutor.

For examples of specific student competencies related to allied health professions, and to midwifery, see Chapters 2 and 6 of this book. Each component mentioned in Table 8.1 is important. In relation to helping an anxious student relax before and during the time they are assessed on a clinical skill, in their study of midwifery students' experiences of objective structured clinical examinations by Kirwan et al. (2022), it emerged that during the assessment phase of OSCEs, students felt 'high levels of nervousness, anxiety, and stress'. The researchers conclude that assessors should manage the various 'controllable factors' that can impact on students' performance during assessment, such as learning the skill in good time in preparation for the assessment, practising with peers, how much the assessor put the student at ease during the assessment, and the noise in the room due to other students being assessed at the same time.

Going beyond Kirwan et al.'s (2022) research, there is another mechanism that is increasingly being instituted for all student assessments, which is known as 'assessment literacy'. Assessment literacy entails incorporating support sessions to enable students to understand how academics judge and decide on a grade or mark for each student's assignment. For the assessment of factual knowledge such as medication calculation, the answers are predetermined, and there is usually only one correct answer, to which the more the student orientates themselves through learning and practice, the more likely they are to give the correct answers. For higher levels of learning, as identified by Anderson, L.W. et al. (2014) and others (see Chapter 2 for details), such as application, analysis and synthesis, students can be shown exemplars of high-achieving submissions; and students can also be helped to gain insight into interpreting the marking criteria by which markers decide on the marks they give.

Assessing students' attitude, values and interpersonal behaviour and skills (the affective domain of learning)

As noted in Chapter 2, each healthcare profession competency consists of three domains of learning, namely (1) a comprehensive knowledge of the competency (cognitive domain), (2) the capability to perform the care intervention safely and effectively (psychomotor domain), and (3) reflecting the appropriate attitude towards the performance and the recipient of the intervention.

The earliest advocate of these domains was Bloom (1956), and later Anderson, L.W. et al. (2014), for example. These domains of learning are very widely applied in several professional learning programmes, be they training programme or educational. The knowledge base and the psychomotor skill components have been discussed already in Chapters 2, 3 and 6 of this book. As for the affective domain, this is also assessed by continuous assessment during care interventions.

The affective component of a clinical intervention refers to the performer's (learner's) attitude and behaviour towards the service user, the service user's health problem, and the intervention itself. It refers to the learner's values, the demonstration of respect, and general behaviour towards service users and the specific patients' conditions, for example. Healthcare professionals' values tend to refer to the individual's acceptance of the service user, truthfulness, equality, dignity, care, compassion, self-discipline, for example, and are closely linked to the profession's code of practice and ethics.

Case Study 8.1, which relates an instance of underachievement in the affective domain by a second-year ODP student, illustrates this, and is also a situation that creates extra demands on practice supervisors' and the practice assessor's time.

─Case study 8.1─

An underachieving second-year operating department practitioner student

Jade is a second-year student on an Operating Department Practitioner programme, undertaking a 12-week placement block in the Day Surgery Unit of a large teaching hospital. She had an uneventful first year of training. However, during the Day Surgery placement, she was involved in an incident alleging her use of unprofessional communication with a senior surgical colleague, and a complaint was made that was immediately dealt with by that Trust's theatre manager. The Unit's link lecturer was also informed.

Five weeks into Jade's placement in the Day Surgery Unit, a placement visit was undertaken by the link lecturer. The lecturer was asked to speak to one of Jade's practice assessors, who discussed the student's progress in detail. The assessor outlined concerns for Jade, noting that her understanding of the role of the operating department practitioner was poor and she had a limited base of knowledge on which to develop from, despite being a second-year student. Jade was not able to meet the criteria for clinical competencies due to this lack of knowledge, and the assessor had grave concerns about her progress, despite her working consistently with different practice supervisors.

Allied to this were further concerns about Jade's professionalism, as concerns were raised that she was overly familiar with senior colleagues, using first names instead of professional titles, made ill-timed jokes at vital times during surgical procedures, and discussed personal matters with patients. Senior clinical staff stated that Jade was unfocused and unaware of the potential problems her behaviour would cause.

Given the nature of both her unprofessional interactions and lack of knowledge related to the role, the link lecturer and assessor felt it necessary to address the issues and had a formal meeting with Jade.

After discussion, it was found that Jade's situation was neither acceptable nor beneficial to her progression and an action plan was drawn up. The action plan incorporated the agreed learning outcomes and included behaviour observations to aid Jade's development, which included those in the action plan in Table 8.2.

Jade's action plan also constitutes a template for action plans in general that is widely utilised, and is, at times, laid out in landscape format.

Examples of practice competencies that ODP students can be required to achieve based on the HCPC (2014b) standards for ODPs, include the following:

- Demonstrates the ability to correctly identify the patient on admission to operating departments, checking documentation in accordance with hospital policy.
- Demonstrates the ability to assist the anaesthetist during the induction, maintenance and emergence from general anaesthesia.

Table 8.2 Jade's action plan

ACTION PLAN

Student's name: Jade ....   Placement Area ......

Student's learning needs	Specific objectives to be achieved	Who will help student achieve the objectives and how?	Other resources required	Achieve-by dates	Evidence of achievement of objectives
1. Understanding professionalism	Ability to display professionalism in clinical practice	Practice supervisor, clinical team and theatre manager		13 February 2023	Displays professionalism in individual attitude, communication and interactions
2. Assisting the Anaesthetist	Be able to assist an Anaesthetist in achieving safe endotracheal intubation	Practice supervisors, clinical team, Anaesthetists	Local policies, procedures and clinical guidelines related to patients undergoing general anaesthesia	7 February 2023	Displays the ability to assist an Anaesthetist in the delivery of endotracheal intubation, understanding the underpinning knowledge related to the procedure.

3. .... (etc)

AGREEMENT OF ACTION PLAN

Practice supervisor's signature: ....   Date: 9 January 2023

Student's signature: ....   Date: ....

Practice assessor's signature: ....   Date: ....

ACHIEVEMENT OF OBJECTIVES

Practice assessor's signature: .... Date: ....

The competencies constitute learning healthcare activities in all three domains of learning. Examples of SOP (HCPC, 2014b) for ODPs from which practice competencies are translated and which ODP students need to achieve by the end of their pre-registration programme, are noted in the box below.

Examples of Standards of Proficiency for ODP Students

14.2 be able to conduct appropriate diagnostic or monitoring procedures, treatment, therapy, or other actions safely and effectively

14.5 be able to undertake appropriate anaesthetic, surgical and post-anaesthesia care interventions, including managing the service user's airway, respiration and circulation

14.9 be able to assess and monitor the service user's pain status and as appropriate administer prescribed pain relief in accordance with national and local guidelines.

In view of Case Study 8.1, about an underachieving ODP student, it is of course necessary for practice supervisors (or practice educators) to be up to date with the actions that they are required to take and those that are recommended for such situations. Accordingly, the HCPC (2017: 8) states, 'Practice educators must undertake regular training which is appropriate to their role, learners' needs and the delivery of the learning outcomes'.

Returning to a person's values, these also include sincerity, respect, the individual's freedom to make their own decisions, and morality. Attitudes, on the other hand, are influenced by the person's positive and negative feelings about certain things, or certain behaviours. For example, if a service user is admitted to hospital with Type 2 diabetes, and is also severely obese, the healthcare professional's values and attitude might be that people in general must maintain a healthy body weight. Towards those who don't, the healthcare professional might harbour negative feelings that may surface spontaneously in their attitude towards the service user, or in their behaviour. As a professional, such negative behaviour is not acceptable, and breaches the healthcare profession's code of conduct (e.g. HCPC, 2016), and therefore the healthcare professional must develop self-awareness of their personal feelings and values, and not allow them to interfere with safe, effective and high-quality care delivery.

Whenever assessing a student's ability to perform a clinical intervention, the practice assessor will also gauge the student's practical knowledge to a good extent, and their attitude. In many PADs, the attitude and behaviour (affective) component is assessed by a list of professional values in practice profile or interpersonal interaction and attitude profile, which are of course integral components of performing service users' care interventions.

The affective domain is enshrined implicitly within SOP under all seven NMC's (2018c) 'platforms'. An example of competence addressing the affective domain of care delivery is: 'Provide and promote non-discriminatory, person centred and sensitive care at all times, reflecting on people's values and beliefs, diverse backgrounds, cultural characteristics, language requirements, needs and preferences, taking account of any need for adjustments' (NMC, 2018c: clause 1.14). Practice assessors have to be confident that pre-registration students are competent in these SOP before signing the corresponding practice outcome in their PAD as a pass.

The above-mentioned competence can be translated into practice competencies to be achieved during practice placement, such as 'Ensures the service user's care is their primary priority, and therefore treats them as individuals and respects their dignity'. The specific students' activities that will demonstrate this were identified under professional values in Chapter 7 of this book.

However, as noted above, assessing students in the affective domain is probably less straightforward than assessing psychomotor skill or the knowledge base. This is because interpreting interpersonal and attitudinal aspects is likely to be clouded by subjectivity, different interpretations and assumptions. Realising this difficulty in relation to paramedic students and learners, Tanner (2014) examined this component and suggests a 12-item framework for this activity, which includes assessing the student's listening skills, body language and appearance, in addition to demonstrating compassion, verbal communication, and so forth. Consequently, the assessor must assess the student's values by:

- making sure that they observe the student's behaviour, not basing their decision only on colleagues' reports
- observing the effect of the student's behaviour on the service user/colleagues
- recording the observed behaviour promptly, to ensure accuracy and to avoid delayed misinterpretation of events
- not being influenced by the 'halo effect'.

Furthermore, the affective aspect of care delivery seems to have been deficient in previous pre-registration healthcare courses, or not valued by registrants, as was pointed out in the Francis (2013) report, which highlighted service users' concerns that healthcare staff lack care and compassion towards them, and that their behaviours and values are inappropriate. The actions taken to prevent such complaints include the new NMC (2018c) standards of proficiency, NHS England's (2016) *Leading Change, Adding Value – A Framework for Nursing, Midwifery and Care Staff*, and HEE's (2014) *Values Based Recruitment Framework* publications.

Making decisions after assessing the student and giving feedback on their performance

Following the assessment of competency, the practice assessor would normally ask the student how effectively they felt they performed the clinical intervention(s) straight (or soon) after their completion of the intervention(s). This is followed by the assessor providing feedback to the student on their performance, and then indicating to the learner whether they have passed or failed the assessment.

The benefits of asking the student how they performed first are that this is likely to make them put aside any anxiety that they might still have about their performance, think more objectively and be more receptive to feedback. So, the practice assessor could ask, 'How do you think you did?' This constitutes a self-assessment undertaken by the learner (which was discussed in Chapter 7), albeit usually only briefly, which should also give the assessor an indication of the learner's insight into their level of competence.

Feedback is also a means of justifying the pass or fail result. Feedback can be: (a) *intrinsic feedback*, which occurs within the performer through self-assessment and reflection (the student often knows how well or not so well they did); or (b) *extrinsic feedback* (or augmented feedback), which is given by the assessor or peers and done concurrently during the skill performance and/or on completion of the performance. Some assessors might find it difficult to give honest feedback on a weak or faulty student performance. This could be tricky for the learner as well, but feedback has to be given honestly and is generally accepted more readily if given constructively.

It is noteworthy that written feedback is also provided by practice supervisors and others on students' learning, behaviour and values in students' PADs. However, at times, teachers' time pressures and administrative issues might negatively affect the nature of the feedback provided. Furthermore, at times, students are given feedback on their clinical performance at end-points such as at the end of a placement, or at mid-placement reviews. Such occasional feedback is of limited benefit to the student who should instead be provided with feedback regularly as and when new skills are learnt and are formatively assessed. Comprehensive and timely feedback can also lead to enhanced student engagement with their learning.

Good practice guidelines for giving feedback that is comprehensive and timely to students are listed in Table 8.3.

Table 8.3 Good practice guidelines for giving feedback

Feedback	Rationales
• Ensure privacy and that adequate time is allocated.	To ensure complete and comprehensive feedback, verbal and written
• Use the sandwich method, which entails starting with comments on the positive points or strengths, discussing areas for improvement, and ending on positive notes.	To encourage further learning
• Give feedback constructively, as the aim of feedback is to enable the learner to learn and improve (feed forward).	To enable student to improve / enhance their practice

(Continued)

Table 8.3   (Continued)

Feedback	Rationales
• Acknowledge good practice.	Positive reinforcement
• Try to be honest and fair, and not over-critical.	Being humane, and applying humanistic theory
• Be clear and concise.	Efficiency
• Allow the recipient of the feedback time to ask questions.	For clarification
• Do not allow anxiety levels to increase unduly.	Anxiety can reduce clear thinking
• Gauge the impact of your feedback on the student's feelings and self-esteem throughout the exercise.	To avoid negative effects on learner
• Respect and treat the recipient as an individual and focus on behaviour and skill performance rather than personality traits.	To ensure feedback is not a personal remark.
• Suggest measures to correct inappropriate practice.	For safe practice
• Remain calm and objective; do not respond in kind to anger, aggression and defensiveness.	Professional behaviour
• Motivate the recipient to consolidate strengths and address limitations through strategies such as action plans.	To build on existing knowledge and competence
• Be empowering by encouraging the recipient to comment on feedback.	Listening to the learner; empathising
• Advise student to develop a positive and open-minded attitude towards feedback despite the mark or grade awarded.	So that they can build on their achievement.

Good general communication skills are essential when giving feedback, including non-verbal communication such as maintaining eye contact, and sitting at an angle. Following feedback, action plans or learning points can be constituted and mutually agreed, as also suggested by the RCN (2017). However, in an ethos of self-directed learning, ultimately it is up to the receiver of the feedback to decide how much of it to heed and act upon, and when, and to be accountable for their decisions.

Various viewpoints discussed so far suggest that appropriate documentation is vital to practice assessor activities. Furthermore, the documentation should be in line with section 10 of the NMC's (2018b) code of practice, and the NMC's (2021b) *Keep Records of all Evidence and Decisions*, when appropriate, as they constitute documentary evidence of the action taken.

━━━━━━━━━━━ **ACTION POINT 8.2** ━━━━━━━━━━━

The student's practice competencies

Look through your copy (the practice assessor's copy) or the student's copy of the practice competencies' document and read the sections where it identifies the roles of the practice learning supervisor, the practice assessor, the academic assessor, and the student during the placement.

A clause in the document usually states the actions that the practice supervisor needs to take if the student is perceived as underachieving or 'failing'. These actions tend to entail drawing on the expertise of colleagues if deemed appropriate, of the PEF and/or the student's personal tutor. There should also be a section on the appeals procedure in the student's Course Handbook. However, for each new course or module being offered, there would have been briefing sessions for prospective practice supervisors and practice assessors to familiarise themselves with the course requirements, and the specific clinical skills to be achieved by students, and to discuss any potential issues.

If you are new to practice assessment, it is very important that, before you conduct any student assessment, you acquaint yourself fully with the student's placement competencies and the healthcare regulator's SOP, and preferably with the overall assessment strategy for the course. Furthermore, you should fully understand the particular summative assessments that you are going to conduct. The action to take in the case of 'failure to achieve required standard' by the learner is discussed later in this chapter.

However, despite careful planning, unfolding day-to-day events can still disrupt the smooth conduct of assessments. The patient could refuse consent to students performing clinical interventions on them, or staff sickness, unexpected emergency admissions or referrals might present as obstacles. Nevertheless, these do not always present as problems, as Neary (2000), for example, recommends 'responsive assessment', which entails taking into account the situational context such as the patient's current physiological or psychological state, and any prevailing resource issues that can mean adjusting to prevailing circumstances.

Action planning

An example of an action plan was presented earlier in this chapter in relation to behaviour issues manifested by ODP student Jade. If action plans are required, they are often constituted at the mid-placement review of students' progress with practice competencies. The competencies to be achieved will have been agreed at the beginning of the placement and might be in the form of a learning contract or learning agreement. The mid-placement review can technically be a formal formative assessment point, which involves dedicated time for a discussion on, and documentation of, the student's progress with placement competencies.

If the student has been progressing mostly as expected, then this is documented, and the student continues as agreed in the learning agreement. If the student has not been achieving as expected in the knowledge, skill and attitude components, then a negotiated action plan needs to be constructed, which the practice supervisor, the practice assessor and the student mutually agree on, and sign. A PEF or the academic link might also be present and sign the action plan accordingly.

In addition to Tanner's (2014) observation that assessing the interpersonal and attitudinal aspects is more problematic than assessing psychomotor skill or the knowledge base, Jervis and Tilki's (2011) qualitative research also previously revealed difficulty with assessing students' attitude and behaviour towards service users and team members accurately, with the undesirable consequence that some practice supervisors or assessors might pass students who are in fact not competent in the attitudinal component of student competence.

Action planning involves specifying all components identified at the top of the six columns related to ODP student Jade's action plan. If such an action plan was not constituted, then the student could have grounds for complaint and appeal if they were subsequently deemed a 'fail' for the placement. This point also indicates the importance of documentation of progress in the achievement of placement competencies.

While there are some similarities between learning contracts and action plans, there are distinct differences between them in that the former are more learning centred and the latter are more assessment centred. The learning contract is a systematic but speculative plan of learning based on the practice competencies to be achieved and anticipated learning opportunities, and may be adjusted during mid-placement progress discussions. The action plan is a 'must-achieve' device that identifies competencies that have to be achieved by an identified date during the practice placement, non-achievement of which would lead to a 'fail' being awarded.

Re-assessing the learner

Once the action plan has been agreed, it must be adhered to, in that the practice supervisor (or the PEF) and the student jointly ensure that the student has access to opportunities to learn those competencies, that continuous assessment is occurring and, when ready, the student is re-assessed summatively and the documentation signed as and when competencies are achieved. The action plan is regularly reviewed and, on the agreed date, a formal review is conducted, which can lead to a further action plan, with more targeted learning support for the student. If, despite these actions, the student still doesn't achieve the identified competencies, then they will be given a fail for those components, and may be allowed a second attempt at those competencies in the same or another practice setting. Depending on the university's policy and circumstances, the student might be allowed a third attempt, and if they still do not achieve the competencies, then they fail the course and do not progress to registration, as also asserted by Gingerich et al. (2020).

The components discussed in the preceding sections have addressed mostly the duties of practice supervisors and practice assessors with regards to assessing students' achievement of their practice competencies. Assessments have to meet the essential criteria of validity and reliability, as discussed in Chapter 7 of this textbook. The next section explores a further dimension of reliability of assessments, namely intra- and inter-assessor reliability.

Intra- and inter-assessor reliability

At practice assessor preparation events, at practice assessors' update sessions and at course reviews, on and off, the question is asked as to how we know that assessors are consistent in their assessment of students' competencies. That is, how do we know and monitor how consistent each assessor is in assessing how students perform specific clinical interventions, and that they are consistent in their expectations and decisions when assessing different students at the same stage of their professional education in performing that particular clinical intervention.

Furthermore, consideration is also given to consistency across assessors, both practice supervisors continuously assessing students, and practice assessors summatively assessing episodes of care. This is the arena of intra- and inter-assessor reliability. Inter-assessor reliability (at times, referred to as inter-examiner or inter-rater reliability, where appropriate) refers to the consistency with which all assessors assess students at the same stage of their programme on each clinical intervention.

The QAA (2018) indicates that assessment criteria have to be 'sufficiently robust to ensure reasonable parity between the judgements of different assessors', which is consistency between different assessors. From their research on whether inter-assessor reliability is feasible for individuals being assessed on basic life support skills following appropriate training, Beck et al. (2016) found that it is indeed achievable between three assessor groups (professionals, medical students and peers) and therefore that the skill can be assessed reliably. However, in Gittinger et al.'s (2022) quantitative research on physiotherapy students being assessed on psychomotor skills by OSCE, it emerged that there is poor inter-assessor reliability.

Furthermore, increasingly, the quality of student performance in practice competencies is graded (e.g. Andre, 2000; Way et al., 2019), and, although grading practice normally requires further appropriate educational preparation for practice assessors, this activity should also enable the achievement of intra- and inter-assessor reliability with more ease.

Additionally, it is only fair to students that assessors are consistent in their expectations of the standard to which students perform care interventions, the highest standard being the healthcare organisation's approved procedure, clinical guidelines or protocol for performing the particular intervention.

Thus, the term intra-assessor reliability refers to how consistently the practice assessor assesses particular categories of students on a particular clinical intervention, that is, that they consistently use the same identified criteria for deciding on whether to give a pass or a fail for that particular intervention, within a responsive assessment approach.

Practice assessor preparation courses and update sessions can incorporate an exploration of ways in which intra- and inter-assessor reliability is achieved and can be monitored in the assessment of practice.

─Reflection point 8.1─

Intra- and inter-assessor reliability

Think of ways in which practice assessors can achieve and monitor intra- and inter-assessor reliability. What are the informal and more structured situations or opportunities that they can utilise to explore these?

As you would have sensed, achieving and maintaining intra- and inter-assessor reliability is a feature of the professionalism of learning supervisors and assessors. There are various ways of monitoring intra- and inter-assessor reliability. The practice assessor update workshops provide suitable opportunities to explore how far consistency within and across practice assessors is achieved. Assessment case studies can be examined in small groups, or these groups can be invited to discuss consistency in the context of situations that they have personally encountered as practice assessors. In these groups, conclusions can be drawn on consistency in the assessments conducted, and, with the help of the facilitator, benchmarks of good practice can be established.

However, monitoring intra- and inter-assessor reliability must not wait for update study days. Informal monitoring is undertaken continuously through reflection by assessors and discussions with peers or team members in the practice setting or unit, with one's line manager, the academic assessor or the assessor's clinical supervisor. So, further ways of achieving intra-assessor reliability are by:

- consistently using approved procedures/clinical guidelines/protocols
- ascertaining that the approved procedures and clinical guidelines are up-to-date
- ensuring that their own competence and skills are up-to-date
- informal monitoring of their own pass/fail rates of students
- ensuring that learners are aware of the level of performance expected of them
- ensuring that the learner is being taught to the same standard and clinical guidelines/procedures by different registrants and practice supervisors
- assessors ensuring an appropriate environment for assessing (so that the learner is relaxed when performing the clinical procedure)
- student feedback such as evaluating how the student feels about the assessment process and decisions

- external feedback from colleagues through reflections on the assessment conducted
- reflection-on-action on the assessment already conducted
- ensuring being aware of the halo effect, being non-judgemental, for instance about the learner as a person; and maintaining objectivity
- being consistent in their own standard of clinical practice.

In addition to the above-mentioned ways of achieving intra-assessor reliability of assessments, inter-assessor reliability is achieved by:

- assessors' meetings within the ward/unit team – formal and informal
- consulting or involving PEF when uncertain
- consulting colleagues on the same ward/unit as appropriate
- auditing the practice assessor's performance of assessments (e.g. by negotiating peer assessment)
- student feedback on practice assessments
- feedback from the university following student evaluations
- monitoring attendance at practice assessor updates, usually trust-based
- knowing and consulting/informing the academic link lecturer
- exploring assessment issues at clinical supervision meetings
- monitoring and recording whether practice supervisors and assessors are up-to-date with the approved procedures and clinical guidelines.

Averting and Resolving Problems in Assessment

Having discussed intra- and inter-assessor reliability of student assessments, this section now examines potential problems related to the assessment of practice competencies. Most problems of assessment can be averted by careful planning, and this is the component wherein practice supervisors' and assessors' leadership is absolutely essential. However, problems with assessments do occur and, when they do, they need to be resolved quickly and efforts made to learn how to avoid them in future.

Potential problems in the assessment of competence

The aims or purposes of assessment are quite clearly identified by several writers on nurse education, as noted in Chapter 7 under 'Why do we assess our students?'. However, how far and how smoothly these aims are achieved in reality vary. We also need to consider exactly what types of problems practice assessors actually encounter in the assessment of students, and what are the potential weaknesses of assessments, including those of written examinations.

━━━━━━━━━━ **ACTION POINT 8.3** ━━━━━━━━━━

Current problems in assessment

1.   Think of the likely weaknesses of assessments and the reasons why
     assessments, even written examinations, are generally unpopular with students
     (assuming that they are). Make brief notes.
2.   Identify the actual problems that tend to occur with student assessment of theory,
     and of practice, in your healthcare profession - ones that you have experienced or
     observed, or that you feel could occur.

Practice supervisors, assessors and learners might encounter various difficulties
with the assessment of clinical skills. For assessment of the knowledge base, for
example, of human physiology, or numerical skills related to drug administration,
written examinations remain a favoured method, because a very high degree of
accurate knowledge is necessary for the healthcare professional. The likely solutions to the problems that you have identified will be explored shortly. A range of
problems with assessment was identified by just one group of students on a previous mentoring course. Many of these are presented in the box.

Problems with Assessment

*   Leaving things to the last minute (i.e. poor time planning)
*   Difficulty with integration of theory and practice, or ineffective application
*   Personality problems/clashes
*   Problems of organisation in the practice setting
*   Lack of time
*   Student disagreeing with the practice supervisor or assessor
*   Attitude problems - student's or practice assessor's
*   Structure of learning programme (e.g. placement is too short)
*   Practice assessor accountable and responsible for how student performs the
    clinical intervention
*   Inconsistency in student performance
*   Student absence
*   Practice assessor's lack of concentration due to preoccupation with other issues
*   Practice assessor changes
*   Student appears indifferent
*   Student's insufficient level of knowledge
*   Lack of resources (e.g. equipment)
*   Non-cooperation or refusal of consent by the healthcare service user.

One of the most cited difficulties encountered in the past has been insufficient time
for student supervision activities. Cognisance of this recurrent problem necessitates

more robust leadership on the part of practice supervisors and assessors in terms of forward planning, prioritising and proactive actions. The substantial empirical study on assessments conducted two decades ago by Phillips et al. (2000) highlighted various problems encountered by assessors, which include the following:

- The quality of assessment varies enormously, depending on staffing levels and workload in the practice setting.
- There can be difficulty in understanding the different levels of practice.
- Few assessors feel well prepared for doing assessments and most express a desire for continuing support after the initial preparation, and a consideration of adequate infrastructure for valid and reliable assessments.

Some of the problems may have been resolved for nursing and midwifery since, with the creation of the practice assessor role, and continuous assessment conducted by practice supervisors. Other problems with assessments have been identified, for example by Rowntree (1987), Lankshear (1990), Gainsbury (2010) and Hughes et al. (2021). Rowntree discusses some of the 'side-effects of assessments', referring to concepts such as 'self-fulfilling prophecy', whereby students who are expected to achieve low grades do tend to end up achieving low grades, which might not necessarily be a reflection of their innate capability.

Gainsbury (2010) reports on a problem with assessment referred to as 'failure to fail' that was identified three decades earlier by Lankshear (1990), and also later by Hughes et al. (2021) and Gingerich et al. (2020), and therefore still prevails. Gainsbury's report reminded universities and their partner healthcare trusts of their accountability with regard to awarding a pass to students only on the basis of evidence of competence, thus signifying fitness for practice.

──────────── **ACTION POINT 8.4** ────────────

Difficulties with student assessment

Thinking about current day-to-day potential problems, and considering them in the context of your own current place of work, first identify at least one clinical assessor who has already conducted quite a few clinical assessments. They do not need to be based solely in your workplace but should work broadly within your specialism. Your task is then to approach the assessor and ask them to explain precisely what steps they take in preparation for, and in actually conducting, the assessment of competence with students. Find out also from the assessor how they anticipate potential problems and avert them. Ask about some of the actual problems encountered and the options that they had for resolving them.

At the same time or afterwards, reflect for yourself on such problems and decide how you would go about managing them if they occurred in your own practice setting.

Alternatively, think for yourself of all the problems that you might encounter in your assessment function as either a practice assessor or a practice supervisor, and then the options that will be available to you to resolve each of them.

Problems of assessment may include differences in the interpretation of the exact meaning of individual placement competencies. There might be problems in conveying the depth of knowledge expected, or the level of skill demonstration. Issues like these can be rectified by open discussion between all personnel directly involved.

Resolving problems with assessment

━━━━━━━━━━ ACTION **POINT 8.5** ━━━━━━━━━━

Resolving difficulties encountered by practice assessors

Refer back to the box titled 'Problems with assessment' and work on the difficulties that you feel could be encountered by practice assessors, by identifying a number of problems of assessment yourself with a particular group of students, and the probable solutions for each of them. This can be done by completing Template 8.1.

Template 8.1   Potential problems of assessments, and actions that can be taken to resolve them

Problems of assessments	Actions that can be taken to resolve them
Leaving things to the last minute	....
Difficulty with integration, or ineffective application, of theory and practice	....
Personality problems/clashes	......
Problems of organisation	....
Lack of time for conducting assessments	....
Student disagrees with practice assessor	....
Attitude problems - student's or practice assessor's	
The service user or patient not consenting to student assessment	
Lack of resources (e.g., equipment)	
Structure of learning programme: variation of experience, e.g. allocation too short	
...... (etc. - add other ones you have identified)	

Chances are that you will be aware of, or have thought of, yet other problematic situations encountered by practice assessors or practice supervisors in the assessment of students, for which similar steps can be taken. They might include passing a student because the practice assessor likes the student or failing the student because they dislike them (at times, referred to as 'halo' and 'horns' effects, respectively), assessors misinterpreting the wording of practice competencies, and signing up clinical competencies as pass.

With some of these problem areas, there could be instances where a practice assessor passes a student on a specific competency when they should be awarding a fail. This cannot be condoned, but failure to fail students has already been identified over the years. If a student is failing, the practice assessor's decision-making comes into play, and action plans are constructed. From their qualitative study of the 'failure to fail phenomenon', Gingerich et al. (2020) conclude that as practice supervisors and practice assessors, we must be reminded to accept that not all students will complete the pre-registration course successfully. The authors also conclude that slow learners are not necessarily under-performers, as a small number of students will require more supervision time than others; and they recommend that a record of student engagement be kept and taken into consideration at summative assessments.

Furthermore, in their research related to students who fail practice competencies, Hunt et al. (2016) found that some students react negatively to feedback that they have not performed to the required standard in their practice assessments, as also noted by Jervis and Tilki (2011) before. In such situations, some students become upset, and others even become angry and threatening. Some say they will take grievances against their assessor. Other students become manipulative by either being charming and obliging or coercive, some blame external factors for failing, while others express open hostility and make personal threats to the assessor, according to Hunt et al. (2016).

Hostile student attitude leads to a breakdown in supervisor–student relationships and trust. However, all practice supervisors and assessors are accountable practitioners, and therefore simply have to abide by the assessment protocol laid down in the students' course curriculum, as well as by their code of practice. The next section considers the ethical aspects of student assessment, particularly in terms of the assessor's accountability.

The Assessor's Accountability in Relation to Assessments

All registrants have to comply with their professional body's code of practice, and this applies also to practice assessment, and supervising juniors and colleagues' learning, of course. 'Being an accountable professional' is one of the seven platforms in the NMC's (2018c) SOP that directly addresses ethical aspects of nurses' and midwives' responsibilities and duties. Similarly, from the collegial stance, 'Professional values' is one of the 'elements' that addresses the ethical and legal aspects of the Physiotherapy Framework (CSP, 2011 – updated 2020), for example.

Thus, practice assessors are already knowledgeable about the ethical aspects of professional practice through their pre-registration preparation, while their students will be developing these through theirs. From a concept analysis of healthcare professionals' 'ethical competence', Kulju et al. (2016) identify a number of factors that are prerequisites for ethical competence for the benefit of service users as well as staff, such as ethical knowledge, moral sensitivity, judgement and behaviour, and supportive surroundings in the organisation, which apply to practice supervisors and assessors as well for effective ethical practice.

'Ethics' tends to refer to the social behaviours, morals and values of individuals and groups in relation to doing good for the greatest number, and to the impact, or end results, of clinical interventions. One widely accepted set of principles of ethics that applies to many spheres of life, including medicine, business and education, has been formulated by Thiroux and Krasemann (2014), which applies directly to instances of practice assessment in the following ways:

- The value of life – can refer to ensuring that students develop the necessary competencies for effective clinical interventions that would restore health and well-being. It can also refer to ensuring that students acquire the necessary knowledge, skills and attitudes to register as a nurse so that they can earn a living.
- Goodness or rightness – refers to the practice supervisors doing good to students and healthcare service users, and doing the right things.
- Justice or fairness – refers to ensuring that all students have the opportunity to acquire the relevant knowledge, skills and attitude in the appropriate detail and depth.
- Honesty and truth-telling – ensuring that incorrect information is not given.
- Individual freedom – means that students have some freedom in deciding on the amount and type of learning, and care service users have a say in the clinical interventions available, where possible.

Other principles of ethics include: (1) being trustworthy; (2) autonomy; (3) beneficence (doing good); (4) non-maleficence (doing no harm); and (5) self-respect. Furthermore, the British Association for Counselling and Psychotherapy's (BACP) (2018) 'ethical framework' for counselling encompasses values, principles and personal moral qualities. Values refer to respecting human rights and dignity, alleviating personal distress and suffering, and fairness. Personal moral qualities include empathy, sincerity, humility and competence.

The codes of practice of healthcare professional regulatory bodies often incorporate ethical principles that registrants have to follow. As for practice assessors' ethical practice related to the assessment of competence, they should, for instance, not award a pass to a student for any particular competency if they are not completely sure that the student can perform the clinical intervention competently and safely.

Furthermore, the NMC's (2018a) SSSA also identifies effective student assessment practices in that it indicates, for example, that practice assessors must 'receive ongoing support and training to reflect and develop in their role' (2018a: clause 8.2), which implicitly suggests that practice assessors have to be fully aware of the knock-on effects of 'pass' decisions on service users' health.

Consequently, if an inexperienced practice assessor finds dealing with the under-performing student a challenge, then they need to recognise this and seek guidance and support from more experienced assessors, or the PEF or academic link, as per local guidelines (see Figure 8.1 later in this section). Other sources of support for clinical assessors might be:

- the student's personal tutor
- the practice assessor's clinical supervisor
- the practice assessor's line manager
- the university's disabilities support officer
- specific guidelines or protocols on ways of managing problematic situations
- retrospectively at assessor update workshops
- employer's and university's intranet
- in-practice supervision team meetings
- own emotional resilience.

One of the legal implications of assessments is that, on being awarded a pass, the individual is being given a licence and the legal right to practise the skill unsupervised when they register with their professional body. Awarding a licence to practise to someone who is not competent is in breach of the law, and the NMC's (2018b) code of practice clearly indicates that all registrants must keep to the laws of the country (clause 20.4).

A feature that frequently surfaces when the legality of the actions of registrants is questioned is the documentation of the actions taken. Andrews and St Aubyn (2015) and various others clearly believe and assert that 'if it is not documented, it was not done'. Alternatively, Kendall-Raynor (2007) reports on the case of a registered nurse who had allegedly failed to supervise a student adequately, which resulted in the wrong dose of medication being given to a service user, who subsequently died. The case was dropped by the Crown Prosecution Service (CPS) 'because of insufficient evidence'. Evidently, this was a situation of unethical practice on two counts, first because the wrong dose of medication resulted in harming a patient, and second, incompetent documentation led to injustice and unfairness.

The three professional bodies most prominently involved in health and social care, namely the HCPC, NMC and GMC, either explicitly or implicitly also incorporate into their codes of practice such ethical components as respect for care service users as individuals, obtaining consent prior to clinical interventions, protecting confidential information, and identifying and minimising risk to patients or service users.

The principles of ethics translate into current healthcare practice by addressing accountability, informed consent, confidentiality (including record keeping), professional misconduct, delegation and supervision.

Accountability and responsibility

All healthcare professionals are accountable for delivering care competently (NMC, 2018b), and also for other components of their roles such as enabling healthcare learners and colleagues to develop their clinical skills. We are accountable to our patients, ourselves, our employers, our professional regulatory bodies, and in fact also to the general public.

To be responsible implies being answerable for one's actions, and it is a component of accountability. However, before the health or care professional can be held accountable for particular clinical interventions or their overall professional competence, they must already have acquired educational preparation in the knowledge, skills and attitudes that underpin their clinical actions, and have been assessed in doing so. In addition, their employment endows them with the authority and responsibility to perform those clinical actions. Furthermore, registrants' teaching and assessment responsibilities are also specified in the healthcare professional's job description (or contract of employment) for the post they occupy; and in clauses in the codes of practice, as well as responsibilities for their own professional updating.

Registrants may not transfer or delegate their accountability to another person. Practice supervisors and assessors also function under legal obligations to know the student's course curriculum and built-in assessment procedures and regulations set out by the relevant HEI, and the appeals system that the student needs to follow if they feel that they are being unjustly treated. Students have a right to appeal against the conduct of the assessment, but not against the practice assessor's decision to pass or fail, or their professional judgement about safe practice.

In accepting the role of practice assessor, the registrant is implicitly accepting responsibility and accountability for maintaining standards of supervision and assessment. Practice supervisors must ensure that students gain the necessary clinical experience to develop their professional competence and that students do 'no harm' to healthcare service users, by teaching them the correct way of performing clinical interventions.

Moreover, making professional judgements about the performance of students and their ability to provide professionally competent and safe care, also constitutes an endeavour to achieve predictive validity and reliability in assessments of competence.

However, Rowntree (1987) indicates that there are times when assessors might intentionally give permission to the learner to perform clinical interventions while supervising them unobtrusively, which can be expected, but, at the same time, assessing their performance without having specified this to them beforehand. This is sometimes referred to as 'hidden assessment' and could be another instance of unethical action by the assessor.

The NMC (2018b) affirms that the interests of the care service user are paramount, that is, accountability to the service user is more important than accountability to the student. However, the legal perspective can be, depending on individual situations, that the student is also answerable for incompetent interventions. Lack of experience or knowledge is not an acceptable reason for incompetent care.

On not being awarded a pass for a clinical intervention that was not performed competently, the learner might feel either merely disappointed or emotionally distraught. The practice assessor then needs to contact the PEF or academic link if further help and support are needed but might also have to use basic counselling skills to help the learner. As for all professional skills, if practice assessors have not had training in counselling skills, then they should refer the student to an appropriate professional or department that does have those skills.

Supporting the Underachieving Student

As mentioned earlier in this chapter, practice supervisors' leadership includes careful planning of practice placement to ensure practice competencies are achieved. However, it is well appreciated that, for a number of reasons, some students could be seen as struggling or even failing to show consistent learning and progress during the placement. So, what are the different reasons for a student failing to learn and achieve the required practice competencies?

Reflection point 8.2

The underachieving student

From your own experience of students who struggle to achieve their clinical competencies, write down as many different reasons as you can think of for this happening during practice placements.

Some students genuinely experience unanticipated obstacles that hinder their achievement of placement competencies. Could this be because they are working extra shifts to supplement their income, and are therefore unable to find sufficient time to give full attention to their practice competencies? There could be placement-based reasons, or personal or domestic ones. The signs that suggest that a student might not progress as expected with the placement competencies can appear quite early on during the placement. Limited interaction with clinical staff, lateness, sickness, absent-mindedness, and inconsistency in standards of care delivery are just a few of them, but when such signs are detected, action should be taken early to ascertain the student's perception of their progress.

ACTION POINT 8.6

Failing to fail the student

So, for one reason or another, a student might not be progressing as expected, and the practice supervisor is not convinced that particular competencies will be achieved.

(Continued)

However, in the past mentors have, on occasion, still decided to award a 'pass' to those students on their practice competencies by the end of the placement, as also asserted by Gingerich et al. (2020), for example.

Consider the whole spectrum of reasons why you think that an assessor might award a pass to a student for a particular competency, even when the student has not provided evidence of competent performance. List as many reasons as you can think of.

You should have been able to think of certain day-to-day circumstances that might lead to the practice supervisor or assessor awarding a pass to the student on specific competencies even without adequate evidence of competent performance, none of which is likely to be a justifiable reason. These could include, for instance, pressure from the student, who indicates that it is the last week of placement and that they have passed all previous placement competencies, and that insufficient time was allocated for assessing competencies. In their meta-analysis of research on failure to fail, Hughes et al. (2021) identify such factors as assessors' workload, giving the benefit of the doubt to the student, and deficient organisational processes such as insufficient support for assessors, for passing under-performing students.

At times, practice supervisors may have done all the planning for the student to achieve competencies, and yet on assessment they might find that the student has not reached the level of competence required to award them a pass for specific competencies. This could mean the student failing the practice placement. Consequently, the student's placement may have to be extended to allow them more time to achieve the competencies, and their course extended.

Individual HEIs usually provide their own specific guidelines on the actions to take to support the struggling student. The necessary steps in such guidelines are sketched out as a simple algorithm in Figure 8.1, and include: meeting with the student as soon as possible to discuss this issue; informing other practice supervisors and the designated PEF; clarifying the area of weakness and advising on how to progress; constituting an action plan with SMART objectives; making provision for any extra support; and keeping careful notes of all discussions and incidents.

Although appearing to be a compact whole-story process, Figure 8.1 does constitute the actions that practice supervisors and assessors should take to facilitate learning and achievement for the underachieving student, each step or stage constituting a concerted intervention that needs to be handled carefully and professionally.

However, the question arises as to how confident practice assessors feel in their judgement and skill at giving a fail for a competency if the student is unable to perform the intervention competently. It is noteworthy that a study conducted by Mead (2011), using a convenient sample of conference attenders as the subject of the study, revealed that mentors had no problem with failing students if the latter could not demonstrate competence in particular service-user care skills. They felt that they had 'sufficient training to enable them to fail nursing students' (2011: 23).

However, Hauge et al.'s (2019) and others' findings were the opposite to Mead's, as they concluded that the preparation and support that mentors received were not adequate for them to be able to fail incompetent students confidently. Nonetheless, Heaslip and Scammell's (2012) research on this issue revealed that

Step	Decision	Action if No
Student was welcomed and orientated to the clinical setting by practice supervisor at the beginning of the placement	→ No →	Orientate student to the practice setting, introduce to key members of the team and co-practice supervisors; give student names of those who he/she should contact to explore their roles
↓ Yes		
Initial interview conducted by practice supervisor, and learning needs and requirements identified	→ No →	Conduct initial interview the same day and identify learning requirements; establish contact with practice assessor
↓ Yes		
Continuous supervision of skill acquisition, and formatively assessed by practice supervisors	→ No →	Student should not be allowed to perform clinical interventions unsupervised
↓ Yes		
Discuss immediately any area of skill acquisition causing concern	→ Not discussed →	Consult other practice supervisors in the team, or PEF, and discuss concern with student
↓ Yes		
If concern persists, formally explore student's perspectives, revisit learning contract	→ Not done →	Student could have grounds for appeal against assessment decisions. Draw on co-practice supervisors support, and PEF/practice assessor/academic link
↓ Yes		
Alert other practice supervisors and PEF of areas of concern	→ No →	Do so, to provide wider support to student
↓ Yes		
Conduct mid-placement interview, including formative assessments conducted; document accordingly	→ No →	Not documented is seen as not done
↓ Yes		
Practice assessor to conduct student assessment on episodes of care related to goals set in learning contract. If student fails, then compose a targeted detailed action plan	→ No →	Action plan with SMART outcomes required for student so that everyone is clear about their responsibilities
↓ Yes		
Monitor student's progress closely, the frequency of which will have been stated in the action plan; and offer help. Keep detailed notes of discussions in own copy of the action plan set	→ No →	Student might be scared of being seen as incompetent by now, and malpractice could occur. Documentation is crucial to justify your decisions
↓ Yes		
Practice assessor awards student pass on specified competencies and attitude components	→ No →	If student is not making progress/achieving, inform student of likelihood of failing identified competencies. Inform co-practice supervisors, PEF and academic link lecturer. Continue with extra support.
↓ Yes		
Final interview, and student passes placement	→ No →	Is preceded by formative assessments, and student fails placement. Students are allowed second attempts at achieving placement competencies/attitude components, therefore discuss likely alternative courses of action, e.g. interruption, extension of placement, another placement in another practice setting, other relevant solutions. Document everything discussed
↓ Yes		
Document in competencies booklet, action plan, etc., and inform parties involved		

Figure 8.1 The underachieving student – actions that practice supervisors and assessors should take

just over half of the 112 mentors who participated in the study indicated that they felt confident to fail students, and also recommended that grading practice may contribute to making it easier because, instead of a pass/fail result, the assessor can give a better indication to the student as to whether their fail was borderline or a more serious fail.

Nonetheless, on conducting a literature review of 'failure to fail', Hughes et al. (2016) found that there were various facets to the concept, and that it remained a real major issue. The review resulted in five themes related to 'Failure to fail', which are:

- failing a student is difficult
- is an emotional experience
- confidence is required
- unsafe student characteristics
- university support is required to fail students.

Still, when the student fails a placement, they are likely to become upset or ashamed of their failure, even if they did all that they could but still did not achieve. The practice supervisor will then need to draw on their helping skills to help the student further. Some registrants/practice supervisors might find the idea of having to use helping skills daunting if they rarely have to use these skills, and consequently may need to know where they can seek advice and guidance from, if required (as discussed throughout this chapter).

Helping and counselling the struggling student

The general and specific communication skills needed to establish a relationship and support the student to develop and achieve competencies, were ascertained in Chapter 7, one of which is the special skill of 'counselling', which is an essential attribute of supervisors of learning and teachers (Hughes and Quinn, 2013: 374). However, it is well recognised that for counselling to be effective, the process should be entered into voluntarily by the person who is the counsellee (in this instance, the health profession student). Indeed, it is generally agreed that unless counselling is actively sought by the student, the interaction might not be as effective, even if the helper uses most of the skills used in counselling. Second, counselling is a therapeutic technique, requiring specialist training. Persons not skilled in its use will, at best, not help the student, and at worst potentially compound the student's problems.

Therefore, unless they are fully qualified as counsellors, supervisors and other teachers in healthcare are more likely to use helping or 'basic' counselling skills. For more intense student problems, students should be referred to the PEF and to specialist services such as the university's counselling service, which is often a section of student services provision.

─── Case study 8.2 ───────────────────────────

The failing student

Bina is a pre-registration student on a 10-week placement at the end of the first year of her course, and the practice learning supervisors in the placement setting have varied roles as part of their managerial functions, and also tend to have to cover extra shifts on both days and nights due to ongoing staff shortages. However, Bina's placement has been marked by her frequent absence from the practice setting due to sickness and occasional tearfulness, claiming to feel depressed. She has been advised to seek help from the Trust's occupational health department and has been made aware that she can access the university's counselling facility if preferred.

Shortly after the placement started, the PEF went on maternity leave, and it took a few weeks to install a replacement for her. The acting PEF contacted the academic link to explain Bina's circumstances, and indicated that Bina was lacking in motivation and 'a real struggle'. In response, the acting PEF was advised that, among other things, a formal review needed to be conducted to ascertain Bina's progress with practice competencies and documented accordingly. In particular, if the competencies were not achieved, then Bina would fail the first year and not progress to year 2 of the pre-registration course.

Due to Bina's continuing absence and health problems, the progress review only took place well after the mid-placement stage, and an action plan was instituted as several practice competencies had still not been achieved. Consider what would be the specialist helping or counselling skills that could be utilised in regular supervisor–student contact if both Bina and her practice supervisors were more available.

───────────────────────────────────────

The most important factor within a counselling situation is the relationship between the counsellor and the counsellee (e.g. the practice supervisor and the student). This was identified initially by Rogers (1983) and later by Rogers and Freiberg (1994). Both identified three key qualities (also known as 'core conditions' of helping) that are required for effective counselling. These key qualities, as detailed under student-centred teaching in Chapter 3, are: genuineness, trust and acceptance, and empathic understanding.

In addition to the generic communication skills, verbal and non-verbal, key helping skills include: self-awareness, attending, active listening, summarising, reflecting, questioning, and using silence. This set of skills can be used as a framework for checking how thoroughly you feel you deal with such situations. By analysing your interactions with others, you will develop a greater awareness of how far you, as a professional, are able to help others.

Furthermore, additional specific communication skills are needed to help students who are struggling to achieve their clinical competencies, or who may be struggling with the nursing course as a whole and are even in danger of failing to become a qualified professional in their chosen career. In addition to the generic communication skills that are necessary for all effective relationships, specialist communication skills are also required by the practice supervisor to manage more complex learner issues, and by assessors to deal with problematic assessment situations.

A communication continuum that spans generic communication at one end to specialist communication at the other is suggested by Scammell (1990), with the associated specific purposes and specific skills for each component on the continuum. These components and their associated purposes and skills are laid out in Table 8.4.

Table 8.4 Scammell's communication continuum

• Primary communications	*Purpose*: initial contacts with others; brief encounters *Skill*: simple interpersonal or social skills, e.g. ability to listen
• Secondary communications	*Purpose*: ongoing relationships – verbal, non-verbal, written; informal support groups *Skill*: interpersonal or social skills, knowledge of how groups work, etc.
• Advice giving	*Purpose*: to offer factual information; to teach, instruct, supervise *Skill*: when to give advice, ability to impart knowledge of subject area, etc.
• Primary counselling	*Purpose*: support for friend or work colleague *Skill*: listen non-judgementally, help with problem-solving, etc.
• Secondary counselling	*Purpose*: therapeutic counselling for specific mental health problems *Skill*: advanced accurate empathy, self-disclosure, etc.

Primary and secondary communication occurs between practice supervisor and learner when exchanging information and establishing a supervisory relationship. Beyond this level, the practice supervisor may need to give direct advice to the student, especially when teaching, as well as when advice is requested. This, however, does not go as far as counselling, for which the individual requires more extensive training.

Primary counselling is a specialised communication skill that the practice supervisor needs to develop to deal with difficult practice supervision situations. Secondary counselling will be required for more intense psychological or behavioural issues, which the practice supervisor can deal with by directing the student to the appropriate support services, or, if trained, by using a systematic approach such as Heron's (2009) six-category intervention analysis (see the box below).

The Six-category Intervention Analysis as a Specialised Communication Skill

Authoritative intervention:

- Prescriptive: giving advice
- Informative: imparting information
- Confrontational: directly challenging.

Facilitative intervention:

- Supportive: understanding and encouraging
- Cathartic: allowing the release of emotions
- Catalytic: encouraging deeper exploration.

Heron's (2009) six-category intervention analysis therefore entails six possible actions that the counsellor can choose from. In difficult supervisor–student situations, for every interaction the practice supervisor may decide which of the six categories is most appropriate. For instance, for a student who frequently claims to be feeling unwell, physically or psychologically, the practice supervisor might use the prescriptive category of helping, and advise the student to consult the occupational health department. They might also give further information about where the department is, and the likely outcomes of this situation. In other situations, the practice supervisor might use another one of the categories, for example cathartic, to enable the learner to elaborate in detail how they feel about a patient whom they have looked after but who has passed away rather suddenly, for instance.

Dedicated time is required for a systematic approach to counselling, which can be done by applying Heron's (2009) six-category intervention analysis model, which identifies six possible interactions between the two parties. In Case Study 8.1, for instance, the practice supervisor could help Bina by utilising components of Heron's framework, whereupon instances of responses by the practice supervisor to the student may be as follows:

- Prescriptive – advise Bina to reduce less important life activities to concentrate on working to achieve her placement objectives as a priority.
- Informative – give specific information on where to access professional and personal support (e.g. the location of the occupational health department).
- Confrontational – ask Bina directly why she behaves the way she does, and how she could behave differently for a more satisfactory placement experience.
- Supportive – allow Bina time and silence to think over the practice supervisor's questions and suggestions.

- Cathartic – allow Bina to verbalise and explain in ample detail why she feels she is struggling in this placement.
- Catalytic – the practice supervisor acts as facilitator to enable Bina to meet her learning needs.

━━━━━━━━━━━━━━ **ACTION POINT 8.7** ━━━━━━━━━━━━━━

An underachieving student whom you have encountered

Think of a student whom you have known to have failed to achieve the required practice competencies, resulting in the student being disappointed, upset or distressed. In case you don't know of a student who has failed a placement, think of such a situation that you might encounter. Describe the situation in up to 75 words. Then, utilising Heron's (2009) six-category intervention analysis framework, identify the specific actions that you could take, using each of the categories to help the student.

Alternatively, consider Mel Alexis' situation (Case Study 1.1) detailed in Chapter 1, and follow the above instructions.

One perspective on how practice supervisors manage underachieving students comes from a study by DeBrew and Lewallen (2014) that explored the thought processes that assessors go through in deciding whether to pass or fail a student on specific competencies. The researchers concluded that when assessors encounter these situations, they might still be wondering afterwards if they have made the right decision. To resolve this feeling, DeBrew and Lewallen recommend that they should afterwards engage in 'deliberate, intentional reflective practices' as a means of checking on the correctness of their decisions and, possibly, needs for professional development. This sounds like a useful recommendation, although such reflective discussions may need to be facilitated by someone who is not closely involved with the assessor's work setting but could be their clinical supervisor, and of course the name of the student being discussed should be withheld.

Hawkins and McMahon (2020) suggest taking an intersubjective approach that focuses on the relationship between the assessor and the student. This notion largely implies using empathy. Universities usually provide a counselling service for any student who is distressed about any issue that is affecting their progress with their course. Becoming a skilled counsellor, especially for dealing with particular psychological problems, requires several years of structured educational preparation. However, Hawkins and McMahon also provide a number of pointers on how supervisors can help, which includes applying their own existing capabilities and qualities, which are noted succinctly in the box.

Qualities of a Good Supervisor

- Flexibility with use of different concepts and intervention methods
- A multi-perspective view (i.e. being able to see the situation from different angles)
- The ability to work transculturally
- The capacity to manage and contain anxiety - their own and that of the supervisee
- Openness to learning from supervision situations
- Sensitivity to the impact of wider contextual issues on the supervision process
- Ability to handle power appropriately
- Humour, humility and patience

Source: Adapted from Hawkins and McMahon (2020: 50)

Proctor's (2011) 'supervision alliance model' is widely accepted as a suitable framework for systematic supervision. As a model of helping that is also acknowledged by Hawkins and McMahon, it comprises three main functions or roles of the helper, namely: normative, formative and restorative (see Chapter 1 of this book for a discussion of Proctor's model of supervision).

Although practice assessors are expected to exercise professional judgement, as also noted by the QAA (2018: 7), and make pass or fail decisions on particular student performances, there are support networks that they can draw on whenever they are unsure. Informal or formal team supervision and peer-consultation facilities might already be in place but, as suggested earlier, the practice assessor should discuss uncertain situations with PEF and the academic assessor.

This chapter has explored ways in which practice supervisors and practice assessors exercise leadership in managing assessments, which includes forward planning, pre-empting issues, and managing those issues that do occur. However, it is useful to note that the leadership role is not just about taking action to avert problems. It is also about taking action to achieve goals, and it is about good practice.

Good practice guidelines for assessments

This final section on student assessment completes the focus on the principal aspects of assessment that were discussed in Chapter 7 and in this chapter by identifying good practice guidelines. The 'principles of assessment' are generally identified by universities and other education providers. For health and care profession students, deriving from the above general principles, together with the profession-specific guidelines (e.g. NMC, 2018a; QAA, 2018), a comprehensive set of good practice guidelines related to practice assessment is presented in the box below.

Good Practice Guidelines Related to Practice Assessment of Health and Care Students

- Practice supervisors and practice assessors ensure that they are fully familiar with the student's practice competencies and standards prior to the start of the practice placement.
- Allocate registrants for teaching specific care interventions and the associated knowledge to the student.
- Agree times and dates for student assessment, diary them, and treat it as 'supported time' (e.g. NMC, 2018a).
- Inform other staff to ensure that they do not interrupt during student assessment.
- Be aware of any urgent issues in the practice setting, e.g. staff sickness, stress, emergencies.
- Inform the service user and obtain permission for student assessment.
- Ensure that all equipment is available.
- Ensure that the learner has had sufficient practice opportunities prior to assessment of the skill.
- Ensure that as assessor you are available and accessible a few minutes before the scheduled time for episodes of assessment.
- Ensure that the learner knows the assessment criteria for the skill.
- Plan the assessment, ensuring you know where procedures and clinical guidelines are located in the practice setting.
- Assessments are conducted in collaboration between practice supervisors, practice assessors and academic assessors, as appropriate.
- Assessments are also informed by service-user feedback and other registrants who have worked with the student being assessed.
- Most care interventions are assessed by direct observations, and other competencies by other methods.
- Practice supervisors create opportunities for formative (or mock) student assessments.
- Incorporate continuous assessment records from practice supervisors and other registrants.
- Consider levels of assessment based on the stage of the pre-registration course the student is at.
- Ensure the assessments you conduct are valid, reliable and fair to students.
- Create an opportunity for the learner to talk through the procedure, if necessary.
- Be sensitive to the student's self-confidence or lack of it.
- Always remain calm and use appropriate interpersonal communication skills.
- If the learner displays awe of the assessor, enable them to relax and build their self-confidence.
- Be and look enthusiastic and motivated.
- Keep the assessment situated (in the context of the practice setting) and responsive.
- Allow the student to work at their own pace as long as this doesn't cause undue discomfort to the service user.
- Allow for holistic/person-centred care.
- Intervene appropriately if unsafe practice is about to occur.
- Encourage self-assessment, allow room for reflection and give feedback as you feel appropriate.
- Incorporate professional judgement when making pass/fail decisions.

- Heed previous potential issues related to assessment, e.g. research identifying 'failing to fail' (Hughes et al., 2021) and 'on-the- hoof' assessment (Phillips et al., 2000).
- Do not be biased by the occasional polarised instances of exceptionally thorough or poor practice during continuous assessment.
- Beware of other factors, e.g. the learner being preoccupied with other course assignments.
- Document results in the student's practice competencies document, etc.
- Take prompt supportive and remedial action if the student is given a fail.

Chapter Summary

This chapter has focused on practice supervisors' and practice assessors' responsibilities in the assessment of healthcare students' competencies, and the challenges that these roles can present in relation to assessments, and has therefore explored:

- The importance of practice supervisors and other assessors exercising leadership through the careful planning and scheduling of student assessments.
- Current difficulties and potential problems in the assessment of students' clinical skills, resolving these problems, including action planning and re-assessment of the learner, and how potential problems are averted.
- The responsibility and accountability of practice assessors in ensuring that pass or fail is awarded based on firm evidence, and the relevant subsequent action taken.
- Use of professional judgement, and how intra- and inter-assessor reliability can be monitored and achieved; and the ethical and legal aspects of student assessment.
- How underachieving students can be supported using communication and helping skills, and more specialist communication skills, including counselling. They constitute skills that would also apply to student assessment situations, and include time management and proactive actions, and the use of support networks with peers, PEFs and academic staff.
- Good practice guidelines related to assessments.

Further Optional Reading

1. For a meta-analysis of factors that lead to failure to fail, and possible solutions to this issue, see:
   - Hughes, L.J., Mitchell, M.L. and Johnston, A.N.B. (2021) 'Moving forward: Barriers and enablers to failure to fail – A mixed methods meta-integration', *Nurse Education Today*, 98(2021): 1–7.

2. For a detailed analysis of grading practice, see:

    • Way S., Fisher, M. and Chenery-Morris, S. (2019) 'An evidence-based toolkit to support grading of pre-registration midwifery practice', *British Journal of Midwifery*, 27(4): 251–257.

3. For further guidance on the ethics of practice supervision and assessment, see:

    • Gopee, N. (2008) 'Assessing student nurses' clinical skills: The ethical competence of mentors', *International Journal of Therapy and Rehabilitation*, 15(9): 401–407.

9

EVALUATING THE EFFECTIVENESS OF PRACTICE LEARNING SUPERVISION, AND CONTINUING LEARNING

INTRODUCTION

Having explored a range of components that should make supervision of practice-based learning and practice assessment of healthcare students effective, this chapter focuses on the question 'How do we know for sure that our teaching and assessment enable students to meet their learning needs fully?' How effective are our facilitation of learning activities for our students, and can they be improved?

Consequently, this chapter directs attention to the evaluation of healthcare professionals' practice learning supervision and practice assessment activities.

Evaluation can be a satisfying experience when we receive positive feedback on our teaching, be it practice-based or classroom-based, and it is usually an eye-opener if it identifies components for further improvement. Evaluation of practice learning entails healthcare professionals self-monitoring the effectiveness and quality of all their supervision of learning activities, as well as heeding external monitoring comments and reports. Evaluation information thus can form a basis for progressive learning for practice learning supervisors.

The chapter therefore examines the different reasons for evaluating supervision of practice learning and practice assessment activities, together with:

- what evaluation is, and precisely what practice supervisors and practice assessors evaluate
- who evaluates practice learning supervision
- how to evaluate, including frameworks for evaluation
- what to do with information gained from the evaluation
- practice supervisors' and practice assessors' continuing professional development.

These areas are discussed in relation to the facilitation of learning and continuous and episodic student assessment, and to the university-based assessment of students on undergraduate and postgraduate healthcare courses.

Chapter objectives

1. Identify and elaborate on a number of reasons for evaluating practice learning supervision activities, including the facilitation of learning and the assessment of competence.
2. Explain the nature and various features of evaluation, and who is involved in evaluating practice learning supervision.
3. Identify the different ways of evaluating clinically based and academically based teaching and assessment.
4. Justify the action that should be taken following evaluation and the likely opportunities for improvement.
5. Explain how the challenges encountered by practice supervisors and assessors also constitute opportunities for reflection and further professional development for them, as well as meeting their continuing learning and updating requirement.

Why Evaluate Practice Learning Supervision and Student Assessment?

The reason for evaluating practice-based supervision of learning activities is that it is logical to do so, to check that our actions are, and remain, effective in meeting learners' learning needs. Healthcare registrants engage in the evaluation of care and treatment continually when on duty, and therefore it is not an unfamiliar activity, as it is also part of pre-registration SOP to be achieved (e.g. NMC, 2018c, Platform 4). Previously, the NMC (2008) identified 'Evaluation of learning' as a key domain of supporting learning in practice settings, which included mentors being receptive to students' evaluation of placement-based learning, and engaging in peer and self-evaluation to facilitate professional and personal development.

━━━━━━ ACTION POINT 9.1 ━━━━━━

Why evaluate?

Other than the evaluation of learning being a required activity, consider for yourself the question why we should evaluate what we do in the course of our duties. Then consider what we can do with the information obtained from evaluations. Make notes of your thoughts on this.

With the problem-solving approach to health and social care, we engage in the assessment of service users' health problems, plan their treatment and care interventions, and implement the plan, and continuously evaluate their effect. More widely, systematic approaches to most novel projects and ventures entail continuing and end-point evaluation of their success, and making decisions about any action that needs to be taken subsequent to evaluation.

There are a number of reasons for evaluation. If practice supervisors do not evaluate how well they are fulfilling their supervisory activities, then they are taking for granted that their actions meet their learners' learning requirements. They are assuming that learners are satisfied with the learning provided, and that they are fulfilling their teaching and assessing duties effectively. Evaluation is an activity that we engage in formally and informally, and, at times, without realising that we are doing so. Formal evaluations provide evidence of the effectiveness of our activities, and often reveal unexpected findings, as the impressions of the recipients of the practice supervision might be different from those anticipated by the supervisor.

In addition to the purpose of identifying improvement points for subsequent supervisory activities, further reasons for evaluating practice supervision and student assessment are:

- to identify any shortcomings or problem areas, and take appropriate action
- to gauge whether the student's learning is pitched at the appropriate level and in sufficient detail
- for continuing self-monitoring of competence in professional practice, which is often a requirement of employment, and a component of staff appraisal (or development and performance review)
- that it is a component of the practice setting's quality assurance mechanism
- to gauge the adequacy of the provision of learning opportunities in practice settings
- that it is professional 'good practice' to evaluate all our work activities.

Evaluation performed for the purposes of quality assurance can be done through looking at structures (e.g. resources), processes, procedures, standards and consistency. It is performed for quality enhancement, which is for improvement through change and development. Evaluation can reveal any problematic aspects and which aspects concerned the individual or group of students most, and it can identify any area of confusion or misunderstanding. Consequently, when problematic areas are uncovered, they also present opportunities for improvement, for creativity, and for novel structures and activities to be suggested and instituted.

The reasons for evaluation can also be categorised as:

1. Evaluation for knowledge – to identify areas of deficiency in care or teaching provision so that action can be taken to rectify the deficiency.
2. Evaluation for development – for engaging in educational or training activities based on evaluation results, and thereby growth and improvement for practice supervisors, team members and the organisation.
3. Evaluation for accountability – to determine whether duties have been performed as required and generate evidence of achievements.
4. Evaluation for management – that is, evaluation conducted as a management activity, with a view to identifying and resourcing any professional development requirement.

For university courses, module leaders and course directors evaluate to identify problems being encountered or foreseen by the students on the education programme, and to solve those problems, or avert them in future. At times, what is seen as an issue by students just needs further explaining or justifying.

Before the evaluation of any activity, it is important to ascertain what the purposes of the activity are. Thus, if we are evaluating our teaching session, what were the specific aims of the session? The purpose of the teaching will have been to arm the recipient with relevant knowledge and to develop competence, and the purpose of the evaluation will be to check if this has happened. In view of the above-mentioned four reasons for evaluation, consider whether you evaluate your teaching for the purposes of accountability, to receive suggestions and explore associated ideas for the further development of your supervision of learning activities, or as a management exercise.

━━━━━━━━━ **ACTION** POINT 9.2 ━━━━━━━━━

How does evaluation of teaching improve learning?

Focusing on the practice supervisor's teaching role, consider the evaluation that you have received on your teaching, requested evaluation or offered voluntarily. Then identify at least two ways in which you can improve or enhance your teaching for more efficacy.

Healthcare course lecturers are required to evaluate their teaching and act on the evaluation comments received, and document them. As for practice supervisors, the NMC (2018d: 11, clause 4.9) asserts that they should 'receive and act upon constructive feedback from students and the people they engage with to enhance the effectiveness of their teaching, supervision and assessment'.

Following evaluation of teaching in the practice setting, the practice supervisor can follow up the teaching component by reflecting on their teaching. Subsequently, further reading materials or information to help rectify or supplement students' learning needs can be offered. Lecturers can arrange further teaching sessions on topics suggested in the evaluation information and can also adjust their subsequent teaching with a view to connecting more fully with learners' learning needs.

Practice assessors also self-evaluate their assessment activities. At university, lecturers often evaluate their structured lessons, be it a knowledge-base component, or teaching a healthcare skill in the skills laboratory. They also evaluate how fit for purpose the modules and courses that they lead are.

As noted in Chapter 5, at the end of each practice placement, students are asked to evaluate the placement, often by the healthcare team in the practice setting, and always by the university. Practice supervisors can ask students to evaluate 'spoke' visits, or they may ask the student to engage in reflective write-ups that the practice supervisor will subsequently read and discuss. All HEIs have their own placement evaluation forms and criteria which students are often invited to complete electronically. Moreover, the RCN (2017: 15–20) provides a comprehensive list of items for inclusion in practice placement evaluation.

What is 'evaluation'?

Evaluation is a key component of a systematic approach to care and treatment, and is also an inherent facet of care pathways.

━━━━━━━━━ **ACTION** POINT 9.3 ━━━━━━━━━

What does the term 'evaluation' itself mean?

Make brief notes on what you understand by the word 'evaluation'. What is it about?

Evaluation of the effectiveness of care given is important, as the goal of providing care is to restore health as much as possible, and we need to know if this has been achieved. The term *evaluation* originates from the French word *evaluer*, meaning to work out the numerical value of something. In current usage in English, to evaluate means to judge or appraise the quality, value or worth of something (Brookes and O'Neill, 2017: 307). Various definitions of evaluation have been offered by interested parties over the years, and generally they indicate that evaluation is essentially about making judgements about the value and worth of something against explicit, justifiable and appropriate criteria.

Thus, evaluation is the process of systematically collecting information with regards to the effectiveness of action taken or interventions that have already been implemented, and then analysing the information received and taking action to enhance care interventions, or rectify any deficiencies. Furthermore, evaluation is also used as an empirical tool in the form of a research method involving in-depth exploration of the component being evaluated through data collection and rigorous analysis (Guba and Lincoln, 1989).

Reflection point 9.1

What do we evaluate?

When evaluating care in clinical practice, exactly what is it that we evaluate, and what are the different ways in which evaluation information is obtained?

Evaluation of care plans and goals is obviously to determine the effectiveness of the plans, which can be supplemented by feedback from the service user. Other terms that tend to have similar or overlapping meanings with evaluation are monitoring, quality appraisal and assessment. The term 'assessment', however, has distinct and specific meanings in healthcare, referring to the assessment of patients' health problems and to assessing students' competence and knowledge. Thus, assessment usually refers to the collection of data against set criteria. It is therefore objective. Evaluation, on the other hand, refers to the values and personal judgement on whether the planned action taken enabled the achievement of specified goals.

Returning to the evaluation of practice supervision, this can also be public evaluation or private evaluation, external or internal, continuous or episodic/intermittent and final or interim (refers to timescale). Moreover, evaluation can be case-specific or generalised/holistic or analytical (see Table 9.1 for a brief explanation of these modes and types of evaluation).

Table 9.1 Who evaluates what?

Type of evaluation	Brief explanation
Public evaluation	Open evaluation of an activity by others
Private evaluation	Self-evaluation by the person who performed the teaching, for instance
External evaluation	Evaluation by others outside the organisation
Internal evaluation	Evaluation by departments or individuals inside the organisation
Continuous evaluation	Ongoing evaluation
Episodic/intermittent evaluation	Evaluation on set or specific dates
Interim/final evaluation	Evaluation at the end of the main activity or a series of activities
Case-specific evaluation	In-depth evaluation of one particular instance of an activity
Generalised (or holistic) evaluation	Inviting and gaining overall impressions
Analytical evaluation	Detailed evaluation, may include numerical data

Furthermore, evaluation can be quantitative or qualitative, formative or summative, formal or informal. Generally, for new topic areas, qualitative evaluation is likely to elicit data that can enable further development of the topic. For more established topic areas, quantitative data are sought to monitor or ascertain the likely ongoing effectiveness of the activity.

As for formative and summative evaluation, formative evaluation of care is a continuous activity, the frequency of which is adjusted according to the dependency level of the patient/service user, or to the criticality of their condition. With some service users who require longer-term care, or those in the community, evaluation may be recorded at longer intervals at specific set periods. Summative evaluations are conducted at end points, i.e. retrospectively, for example the evaluation of a practice placement experience or a module.

Evaluation is also one of the four stages of the regular development review process of healthcare professionals identified in the NHS KSF (DH, 2004; CIPD, 2021b). The first stage is the joint review of the individual's work against the requirements of the post. This is in the context of the six core dimensions of healthcare work. The second is the personal development planning stage (PDP), the third is the learning and development stage, and the fourth is the evaluation stage. At the evaluation stage, the individual:

- reflects on the effectiveness of their learning and the development of their knowledge and skills
- identifies how their learning has improved the application of their learning to their post
- feeds back to the organisation on how the learning and development can be improved.

In the context of evaluating practice supervision, this chapter addresses all the above aspects of evaluation except evaluation as a research method. Having examined why we need to evaluate practice supervision and practice assessor activities and exactly what evaluation is, it is also important to consider who evaluates before moving on to how practice supervisors evaluate their supervision of practice-based learning.

Who evaluates teaching and learning?

As mentioned earlier, evaluation can take different forms (see Table 9.1). Formative evaluation of practice-based teaching and learning is conducted through informal and formal mechanisms. It is a micro-level evaluation that practice supervisors perform informally when teaching clinical interventions, either in the clinical area or in university settings. It is a valuable internal mechanism for monitoring one's own competence through a continuous process of observation and sensory feedback.

There is also the formal evaluation mechanism that requires more criteria-based evidence to be gathered and then analysed. Formal evaluation mechanisms can reveal patterns of good or poor teaching delivery. These formal evaluation exercises take place periodically and allow scrutiny of the quality of theoretical and clinical learning. For instance, during practice placements, students also engage in a continuous process of informal evaluation of the extent to which the practice setting is also an effective learning environment. Furthermore, evaluation can be conducted by individual professionals, by clinical teams or by the organisation's audit team.

—Reflection point 9.2—

Evaluation of teaching in the practice setting

Who, in your experience, evaluates the effectiveness of teaching, both planned and informal or opportunistic, in health and care settings?

In general, it is the recipient of the teaching, that is, the learner, who is best placed to evaluate the effectiveness of the teaching. The result of the teaching will usually emerge as the knowledge and skill acquired by the learner and is ultimately reflected in the effectiveness and quality of care they deliver to service users. In addition to practice supervisors and practice assessors engaging in self-evaluation or self-monitoring of the quality of their work-based teaching and assessment, quality and effectiveness can also be ascertained through peer evaluation.

Generally, there are at least two parties interested in the quality of a service or education provision: the provider, and the consumer or user (who is, at times, referred to as the customer). The consumers of practice supervision activities are the students on practice placement, and the university whose students' learning they supervise, as well as healthcare service users.

The quality of healthcare courses is of interest to both purchasers and consumers of the provision. Purchasers of education are generally students who directly or indirectly pay course fees. NHS Trusts may be regular purchasers of certain post-registration courses, often when they receive extra funding for registrants to attend specified courses. The quality of courses is also of interest to ward managers and other qualified colleagues, directly enabling students to learn, and who have certain expectations of them during and after the course; it will also interest the public who expect expert professional care.

Therefore, as professional learning takes place in clinical as well as university settings, learning is a tripartite partnership agreement between healthcare providers, education providers and students, to enable learning that ultimately benefits service users' health. Practice supervisors and assessors should seek to have some knowledge of a number of ways in which university-based healthcare education programmes are monitored by external organisations, such as the QAA and the NMC to ascertain the programme's rigour.

Other stakeholders interested in the quality of educational provision are the HEI's internal audit or quality enhancement mechanisms, and, externally, the QAA, the NMC, the HCPC, Ofsted (for apprenticeship programmes) and other relevant regulatory bodies. Other universities who specialise in education in the subject being evaluated might also be involved, usually by invitation.

How Practice Supervisors Evaluate Learning Provision

Having ascertained why we evaluate, what evaluation is and who evaluates, this section explores the different ways in which evaluation is conducted and performed. As noted above, evaluation data can be obtained informally and formally. In general, informal evaluation can be performed by:

- observation of the learner performing care interventions independently
- casual quasi-social conversation
- overhearing casual in-class evaluation

- anecdotal accounts (e.g. from recent students)
- information leaks through the 'grapevine' (the organisation's informal sub-groups) and social media mechanisms.

Formal evaluation can be conducted by student surveys – national or local (i.e. at own university); via module and course evaluation questionnaires; by asking the patient directly about the quality of care they received (maybe asked via an electronic device); and through focus group conversations (see also Table 9.1 regarding who evaluates).

The formal evaluation tools used, however, need to be 'fit for purpose', preferably ones that have already been tested for validity, rather than applying convenient tools that happen to be readily available. 'Fit for purpose' means exactly what the term states, that is, the evaluation mechanism has to be appropriate for the activity being evaluated, and the criteria in the tool must be fully relevant and comprehensive.

Quantitative and qualitative evaluation information can be obtained through the use of structured or semi-structured forms, with a purpose-designed set of questions. Such information can also be obtained through verbal or written means. Teaching sessions in practice settings can be evaluated from a number of viewpoints or conducted in various ways. As an internal evaluation mechanism, the learning supervisor can decide which evaluation tool or model is the most appropriate to gain the necessary information. For various methods of evaluating teaching in practice settings, see the Methods box below.

Methods of Evaluation of Teaching in the Practice Setting

- General brief discussion at the end of the teaching session
- Verbal feedback - requested/volunteered
- Verbal questions and answers
- Feedback from the university, probably through link lecturers or PEFs from the particular module leader
- Feedback from colleagues or peers
- A specific set of questions constituted by the teacher on a returnable sheet of paper
- Observing how other teachers teach the skill
- Self-evaluation/reflection
- Using questionnaire(s), e.g. a placement evaluation questionnaire
- Monitoring whether instructions are being followed
- Directly observing clinical skill performance
- Continuous monitoring of the student's general clinical competence and motivation to learn
- Checking whether objectives are being met
- Reflection/reflective account
- A short multiple-choice-type test
- Discussing achievement/progress with items in the practice assessment document
- Asking the student to teach others, e.g. a patient or junior staff
- Service-user feedback received about the student.

However, evaluation is not always a favoured exercise as, according to Handy (1989), the highest quality service is not always easy to achieve, since it needs the right equipment, the right people and the right environment, which might not always be fully available. It should, however, elicit opinions from all interested parties, and could influence the content and mode of delivery of teaching.

Evaluating learning using models of evaluation

There are several published as well as some internally designed frameworks for evaluation that individuals or organisations can use for evaluating the quality of learning provision systematically. Maxwell's (1984) six elements or dimensions of quality is one of them. The six dimensions are: accessibility, acceptability and appropriateness (3 As) of the teaching; and its efficiency, effectiveness and equity (3 Es).

Healthcare course providers can develop their own criteria using Maxwell's model for the formal evaluation of quality of learning by asking questions related to each of the six dimensions, such as whether the provision was appropriate, and efficient. Yet another useful framework for evaluation which practice supervisors, nurse lecturers and other education facilitators can use to evaluate their learning facilitation, is the popular Donabedian (1988) model of quality assurance, which uses standard statements, and structure, process and outcome criteria, as noted in Chapter 6.

Formal evaluation is also conducted using the regulatory body's (e.g. HCPC) published quality criteria. The education provider that aims and claims to offer a quality service should meet all the pre-set criteria. Some manage to do so explicitly, while others may be at different stages of development. Furthermore, the criteria against which the CQC (2022) reviews care provision sites also constitute the criteria by which decisions are made regarding the suitability of the setting for students' practice placement, such as whether person-centred care is practised, and confidentiality is maintained all the time.

However, an evaluation of professional healthcare courses and modules performed by the university generally uses items under standard headings such as teaching, assessment and feedback, academic support, organisation and management, resources, personal development, and any other comments. An example of evaluation in healthcare is the evaluation of a preceptorship programme by Forde-Johnston (2017), who found that the programme had several benefits for newly qualified nurses and nurse managers, and their feedback on the programme was positive.

Evaluating practice placements

Standards of teaching in practice settings are closely related to the quality of service-user care, to the quality of student supervision and the expertise of practice supervisors. For students' learning experiences during placements, the student may be asked informally at the end of the placement how good and useful they feel that the placement has been, maybe at the same time as the final interview at the end of the placement, or they may be given an evaluation form to complete after the final interview. On returning to university for lectures after the placement, they are asked to complete a practice placement evaluation form, electronically or on paper, along with further verbal evaluation.

The written placement evaluation form asks students to give feedback on various aspects of the experience, such as whether they had adequate preparation for the placement and were given an orientation to the clinical setting on the first day of placement. They may be asked to comment on whether their practice supervisors had been tentatively identified by the tme they started the placement, whether their learning needs and placement objectives were agreed in good time, a range of learning opportunities identified, feedback on performance of clinical skills given, the inter-disciplinary practice supervisors they worked with, and whether evidence-informed, person-centred practice was prevalent. There could also be questions on the amount and nature of personal support available to them.

However, it is noteworthy that since modules and course evaluation have moved from anonymous paper copies to electronic form, the return rates have been very low. Chan et al.'s (2017) study of student evaluations revealed that students are dubious about completing evaluation forms because they indicate that electronic versions contravene anonymity, that is, the university will have some way of identifying which student made negative comments about the specific module or the course.

Evaluation information on the quality of the learning experience is imparted to the placement areas by the university afterwards. Practice supervisors may have obtained qualitative evaluation information from the student prior to the end of the placement. Placement evaluations also form a basis for communication between professionals in practice settings and university lecturers, and an additional benefit of the process is that any further training and development needs of clinical staff can be identified both for more effective clinical care and for more competent practice supervision. Problems reported after the placement are generally investigated by PEFs/CHEFs.

As indicated in Chapter 5 of this book, you are strongly encouraged to take a close look at the latest completed educational audit form for your workplace, which might reassure you that it constitutes an effective clinical learning environment, but also to aid your own ideas about student placement in the setting.

Evaluation of assessments

Practice supervisors generally contribute to student assessment of competencies continuously, and practice assessors perform various episodes of assessment of student competencies during students' practice placements. How are the quality and efficacy of assessments performed by assessors monitored? Practice assessors' professional judgement comes into play to some extent, as they have to be able to justify the decisions they make about each student's competence, in that the responsibility normally lies with the assessor to seek all information relevant to assessments so that their pass/fail decisions are as well-informed as can be.

Furthermore, if a student feels that the result of an assessment was unfair or incorrect, then they can appeal following the appropriate procedures. This is usually only for the conduct of the assessment and any technical or practical hindrances during the assessment, but not against the professional judgement of the practice assessor.

Practice assessors' accountability has a major role to play in ensuring that their own knowledge and competence in assessing students remains up to date, valid and reliable. One reason for this is that individuals can lose their ability to perform most skills and competencies if those skills are not performed over several years, and as Garside and Nhemachena (2013) note, even our qualifications can become meaningless if the knowledge and skills acquired during the education programme are not maintained by periodic updating. Assessors can keep their assessing skills up to date by:

- carrying out discussions on assessor update study days regarding, say, intra-assessor and inter-assessor reliability
- consulting an academic assessor, PEF and/or a senior colleague (e.g. a ward sister).

Ways of achieving intra-assessor reliability were examined in Chapter 8, and grading practice was discussed in Chapters 6 and 8.

ISSUES RELATED TO EVALUATIONS, AND PROFESSIONAL DEVELOPMENT OPPORTUNITIES

Accurate evaluation is a complex skill to acquire, especially if making subsequent changes to the provision is being speculated. It is also, at times, an uncomfortable exercise as it may reveal some unanticipated or perceived flaws, which could depend on the evaluator's own state of mind and general outlook. There might be other biased views stated or some practical problems related to the evaluation of teaching highlighted, and issues around whether the teaching should be clinically based or in university classrooms.

Following on from these observations, the remainder of this chapter explores some of the issues related to evaluations, and the consequences of evaluations, such as practice supervisors' and practice assessors' identifying further learning needs. Practice supervisors and assessors as career-long learners, as well as the utilisation of professional development plans, are also discussed.

As indicated throughout this book, the practice supervision role of health professionals has various facets. Consequently, each facet involves a set of activities in itself which requires relevant knowledge and competence. To ascertain how well each role is being performed, practice supervisors self-monitor their performance and also obtain comments from their students, peers and their own clinical supervisors. How much and how comprehensively do practice supervisors do this, and what do they do with the information obtained?

Mostly, this is not an issue because, as accountable professionals, practice supervisors and practice assessors continually endeavour to rectify any weakness in their performance and knowledge, and strive to improve their practice at all times. However, there can be problems with the evaluation of these roles.

─Reflection point 9.3─

Issues with evaluation

What do you feel are the likely problems associated with the evaluation of practice learning supervision activities?

A possible problem area or danger related to the evaluation of a teaching session (practice or knowledge based) is that the consequent perceived criticisms of one's teaching sessions could be interpreted by the teacher as meaning that they are not quite cut out for teaching. Despite this, teaching is one of the competencies of all qualified nurses and, like many other skills, can be learned and subsequently mastered with ample practice. It is also usually one of the items in healthcare professionals' job description, at times worded as 'contribute to the professional development of other staff'. On self-evaluation of their practice supervision functions, which is also referred to as 'post-hoc evaluation' by Rogers and Horrocks (2010), practice learning supervisors may encounter weaknesses that they may or may not wish to reveal to others, and choose to rectify themselves by trial and error, or by applying published guidance and/or research.

Practice placement evaluations might also highlight serious problems with practice learning supervision and student assessment, as was found by Hamshire et al. (2019), for instance, which might not prove easy to resolve. The practice supervisor needs to be able to differentiate between progress and the levels and speed of attainment by learners. All learners may be making progress, but they could be achieving at different levels, depending on the availability of learning opportunities, their educational background, and the effort and time that they invest in learning. Some of the likely problems of evaluation are as follows:

- Individuals raising and arguing certain points with the aim of influencing peers' opinions.
- Just one incident could colour statements made about the whole placement experience, session or module.
- The teacher may be a perfectionist and may feel very disappointed if any weakness is pointed out.

- Points identified by students might not be seen as positive statements.
- Evaluation comments may be seen as 'some you win, some you lose', with no action taken on the suggested weaknesses.
- The person might genuinely not appreciate the weaknesses pointed out.
- It might occasionally be tricky to be entirely objective when assessing students' work or clinical skill performance.

Evaluative research on student assessment has sporadically identified the problems of students not being fit for practice at the point of registration, because, in the past, assessors had awarded a pass to students on their practice competencies without full evidence of their competence (e.g. Bachmann et al., 2019). Furthermore, it has, at times, been pointed out by universities that students report having been 'under extreme pressure' to achieve competencies due to placement-based issues (Duffin, 2005: 4); and also in relation to student attrition because of negative placement experience (Hamshire et al., 2019).

Recently, the NMC indicated that HEIs/AEIs can allow students to undertake up to 300 of the 2,300 hours of practice learning within simulated learning environments, such as in skills laboratories (RCN, 2021), but also emphasised the need for 'protected time' or 'supported learning time' for the student (NMC, 2018a, 2022b). The learning-by-simulation hours were increased to 600 in 2021, but universities have to make a case to the NMC for this new 'discretionary standard' (NMC, 2021a) (see Chapter 4 for a detailed analysis of learning by simulation).

Students raising concerns related to practice placement

As noted already under 'Evaluating practice placements', on returning to university following a practice placement, and even during placement, students might voice concerns in relation to aspects of the placement. This therefore forms a basis for further communication between university staff and staff in the practice setting, and can result in identifying the need for adjustments to be made.

Students of course should not wait till the end of the placement to raise concerns – they should do so straightaway, and as the NMC (2022c: 6–7, clause 8) indicates, 'The principles (of raising concerns) … apply to student nurses, midwives and nursing associates in the same way that they apply to registered nurses, midwives and nursing associates'. Examples of issues that might cause concern include neglect of service users and acts of omission, physical or psychological abuse, and discriminatory abuse (NMC, 2022c: 2). However, when a disagreement situation occurs, this can sometimes be due to misunderstandings between the two parties or to deficient communication.

Furthermore, dedicating just a few minutes to identify the various avenues or media, informal and formal, that students are likely to use to express their dissatisfaction or concerns, reveals several powerful ways of doing so, but there are also some misleading ways. It may well be that students, at times, just 'have a moan' with their close friends with regard to what they were unhappy about in relation to the placement, and the matter goes no further. Alternatively, students can report their concerns through various channels, such as:

- directly to those whose practice they are not content with
- at workshops for students held by PEFs during the placement
- at post-placement evaluation, as already mentioned
- to their university personal tutor or link lecturer
- through the Student Union department at the university
- at organised termly student forums at the university.

Some students even resort to social media (such as Facebook), which is widely discouraged by universities. Others may even venture to mention their concerns at QAA or NMC periodic reviews when students are invited to meet reviewers to comment on their programme of study. The NMC (2018d: 6, clause 1.5) re-emphasises the point that students should be encouraged and supported to raise concerns or complaints 'without fear of adverse consequences'.

The NMC (2022c) publication *Raising Concerns* and the HCPC's (2016) code (standards of conduct) provide guidance for qualified nurses and midwives on raising concerns, albeit at the level of broad principles that can be applied as felt appropriate in each situation. They also include information on legal protection for whistleblowers and information on organisations that nurses and midwives can go to for further advice.

In a review of 23 research papers on support for health professionals who raise concerns related to quality of care, Milligan et al. (2017) deduced that students are fully aware of the need to report concerns, but they fear there could be negative repercussions for their practice assessment results if they do so, especially as they are unclear about how, when and to whom students should report.

As just indicated, an evaluation of practice supervision activities might highlight areas that are problematic and warrant further learning. The practice supervisor also has a duty to be up to date in all aspects of practice learning supervision. Thus, of necessity, practice supervisors have to engage in ongoing updating and in new learning in relation to their day-to-day work duties.

Updates for practice supervisors and assessors

Update sessions for practice supervisors and assessors provide them with the opportunity to meet and explore learning supervision and assessment issues with other supervisors and assessors (face to face or online), and to explore as a group the validity and reliability of judgements made when assessing practice in challenging circumstances.

━━━━━━━━━━ **ACTION** POINT 9.5 ━━━━━━━━━━

Updating for practice learning supervisors and assessors

Think about how you keep yourself up to date with new developments in professional knowledge in relation to the supervision of learning and student assessment. Discuss this with a colleague or with your own clinical supervisor.

Which areas would practice supervisors and assessors themselves wish to see covered in the update sessions?

Practice learning supervisors' and assessors' update events are usually one-day or half-day events, conducted by PEFs/CHEFs usually within the healthcare trust premises. At the update sessions, issues related to the reliability and validity of assessments should also be discussed so that a certain level of parity is achieved in the locality or, better still, examined in small-group workshops, which could include group activities, to explore the exact ways in which intra- and inter-assessor reliability is achieved and monitored. Previous NMC (2008) suggestions for activities to be addressed in update sessions include:

- ensuring knowledge of current NMC-approved programmes
- the opportunity to discuss issues related to the supervision of practice-based learning
- the assessment of competence and fitness for safe and effective practice
- discussion on issues, which may include exploring the support mechanisms available for dealing with under-achieving students
- any new NMC rules and guidelines related to supervision of learning and student assessment in practice, and their implications.

Alternatively, NHS Education for Scotland (2019: 4–5) indicates that both preparation programmes and updates tend to be 'available, delivered and supported by key persons in both practice and education environments ... (but) will be flexible and designed to meet the needs of (individual) practice supervisors from various professions and those practice supervisors supporting different student groups'. Both preparation and update can include, for example:

- details of the pre- or post-registration programme the supervisor will be supporting students for
- information in relation to the practice supervisor's contribution to the student's PAD
- the relationship between the roles of the practice supervisor, practice assessor and academic assessor – for all programmes for which the supervisor is supporting students.

In addition to continuing learning for revalidation purposes and for updating one's knowledge related to practice supervisor and assessor duties, which are essentially for keeping one's registration and employment, registrants are often also career-long learners and lifelong learners. Career-long learning can develop into more management posts, or towards specialist or advanced practice roles. Lifelong learning, however, extrapolates beyond the day-to-day duties and is about personal aspirations for their profession and for themselves, that is, career-cum-leisure pursuits. The NMC (2018d: 9) asserts that students should be empowered and supported to become resilient and reflective lifelong learners who are capable of effective inter-agency team-working.

Consequently, lifelong learning is more about a state of mind and about professionalism, that is, about always seeking improvement or enhancement in care delivery for service users. There are several reasons for healthcare professionals being lifelong learners, including increasing technological advances in treatment and care, and more person-centred and values-based approaches to care. The characteristics of lifelong learners include:

- a positive view of the value of learning
- good self-management skills, such as being well organised and managing time effectively
- knowing when and how to seek help and when to collaborate with peers
- the motivation to learn, self-knowledge, self-confidence and persistence
- having positive feelings about themselves as learners
- the ability to manage their feelings during the highs and lows of learning
- the ability to apply a set of learning strategies (e.g. when to dedicate time to study and where to learn).

Other known characteristics can be added to the above list such as external motivators and situational support. Additional characteristics such as enjoying learning, being reflective, asking questions and tracking down answers, were identified from research into lifelong learning by Davis et al. (2014). The learning activity undertaken is of course also based on self-assessment, and members of healthcare professions need to be responsible for identifying their own learning needs, maybe at appraisal sessions or during clinical supervision sessions.

Continuing Learning For Practice Supervisors and Assessors

Healthcare professionals having to continue to develop their own knowledge and competence is a statutory requirement; and as the NMC (2018d: 11) states, 'all educators and assessors (must) act as professional role models at all times'. Career development avenues for healthcare professionals have been identified, for example, by the Welsh Assembly Government (2009); and the likely progression of teaching roles may develop, as illustrated in Figure 9.1.

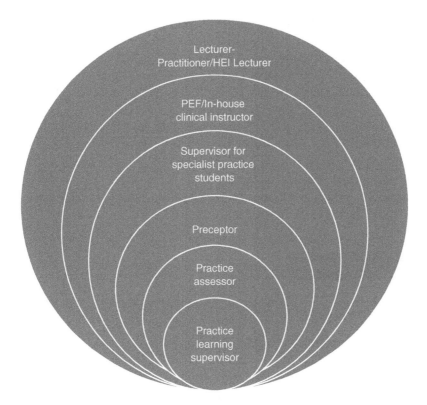

Figure 9.1 Progressive development of the registrant's teaching role

Intercalated between these teaching positions are likely to be other education facilitation and assessor of competence titles, such as clinical instructor, clinical education coordinator and practice educator. These various teaching and assessing duties require our own ongoing professional development, and the NMC (2018a: 10, clause 8.2) indicates that assessors should 'receive ongoing support and training to reflect and develop in their role', which can often also be achieved by self-directed, practice-related, career-long learning.

The practice supervisor may be required to take on the preceptor role for new registrants, and to oversee the clinical learning of those who are new to the clinical specialism or the practice setting (the preceptor role was discussed in some detail in Chapter 1). They might benefit from the availability of clinical supervision.

Practice supervisors and assessors may also be required to assess competence for RNs on post-qualifying clinical short courses. Naturally, they will need to hold the same post-qualifying short-course qualification themselves in the first place. However, to facilitate learning and assess students on postgraduate specialist or advanced practice educational programmes, they will need to hold the particular specialist or advanced practice qualification and/or proven expertise themselves, as well as having kept up to date with the latest developments in all aspects of their post.

Furthermore, self-evaluation, along with personal research and clinical audits, can highlight issues that may present opportunities for further development for practice supervisors and assessors.

Regarding the development of specialist practitioners, however, research conducted by Barton (2006) on the experiences of doctors supervising learning for students on nurse practitioner courses, concluded that medical clinical educators experience conflict in that, as the students acquire new clinical skills and roles, this also amounts to the supervisors feeling that their traditional medical authority is being challenged. This has led to a renegotiation of professional boundaries between nurse practitioners and doctors.

Case Study 9.1 is a brief account of a registrant who progressed from being a new NMC registrant to becoming a university lecturer just a few years later.

—Case study 9.1—

Career progression from practice learning supervisor to nurse lecturer

Straight after qualifying as an RN, Ellie took up a post as a community nurse as she felt that in the community setting, she would be in a better position to provide holistic care, see patients' health improve in their own home setting, and also advise on preventing health problems recurring. This in turn enabled Ellie to build good relationships with patients and families, and therefore Ellie felt it was a very rewarding job.

Ellie had achieved good marks in her course assignments during her pre-registration course, and felt that overall she had enjoyed her course. Students are regularly on practice placement with the community team, and Ellie has enjoyed teaching all about how to provide person-centred care for service users safely and effectively in their own home. During a conversation with the community PEF, Ellie found out that the partner university was receptive to practitioners coming to teach specific clinical skills to student nurses in the university setting periodically, for a few pre-agreed hours.

Approximately three years after qualifying, Ellie negotiated with the university to participate in co-teaching manual blood pressure measuring skills in the university's skills laboratory. Despite some initial anxiety, Ellie realised that she enjoyed imparting this clinical skill to student nurses in the university setting as well. On further taking up such opportunities related to other clinical skills, Ellie later acquired a post as a lecturer-practitioner at the university, and soon secured a place on the postgraduate certificate in higher education course. Eighteen months after her successful completion of the course, Ellie took up an appointment as a lecturer in clinical practice and simulation at a UK university's Faculty of Health, and is loving the experience, and is also hoping to engage in research on simulation-based education in the very near future, as well as completing a Master's degree in the same field.

In relation to healthcare professionals' own ongoing professional development, a brief overview of what continuing professional development (CPD) and career-long learning entail is provided next in this chapter, and is followed by a brief on specific CPD requirements for revalidation.

Continuing professional development and revalidation requirements

Continuing professional development, as the term implies, signifies the continuing learning (development) that professionals engage in throughout their careers, and is defined by the HCPC (2018: 1) as 'the way in which registrants continue to learn and develop throughout their careers so they keep their skills and knowledge up-to-date and are able to practise safely and effectively'. The definition emphasises that continuing learning eventually benefits service users. However, CPD for healthcare professionals is also an inherent component of lifelong learning, a state of mind, and an attitude that requires personal decision-making by responsible individuals, proactive planning and the taking of action.

Furthermore, CPD is a term associated with adult learning (i.e. not children), and usually refers to learning by professionals after the point of qualification and registration with an appropriate national representative body. Organisations tend to implement one or other of two main approaches to CPD: the sanction model or the benefit model. The sanction model of CPD implies that if the required learning is not taken by the employee, then there may be some penalty involved for the individual for not engaging in the work-related learning.

The sanction model furthermore comprises of two sub-types of CPD: statutory and mandatory. While there is some overlap between statutory and mandatory learning, statutory CPD is that which is undertaken as a result of statute or legislation. Mandatory CPD has a similar meaning, in that it is instigated by employing organisations, and employees are required to complete them. Mandatory CPD is therefore based on a mandate by employers or national bodies which has to be executed but no penalty is attached immediately to the individual if not fulfilled. In summary, 'Statutory training is required by law, and mandatory training is determined by the organisation – based on local risk assessments and training needs analysis' (LearnPac Systems UK, 2020: 9).

The benefit model of CPD, on the other hand, does not threaten employees with sanctions but reinforces and, where possible, rewards individuals for self-directed or voluntary learning, or for the uptake of recommended or suggested CPD. With self-directed CPD, the individual has choices, as self-directed continuing learning can take diverse forms that suit individuals personally, and is not time-bound. It is intentional learning as well as incidental learning in healthcare settings, and includes experiential learning combined with self-reflection, and peer-supported discussion where available (see the illustration in Figure 9.2).

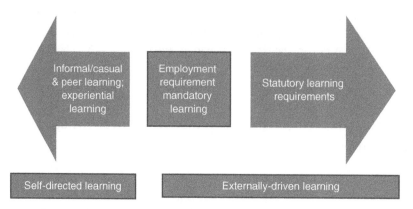

Figure 9.2   Spectrum of career-long continuing learning

In this context, research reveals that although learning needs are often identified through appraisal and personal development planning, it is CPD based on the 'individual personal drive and enthusiasm of practitioners' that results in contributing to implementing change in clinical practice more effectively, while change that is policy-driven or is a national health target is less easily achieved (Lee, 2011: 390). The finding is supported further as 'practitioner driven CPD' in healthcare is found to be effective within organisations that support and facilitate workplace learning and effective organisational learning cultures (Manley et al., 2018: 134), for example.

Employment-required mandatory learning is to some extent personal to the employee, in that if they do not fulfil this learning they may be urged to do so via reminders from line managers or the personnel department (e.g. fire safety, manual handling, CPR training; teaching peer observation for lecturers). The statutory learning requirement is a national requirement for all those registered with a regulatory body, such as professional revalidation, and if not adhered to by the cut-off date then the individual loses the title (e.g. Registered Nurse) and their right to practise under that title. Both mandatory and statutory learning can be accessed in the workplace, possibly in the in-service training department, and certain components can be completed by online learning and assessment.

Another perspective on CPD is that care practitioners should be able to 'demonstrate maintenance of competence' or continuing clinical competence, as noted by Hegarty (2017), and this has already been implemented in other countries. The concept extends the notion of CPD to practitioners specifically being able to prove their competence when required, whether it is by spot-check or a supervision requirement.

Numerous healthcare reports and problematic incidents indicate that healthcare registrants need to be receptive to new learning all the time (e.g. Francis, 2013). Continuing learning is also a feature of healthcare professionalism, which has been converted into policy and requirements by healthcare regulatory bodies (e.g. GMC), and is known as revalidation. Revalidation has become a requirement for different professions at different times, and for nurses and midwives from April 2016, and it has replaced the previous requirement for the renewal of healthcare professionals' registration.

Revalidation requirements for registrants

One instance of the statutory model of CPD is the revalidation requirement for healthcare professionals across the UK and other countries; the sanction for not fulfilling this requirement being the loss of registration with the regulatory body, and therefore loss of employment in that capacity. The NMC (2021c), for instance, indicates that to meet revalidation requirements, every practising nurse, midwife and nursing associate must have evidence of having undertaken a minimum of 35 hours of CPD, among other requirements, that is relevant to their practice during every three-year cycle, to be able to renew their registration. The registrant must also have worked in some capacity by virtue of their professional qualification during the previous three years for a minimum of 450 hours. The GMC and the HCPC have similar requirements.

The NMC (2021c: 1) indicates that 'Revalidation is about promoting good practice, as well as strengthening public confidence in the nursing and midwifery professions' ... [because it] helps to encourage a culture of sharing, reflection and improvement' and provides benefits for the nurse, midwife or nursing associate as well as for service users. Indeed, the NMC's (2018b: 20, clause 22.3) code of professional standards states that registrants must 'keep your knowledge and skills up to date, taking part in appropriate and regular learning and professional development activities that aim to maintain and develop your competence and improve your performance'.

Despite revalidation being a statutory requirement, it is also reasonable to expect healthcare professionals to take a planned career route, or a rewarding vocation, by continually ensuring that their practice is evidence-informed, and of the safest and highest quality that they can provide. CPD thus reflects a proactive and responsible approach to one's own professional learning and practice-related research (with a small r or a big R). It thereby also involves an attitude to life and work that allows for creativity in one's professional activities.

The CPD for meeting revalidation requirements has to be in relevant areas of practice and can be in one or more of the key components of healthcare interventions, aptly categorised in the NHS KSF (DH, 2004; CIPD, 2021b) under six core dimensions – as noted in Chapter 6 – and applying to all NHS employees (except doctors, dentists and some board-level managers). More specific details on each of these dimensions of healthcare interventions can be found in the NHS KSF document.

For revalidation however, registrants are required by the NMC, HCPC, GMC and other regulatory bodies to accumulate evidence of having engaged in a predetermined minimum number of hours of learning activity over a specified period of time for revalidation purposes. The 35 hours of CPD advocated by the NMC is the minimum requirement for safe and effective practice, but it is recognised that the practitioner generally engages in substantially more learning than this minimum.

Despite revalidation being a statutory requirement, there is substantial scope for self-directed learning in that the topic areas and the areas of professional practice updating can be entirely self-chosen by the registrant, as long as the 35 hours include 20 hours of participatory learning. Relevant university-based courses may meet quite a few of the NMC requirements, but for most registrants, learning from short courses (in-house or at external venues), practice-related training, workshops, attending conferences for updating knowledge, based on either self-directed or peer learning, can all easily contribute to these requirements. Self-directed learning is explained in detail in Chapter 2 under andragogy and the work of Knowles (2020) and Rogers and Horrocks (2010). Peer learning is also well documented, in particular in the context of human and social capital (see, for instance, Gopee, 2002).

Many healthcare trusts periodically offer workshops for their employees to facilitate the building and presentation of portfolio evidence of their updated clinical practice and of their supervision of practice-based learning activities, that in turn contributes to meeting revalidation requirements. In such workshops, attendees can work in groups to identify a range of activities that comprise items that are pertinent evidence of learning activities. Evidence may also include the achievement of annual performance review or personal development plan (PDP) objectives, evaluation or feedback from any related presentations (in-house, or at local or national conferences), any EBP initiative implemented or disseminated, and incidental learning.

To revalidate with the NMC, registrants have to provide evidence of continuing learning every three years (in addition to paying an annual fee to the NMC) by compiling the following:

1.   450 practice hours or 900 hours if revalidating two registrations, e.g. as both nurse and midwife
2.   35 hours of CPD (including 20 hours of participatory learning)
3.   Five pieces of practice-related feedback
4.   Five written reflective accounts
5.   Reflective discussion
6.   Health and character declaration
7.   Professional indemnity arrangement
8.   Confirmation.

Each item of evidence has to be cross-referenced against themes of the NMC's (2018b) code of practice. Practice supervisors also have to meet revalidation requirements, and, when appropriate, facilitate other registrants to meet theirs, and some of the learning can occur at update sessions for practice learning supervisors and assessors. Both the NMC and subsequent publications in professional journals elaborate on ways in which revalidation requirements can be met (e.g. Middleton and Llewellyn, 2016). For ample details on the ways in which revalidation requirements can be met, see 'Revalidation' on the NMC's or HCPC's website.

Organisational support for continuing learning

Usually, all university–healthcare trust partnerships already have an infrastructure of support for professionals in supervisory or assessment roles, usually from PEFs/

CHEFs, placement co-ordinators, and academic assessors. Such support implies a network of personnel and other resources that can be accessed to discuss, or to reflect on, the decisions that they are about to make on their student's performance of clinical skills, or to consult. Support is also available from peers and colleagues within their practice setting or department, and also from link lecturers and the student's personal tutor, which invariably results in further learning. Further support can be gained through professional networks, some of which are formed informally at conferences, and when exploring issues at regular update sessions, followed by self-reflection.

Clinical supervision is another mechanism that practice supervisors and assessors can draw on for regular structured support and for identifying learning needs. However, one of the key sources of such support for continuing learning is the study days and workshops that the PEF team offers.

Funding might also be available for registrants to undertake CPD related to their employment, although such funding is usually meagre. Health Education England is the organisation that has taken responsibility for the education, training and CPD of healthcare staff since April 2013, and spends more than £4 billion a year (HEE, 2022e) on a range of education and training activities, working with NHS Trusts and education providers (e.g. HEIs). Therefore, HEE funding might be available to support your career aspirations.

Health Education England thereby supports a few undergraduate programmes (e.g. trainee nursing associates and undergraduate medical placements), but mostly it funds post-registration programmes such as advanced practitioners, community specialist practitioners and mental health specialists (HEE, 2022e). It also supports funding for workforce development in relation to the 42 ICSs (Integrated Care Systems) that constitute the very recent organisational methods of providing healthcare in England.

Reflections on practice learning supervision

Teaching transforms careers and lives. Practice learning supervision duties give you the opportunity and permission to teach and impart your knowledge and care intervention skills to learners and colleagues. It is a career-long journey, whether it's to do with facilitating learning for learners of our own healthcare profession, of allied health professions, medical students, nursing associates or healthcare assistants. It is a journey that begins from the time you are a preceptee.

One of the strengths of most healthcare professions is the holistic approach that professionals intend, endeavour and usually succeed in taking in their day-to-day practice. Some clinical settings have students all the time, others occasionally but they always have learners, and the actions that learning supervisors take stay in the minds of learners for several years afterwards, as they shape their careers and quality of care for service users. The practice learning supervisor's actions are therefore seminal in shaping the attitudes of practitioners for years to come.

On the other hand, as Rogers and Freiberg (1994: 375) indicate, 'not all journeys are trouble-free ... but the process alone makes us a bit wiser. Gaining wisdom comes not with time or age, but from living the challenges of life, learning from any mistakes we make, and building on experiences'. This book on supervision of learning was designed to achieve the objectives outlined in the introductory section, which are predominantly to examine the knowledge and understanding necessary for supervising learners' learning and assessing their practice competencies. A precondition to these is effective and safe, evidence-informed, person-centred practice as well as effective leadership by registrants.

The knowledge and skills that you develop can be built upon by further pursuing opportunities for imparting knowledge and skills. They could play a significant role along your career path, be it as a much more senior clinical practitioner or in a part- or full-time educational role. What are the next steps that you will take to facilitate and supervise learning as you further develop your expertise by seizing the multifarious opportunities that will come your way from now on?

Personal development plans

Systematic CPD and career-long learning for health and care professionals can be further effectively supported through the utilisation of personal development plans (PDPs), as have been advocated for a number of years in the UK through key NHS and education policy documents such as *The Dearing Report* (NCIHE, 1997), the NHS KSF (DH, 2004; CIPD, 2021b) and PDP guidance (QAA, 2009). The NHS KSF advocates the use of PDPs by all NHS healthcare professionals for their professional development throughout their careers. Other than education and health policies, influential writers on self- and staff management such as Lancer et al. (2016) also advocate the use of PDPs.

PDPs provide individuals with the opportunity to focus attention on their career aspirations and are a mechanism for recording and reviewing career decisions periodically. However, PDPs should not be part of the performance and development review (or appraisal) process, which is a managerial activity more focused on work productivity. They are however powerful agreements that can be stored locally, or preferably by the employee only (i.e. they are not centrally recorded). PDPs are nevertheless also a component of effective learning organisations (a concept discussed in Chapter 5).

A PDP is also often an NMC requirement for reinstatement to the professional register where a registrant's competence has been in question, and it suggests that, in future, PDPs can be easily linked to revalidation. However, a PDP is not a punitive activity, as it can be beneficially utilised in conjunction with annual development and performance reviews. It is feasible to implement PDPs so that they are discussed as part of annual development reviews, with only an agreed selection of objectives being incorporated into the performance review and the remaining PDP objectives being supported by clinical supervision.

Template 9.1 A professional development plan

Name: .... **[Other relevant details, e.g. clinical supervisor's name]**

Objective and development need/interest	Relevant dimension of my work and career	Hours required and date objective to be achieved	What will I do to achieve this development need/interest? Resources and support required	How will I apply this learning to my work?	How will I know I have completed the development activity successfully?	How will I share this learning with relevant others?
1. Establish supported learning time for practice supervision	Teaching learners	One hour every week, achieve throughout the student's practice placement	Duty roster planned in advance. Team members aware. Two alternative protected times identified each week	Spend the protected time focusing on practice supervision activities. Monitor and record use of protected time	An appropriate record of practice supervision activities	Item on team meeting agenda. Present at local conference
2. Develop teaching skills in in-house short courses	.....	.....	.....	.....	.....	.....

The QAA (2009: 2) defines a PDP as 'a structured and supported process undertaken by a learner to reflect upon their own learning, performance and/or achievement and to plan for their personal, educational and career development'. Thus, PDPs can be separated as either personal or professional development, except that for most individuals these two components are either intertwined or experienced on a continuum in day-to-day activities. An example of a PDP for practice supervisors – which has been constructed from prevailing guidance and other literature on the topic, and can be constituted in landscape or portrait format – is presented as template 9.1.

The two development needs mentioned in Template 9.1 are part of the education component of nurses' and midwives' roles, other components being clinical practice, research and management, as noted at the beginning of Chapter 3. Various components of required knowledge and competence can be acquired through in-house and in-service training, but for paid time for study, funding and support from managers for HEI-based courses, this can be an issue (RCN, 2012 [Willis Report]) and therefore needs forward planning.

Chapter Summary

This chapter has provided a comprehensive analysis of the evaluation of practice supervisor and assessor activities, and of continuing learning requirements, and having completed this chapter you have explored:

- Why we should evaluate the effectiveness with which practice supervisors facilitate learning and engage in continuous assessment, while they also fulfil their other duties.
- What evaluation is, i.e. the nature and various aspects of evaluation, and who evaluates the practice supervisor's teaching activities.
- Different ways of evaluating clinically based and academically based teaching and assessment; and how practice supervisors evaluate learning provision and assessments during practice placements. The use of models of evaluation, including heeding the findings of audits by external organisations such as the QAA and the NMC.
- The likely problems of evaluation, the results of evaluations, issues ensuing from them, the related consequences and the subsequent actions that can be taken.
- The opportunities and scope for ongoing learning arising from the results of evaluations, practice learning for RNs on specialist practice courses, and the requirement for CPD in one's practice supervisor role, ways of meeting NMC revalidation requirements, as well as practice supervisors as lifelong learners.

Further Optional Reading

1. For a current textbook explaining learning supervision, see:

    - Johnson, E.A. (2017) *Working Together in Clinical Supervision: A Guide for Supervisors and Supervisees*. New York: Momentum Press Health.

2. For more details on HEE funding for healthcare professionals' CPD and for some undergraduate programmes, see:

    - Health Education England (2022e) *NHS Education Funding Guide 2020–2021 Financial Year*. Available at: www.hee.nhs.uk/our-work/education-funding-reform/nhs-education-funding-guide (accessed 2 June 2021).

GLOSSARY

Academic assessor Assigned to collate and confirm the student's achievement of proficiencies and programme outcomes for each part / year of the programme; works closely with practice assessors

Academic link lecturer A university lecturer who singly or as part of a team of lecturers is the named academic contact who staff in specific practice settings can contact for information, clarification, etc., about student matters

Andragogy An approach to teaching adults that is different from teaching children and adolescents whereby the teacher takes a facilitator of learning role, rather than being an authoritarian who has all the knowledge and the answers to all issues

Clinical (or care) intervention Any action taken by healthcare professionals to improve the health of patients or service users, or to enhance their health and prevent health problems

Clinical learning environment (CLE) The practice setting as an environment where learning is valued and encouraged, and occurs among staff and students, alongside safe and effective care delivery; the term is used interchangeably with 'practice learning environment'

Collaborative Learning in Practice (CLiP) A novel model of nursing and midwifery practice learning supervision, whereby the identified clinical educator supports, coaches and mentors learners, and is available to actively contribute to the ward learning environment; and also acts as a source of expert advice in such circumstances as when students are struggling to pass their practice competencies

Competency The skill and associated practical knowledge required to perform a clinical intervention

Educational audit An audit that is normally conducted jointly by senior staff in a practice setting and a university academic to ensure the practice setting is suitable for healthcare students' practice placement as part of their professional learning

Ethical competence Refers to the ability of the healthcare professional to deliver safe and effective care that is based on full accountability, and whose practice and social behaviour are based on the principles of ethics and on moral values such as doing good, demonstrating respect for human rights and dignity, etc.

Evidence-based practice (EBP) Practice that is based on evidence, which can be research evidence

Facilitation of learning An idea that is different from the term teaching in that it signifies a practice-based teacher or lecturer structuring activities that enable students to learn by themselves, as individuals or in groups. The concept can be applied to acquiring the required healthcare knowledge base, as well as to clinical competencies

Forcefield analysis An analysis that applies to a proposed change, and entails identifying the factors that are indicating the need for the change, and also factors that are hindering the implementation of the change

Haptic gloves A wearable device that stimulates tactile sensation of virtual objects allowing the user to experience realistic human touch in a computer-generated scene or surgical intervention

Healthcare organisations NHS Acute Trusts, primary care, private hospitals, nursing homes, day care settings, etc., involved in the provision of care and treatment

Healthcare provider A healthcare organisation in the public or independent sector that directly provides care and treatment to individuals with health problems

Informal learning Learning that occurs ad hoc, often based on seizing learning opportunities as they arise

Learning pathway A structured plan of learning based on patients' or service users' journeys through health and/or social care

Neurodiversity An individual can claim to be neurodivergent if their brain works differently from the average (neurotypical) person, and therefore have diverse ways of thinking, learning, processing information, communicating, etc., for example someone with autism

Person-centred care Is an approach to practice that is holistic and underpinned by such values as respect for the person, for individuals' rights, and a culture of empowerment for the patient

Practice assessor A healthcare professional who is assigned for the conduct of students' practice assessments to confirm student achievement of practice objectives and proficiencies, and whose assessment decisions are also informed by comments sought and received from practice supervisors

Practice learning Learning that occurs during practice placements

Practice setting Any NHS or independent sector setting where health and/or social care is provided in accordance with Department of Health and Social Care guidelines

Practice supervisor A registered health or social care professional who supports and supervises learning in practice in line with their competence (also referred to as practice learning supervisor in this textbook)

Preceptorship A role allocated to an appropriately qualified and experienced healthcare professional for the supervision of the professional development of a newly qualified registrant in the practice setting

Pre-registration A term used interchangeably with pre-qualifying and pre-licensure professional education to signify health or social care profession students' education programmes that lead to students becoming eligible to have their names entered on the NMC or HCPC professional registers

Registrants Refers predominantly to qualified healthcare professionals on either the NMC or the HCPC professional register

Regulatory body Organisations such as the HCPC, GMC, NMC, etc., who hold the register of all profession-specific registrants who can legitimately practise with their professional title in the UK

Supernumerary status Health profession students are deemed supernumerary if they are not part of the paid workforce in a practice setting, but are expected to engage in learning healthcare knowledge and skills by participating in the care of patients or service users

Task trainers Are specialised simulators or lifelike models of human anatomy designed to help learners practise a specific skill; these devices are designed to teach competency-based and procedural skills such as airway management, naso-gastric tube placement, lumbar puncture and IV procedures

Theoretical knowledge Stands for background knowledge that is necessary for a deeper understanding of rationales/reasons for specific clinical interventions

REFERENCES

Abulebda, K., Auerbach, M. and Limaiem, F. (2022) Debriefing techniques utilized in medical simulation. In: *StatPearls*. StatPearls Publishing, Treasure Island (FL). Available at: https://pubmed.ncbi.nlm.nih.gov/31536266 (accessed 30 June 2022).

Academy of Medical Royal Colleges (2017) *Joint Professions' Statement*. Available at: www.aomrc.org.uk/statements/joint-professions-statement (accessed 14 June 2022).

Adelman-Mullally, T., Mulder, C.K., McCarter-Spalding, D.E., Hagler, D.A., Gaberson, K.B., Hanner, M.B., Oermann, M.H., Speakman, E.T., Yoder-Wise, P.S. and Young, P.K. (2013) 'The clinical nurse educator as leader', *Nurse Education in Practice*, *13*(1): 29–34.

Advance HE (2020) *Equality Act 2010: Implications for Colleges and HEIs*. Available at: www.advance-he.ac.uk/knowledge-hub/equality-act-2010-implications-colleges-and-heis-revised (accessed 20 June 2022).

Agnew, T. (2018) 'New Standards will prepare students for the rigours of modern nursing', *Nursing Standard*, *33*(1): 14–17.

Akhnif, E., Macq, J. and Meessen, B. (2017) 'Scoping literature review on the Learning Organisation concept as applied to the health system', *Health Research Policy and Systems*, *15*(16): 1–12.

Amy, A.H. (2008) 'Leaders as facilitators of individual and organizational learning', *Leadership & Organizational Development*, *29*(3): 212–234.

An, D. and Carr, M. (2017) 'Learning styles theory fails to explain learning and achievement: Recommendations for alternative approaches', *Personality and Individual Differences*, *116*: 410–416.

Anderson, A., Cant, R. and Hood, K. (2014) 'Measuring students' perceptions of inter-professional clinical placements: Development of the Inter-professional Clinical Placement Learning Environment Inventory', *Nurse Education in Practice*, *14*(5): 518–524.

Anderson, E.E. (2009) 'Learning pathways in contemporary primary care settings – student nurses' views', *Nurse Education Today*, *29*(8): 835–839.

Anderson, L.W., Krathwohl, D.R. and Airasian, P.W. (2014) *A Taxonomy for Learning, Teaching, and Assessing: A Revision of Bloom's Taxonomy of Educational Objectives*. Harlow: Pearson Education.

Andre, K. (2000) 'Grading student clinical practice performance: The Australian perspective', *Nurse Education Today*, *20*(8): 672–679.

Andrews, A. and St Aubyn, B. (2015) 'If it's not written down; it didn't happen…'. *Journal of Clinical Nursing, 29*(5): 20–22.

Argyle, M. (1994) *The Psychology of Interpersonal Behaviour,* 5th edn. London: Penguin.

Ashenafi, M.M. (2017) 'Peer-assessment in higher education: Twenty-first-century practices, challenges and the way forward', *Assessment & Evaluation in Higher Education, 42*(2): 226–251.

Ausubel, D., Novak, J. and Hanesian, H. (1978) *Educational Psychology: A Cognitive View.* New York: Rinehart & Winston.

Axley, L. (2008) 'Competency: a concept analysis'. *Nursing Forum, 43*(4): 214–222.

Bachmann, L., Groenvik, C.K.U., Hauge, K.W. and Julnes, S. (2019) 'Failing to Fail nursing students among mentors: A confirmatory factor analysis of the Failing to Fail scale'. *Nursing Open, 6*(3): 966–973.

Baillie, L. and Fish, J. (2021) 'An evaluation of a unified practice assessment document for student nurses: Students', mentors' and academics' views and experiences', *Journal of Practice Teaching and Learning, 18*(1–2): 24–37.

Ballantyne, H. (2017) 'Undertaking effective handovers in the healthcare setting', *Nursing Standard, 31*(45): 53–61.

Bandura, A. (1996) *Social Learning Theory.* Harlow, UK: Pearson.

Barnett, J.E. (2008) 'Mentoring, boundaries, and multiple relationships: Opportunities and challenges', *Mentoring & Tutoring: Partnership in Learning, 16*(1): 3–16.

Baron, S. (2009) 'Evaluating the patient journey approach to ensure health care is centred on patients', *Nursing Times, 105*(22): 20–23.

Barr, H. (2003) 'Inter-professional issues and work-based learning', in J. Burton and N. Jackson (eds), *Work-Based Learning in Primary Care.* Oxford: Radcliffe Medical.

Barron, A.B., Hebets, E.A., Cleland, T.A., Fitzpatrick, C.L. and Hauber, M.E. (2015) Embracing multiple definitions of learning. *Trend in Neurosciences, 38*(7): 405–407.

Barton, T.D. (2006) 'Clinical mentoring of nurse practitioners: The doctors' experience'. *British Journal of Nursing, 15*(15): 820–824.

Bear, S. and Jones, G. (2017) 'Students as protégés – factors that lead to success', *Journal of Management Education, 41*(1): 146–168.

Beck, S., Ruhnke, B., Issleib, M., Daubmann, A., Harendza, S. and Zollner, C. (2016) Analyses of inter-rater reliability between professionals, medical students and trained school children as assessors of basic life support skills. *BMC Medical Education, 16*(2016): 1–8.

Benner, P. (2001) *From Novice to Expert: Excellence and Power in Clinical Nursing Practice.* London: Addison-Wesley.

Bennett, S., Mohr, J., Deal, K.H. and Hwang, J. (2012) 'Supervisor attachment, supervisory working alliance, and affect in social work field instruction'. *Research on Social Work Practice, 23*(2): 199–209.

Berger, P. and Luckmann, T. (1967) *The Social Construction of Reality.* Middlesex: Penguin Books.

Bergsteiner, H., Avery, G.C. and Neumann, R. (2010) 'Kolb's experiential learning model: Critique from a modelling perspective', *Studies in Continuing Education*, *32*(1): 29–46.

Biggs, J. and Tang, C. (2022) *Teaching for Quality Learning at University*, 5th edn. Maidenhead: Open University Press.

Bijol, V., Byrne-Dugan, C.J. and Hoenig, M.P. (2015) 'Medical student web-based formative assessment tool for renal pathology', *Medical Education Online*, *20*(1): 26765.

Bloom, B. (ed.) (1956) *Taxonomy of Educational Objectives: The Classification of Educational Goals, Handbook One: Cognitive Domain*. London: Longman.

Boitel, C.R. and Fromm, L.R. (2014) 'Defining signature pedagogy in social work education: Learning theory and the learning contract', *Journal of Social Work Education*, *50*(4): 608–622.

Bondy, K.N. (1983) 'Criterion-referenced definitions for rating scales in clinical evaluation', *Journal of Nursing Education*, *22*(9): 376–382.

Boud, D. (2016) *Enhancing Learning through Self-assessment*. London: Routledge.

Bray, L., O'Brien, M.R., Kirton, J., Zubairu, K. and Christiansen, A. (2014) 'The role of professional education in developing compassionate practitioners: A mixed methods study exploring the perceptions of health professionals and pre-registration students', *Nurse Education Today*, *34*(3): 480–486.

British Association for Counselling and Psychotherapy (BACP) (2018) *Ethical Framework for the Counselling Professions*. Available at: www.bacp.co.uk/media/3103/bacp-ethical-framework-for-the-counselling-professions-2018.pdf (accessed 9 March 2022).

British Association of Social Workers (BASW) (2019) *Practice Educator Professional Standards for Social Work*. Available at: www.basw.co.uk/system/files/resources/peps-for-social-work.pdf (accessed 8 March 2022).

Brook, J. and Kemp, C. (2021) 'Flexible rostering in nursing student clinical placements: A qualitative study of student and staff perceptions of the impact on learning and student experience', *Nurse Education in Practice*, *54*(July): 1–8.

Brookes, I. and O'Neill, M. (eds) (2017) *Collins English Dictionary*, 2nd edn. Glasgow: HarperCollins Publishers.

Bruner, J. (1960) *The Process of Education*. Cambridge, MA: Harvard University Press.

Buring, S.M., Bhushan, A., Broeseker, A., Conway, S., Duncan-Hewitt, W., Hansen, L. and Westberg, S. (2009) 'Inter-professional education: Definitions, student competencies, and guidelines for implementation', *American Journal of Pharmaceutical Education*, *73*(4): 59.

Burrows, D. (2008) 'Facilitation: A concept analysis', *Journal of Advanced Nursing*, *25*(2): 396–404.

Campbell, C. and Evans, P. (2016) 'Reciprocal benefits, legacy and risk: Applying Ellinger and Bostrom's model of line manager role identity as facilitators of learning', *European Journal of Training and Development*, *40*(2): 74–89.

Campbell, D., Lugger, S., Sigler, G.S. and Turkelson, C. (2021) 'Increasing awareness, sensitivity, and empathy for Alzheimer's dementia patients using simulation', *Nurse Education Today*, *98*(2021): 1–6.

Cant, R., Ryan, C., Hughes, L., Luders, E. and Cooper, S. (2021) 'What helps, what hinders? Undergraduate nursing students' perceptions of clinical placements based on a thematic synthesis of literature', *SAGE Open Nursing*, 7(Jan.): 1–20.

Care Quality Commission (CQC) (2022) *The Fundamental Standards*. Available at: www.cqc.org.uk/what-we-do/how-we-do-our-job/fundamental-standards (accessed 6 March 2022).

Carlisle, C., Calman, L. and Ibbotson, T. (2009) 'Practice-based learning: The role of practice education facilitators in supporting mentors', *Nurse Education Today*, 29(7): 715–721.

Carlson, E. and Idvall, E. (2014) 'Nursing students' experiences of the clinical learning environment in nursing homes: A questionnaire study using the CLES + T evaluation scale', *Nurse Education Today*, 34(7): 1130–1134.

Carnwell, R., Baker, S., Bellis, M. and Murray, R. (2007) 'Managerial perceptions of mentor, lecturer practitioner and link tutor roles', *Nurse Education Today*, 27(8): 923–932.

CASP UK (2022) *Critical Appraisal Skills Programme*. Available at: https://casp-uk.net/casp-tools-checklists (accessed 22 June 2022).

Centre for Policy on Ageing (2014) *The Effectiveness of Care Pathways in Health and Social Care*. Available at: www.cpa.org.uk/information/reviews/CPA-Rapid-Review-Effectiveness-of-care-pathways.pdf (accessed 15 June 2022).

Centre for the Advancement of Inter-professional Education (CAIPE) (2017) *CAIPE Inter-professional Education Guidelines*. Available at: www.caipe.org/resources/publications/caipe-publications/caipe-2017-interprofessional-education-guidelines-barr-h-ford-j-gray-r-helme-m-hutchings-m-low-h-machin-reeves-s (accessed 14 June 2022).

Cervera-Gasch, A., González-Chordá, V.M., Ortiz-Mallasen, V., Andreu-Pejo, L., Mena-Tudela, M. and Valero-Chilleron, M.J. (2022) 'Student satisfaction level, clinical learning environment, and tutor participation in primary care clinical placements: An observational study', *Nurse Education Today*, 108(2022): 1–6.

Chan, Z.C.Y., Stanley, D.J., Meadus, R.J. and Chien, W.T. (2017) 'A qualitative study on feedback provided by students in nurse education'. *Nurse Education Today*, 55 (August 2017): 128–133.

Chartered Institute of Personnel and Development (CIPD) (2021a) *Coaching and Mentoring*. Available at: www.cipd.co.uk/knowledge/fundamentals/people/development/coaching-mentoring-factsheet#6995 (accessed 8 March 2022).

Chartered Institute of Personnel and Development (CIPD) (2021b) *Knowledge and Skills Framework in the NHS*. Available at: www.hr-inform.co.uk/employment_law/knowledge-and-skills-framework-in-the-nhs (accessed 9 May 2022).

Chartered Society of Physiotherapy (CSP) (2011 – updated 2020) *Physiotherapy Framework (condensed version): A resource to promote and develop physiotherapy practice*. Available at: www.csp.org.uk/professional-clinical/cpd-education/professional-development/professional-frameworks/physiotherapy (accessed 11 April 2022).

Chartered Society of Physiotherapy (2020) *Learning and Development Principles. CSP Accreditation of Qualifying Programmes in Physiotherapy.* Available at: www. csp.org.uk/system/files/publication_files/L%26D%20Principles%202020.pdf (accessed 22 June 2020).

Chernikova, O., Heitzmann, N., Stadler, M., Holzberger, D., Seidel, T. and Frank Fischer, F. (2020) 'Simulation-based learning in higher education: A meta-analysis', *Review of Educational Research, 90*(4): 499–541.

Choe, K., Park, S. and Yoo, S.Y. (2014) 'Effects of constructivist teaching methods on bioethics education for nursing students: A quasi-experimental study', *Nurse Education Today, 34*(5): 848–853.

Choi, Y., Kim, J.Y. and Yoo, T. (2016) 'A study on the effect of learning organisation readiness on employees' quality commitment: The moderating effect of leader–member exchange', *Total Quality Management & Business Excellence, 27*(3): 325–338.

Christiansen, B., Averlid, G., Baluyot, C., Blomberg, K., Eikeland, A., Finstad, I.R.S., Larsen, M.H. and Lindeflaten, K. (2021) 'Challenges in the assessment of nursing students in clinical placements: Exploring perceptions among nurse mentors', *Nursing Open, 8*(3): 1069–1076.

Cleak, H. and Smith, D. (2012) 'Student satisfaction with models of field placement supervision', *Australian Social Work, 65*(2): 243–258.

Cochrane Collaboration (2022) *Cochrane Handbook for Systematic Reviews of Interventions.* Available at: https://training.cochrane.org/handbook/current/chapter-i.

Coleman, M. and Glover, D. (2010) *Educational Leadership and Management.* Maidenhead: Open University Press.

Collier, A. (2018) Characteristics of an effective nursing clinical instructor: the state of the science. *Journal of Clinical Nursing, 27*(1–2): 363–374.

Connor, M. and Pokora, J. (2017) *Coaching and Mentoring at Work: Developing Effective Practice*, 3rd edn. London: Open University Press.

Council of Deans of Health (2017) *Apprenticeships in Nursing and The Allied Health Professions – Briefing Paper Version 5.* Available at: https://councilofdeans.org.uk/wp-content/uploads/2017/01/Apprenticeships-paper-version-5-June-2017.pdf (accessed 3 July 2022).

CTC Training (2022) *Level 3 Certificate in Assessing Vocational Achievement (CAVA).* Available at: https://ctccourses.org/product/level-3-certificate-in-assessing-vocational-achievement-rqf/?gclid=CjwKCAjw0a-SBhBkEiwApljU0k3bsSxc4TLglJNrUL-aH7ZBjNTbuxyu8Mb-yPvnCcK3nBC9pyCsghoCujEQAvD_BwE (accessed 5 April 2022).

Curtis, K., Horton, K. and Smith, P. (2012) 'Student nurse socialisation in compassionate practice: A Grounded Theory study', *Nurse Education Today, 32*(7): 790–795.

Curzon, L.B. and Tummons, J. (2013) *Teaching in Further Education: An Outline of Principles and Practice*, 7th edn. London: Bloomsbury Academic.

Daloz, L.A. (1989) *Effective Teaching and Mentoring: Realizing the Transformational Power of Adult Learning Experiences.* San Francisco, CA: Jossey-Bass.

Darling, L.A.W. (1984) 'What do nurses want in a mentor?', *Journal of Nursing Administration, 14*(10): 42–44.

Darling, L.A.W. (1985) 'What to do about toxic mentors?', *Journal of Nursing Administration*, 15(5): 43–44.

Davis, L., Taylor, H. and Reyes, H. (2014) 'Lifelong learning in nursing: A Delphi study', *Nurse Education Today*, 34(3): 441–445.

DeBrew, J.K. and Lewallen, L.P. (2014) 'To pass or to fail? Understanding the factors considered by faculty in the clinical evaluation of nursing students', *Nurse Education Today*, 34(4): 631–636.

Department for Education & Department of Health and Social Care (DHSC) (updated 2020) *Special Educational Needs and Disability Code of Practice: 0 to 25 Years*. Available at: www.gov.uk/government/publications/send-code-of-practice-0-to-25 (accessed 18 June 2022).

Department of Health (2004) *The NHS Knowledge and Skills Framework (NHS KSF) and the Development Review Process*. Available at: www.nhsemployers.org/sites/default/files/2021-07/The-NHS-Knowledge-and-Skills-Framework.pdf (accessed 24 May 2022).

Department of Health (2010) *Preceptorship Framework for Newly Registered Nurses, Midwives and Allied Health Professionals*. Available at: www.networks.nhs.uk/nhs-networks/ahp-networks/documents/dh_114116.pdf (accessed 17 June 2022).

Department of Health (2013) *Education Outcomes Framework for Healthcare Workforce*. Available at: https://assets.publishing.service.gov.uk/government/uploads/system/uploads/attachment_data/file/175546/Education_outcomes_framework.pdf (accessed 19 June 2022).

Department of Health and Social Care (DHSC) (2012) *Health and Social Care Act 2012*. Available at: www.gov.uk/government/publications/health-and-social-care-act-2012-fact-sheets (accessed 19 June 2022).

Department of Health and Social Care (2021) *NHS Constitution for England*. Available at: www.gov.uk/government/publications/the-nhs-constitution-for-england/the-nhs-constitution-for-england (accessed 14 May 2022).

Dixon-Woods, M., Baker, R., Charles, K., Dawson, J., Jerzembek, G., Martin, G., McCarthy, I., McKee, L., Minion, J., Ozieranski, P., Willars, J., Wilkie, P. and West, M. (2014) 'Culture and behaviour in the English National Health Service: Overview of lessons from a large multimethod study', *BMJ Quality and Safety*, 23: 106–115.

Donabedian, A. (1988) 'The quality of care: How can it be assessed?', *American Journal of Public Health*, 260(12): 1743–1748.

Donaldson, J.H. and Carter, D. (2005) 'The value of role modelling: Perceptions of undergraduate and diploma nursing (adult) students', *Nurse Education in Practice*, 5(6): 353–359.

Drayton, L. and Edmonds, M. (2020) 'Understanding the role of the academic assessor', *Nursing Standard*, 35(9): 41–45.

Du Toit-Brits, C. and Van Zyl, C. (2017) 'Self-directed learning characteristics: Making learning personal, empowering and successful', *Africa Education Review*, 14(3–4): 122–141.

Duane, B.T. and Satre, M.E. (2014) 'Utilizing constructivism learning theory in collaborative testing as a creative strategy to promote essential nursing skills', *Nurse Education Today, 34*(1): 31–34.

Duffin, C. (2005) 'Pre-registration education to undergo major review', *Nursing Standard, 19*(26): 4.

Education and Training Foundation (2022) *Taking Teaching Further.* Available at: www.et-foundation.co.uk/professional-development/taking-teaching-further (accessed 3 July 2022).

Eick, S.A., Williamson, G.R. and Heath, V. (2012) 'A systematic review of placement-related attrition in nurse education', *International Journal of Nursing Studies, 49*(2012): 1299–1309.

Eller, L.S., Lev, E.L. and Feurer, A. (2014) 'Key components of an effective mentoring relationship: A qualitative study', *Nurse Education Today, 34*(5): 815–820.

Embo, M., Driessen, E., Valcke, M. and van der Vleuten, C.P.M (2014) 'A framework to facilitate self-directed learning, assessment and supervision in midwifery practice: A qualitative study of supervisors' perceptions', *Nurse Education in Practice, 14*(4): 441–446.

Encyclopaedia Britannica (2022) *Herbartianism – Education.* Available at: www.britannica.com/topic/Herbartianism (accessed 13 June 2022).

Falender, C.A. (2014) 'Clinical supervision in a competency-based era', *South African Journal of Psychology, 44*(1): 6–17.

Field, J. (1999) 'Participation under the magnifying glass', *Adults Learning, 11*(3): 10–13.

Finnerty, G. and Collington, V. (2013) 'Practical coaching by mentors: Student midwives' perceptions', *Nurse Education in Practice, 13*(6): 573–577.

Fitts, P.M. and Posner, M.I. (1973) *Human Performance.* London: Prentice-Hall.

Forde-Johnston, C. (2017) 'Developing and evaluating a foundation preceptorship programme for newly qualified nurses', *Nursing Standard, 31*(42): 42–52.

Foronda, C., MacWilliams, B. and McArthur, E. (2016) 'Inter-professional communication in healthcare: An integrative review', *Nurse Education in Practice, 19*(July): 36–40.

Foster, H., Ooms, A. and Marks-Maran, D. (2015) 'Nursing students' expectations and experiences of mentorship', *Nurse Education Today, 35*(1): 18–24.

Francis, R. (2013) *Report of the Mid Staffordshire NHS Foundation Trust Public Inquiry (Francis Report).* Available at: www.gov.uk/government/publications/report-of-the-mid-staffordshire-nhs-foundation-trust-public-inquiry (accessed 15 May 2022).

Freire, P. (2005) *Pedagogy of the Oppressed.* London: Continuum International Publishing Group. [First published 1970]

Fretwell, J.E. (1980) 'An inquiry into the ward learning environment', *Nursing Times, 76*(16): 69–75.

Gagné, R.M., Wager, W.W., Golas, K.C. and Keller, J.M. (2005) *Principles of Instructional Design,* 5th edn. Belmont, CA: Wadsworth Publishing.

Gainsbury, S. (2010) 'Mentors passing students despite doubts over ability', *Nursing Times, 106*(16): 1–3.

García-Mayor, S., Quemada-González, C., León-Campos, A., Kaknani-Uttumchandani, S., Gutiérrez-Rodríguez, L., del Mar Carmona-Segovia, A. and Martí-García, C. (2021) Nursing students' perceptions on the use of clinical simulation in psychiatric and mental health nursing by means of objective structured clinical examination (OSCE). *Nurse Education Today*, *100*(May): 1–6.

Garside, J., Nhemachena, J.Z.Z, Williams, J. and Topping, A. (2009) 'Repositioning assessment: Giving students the "choice" of assessment methods', *Nurse Education in Practice*, *9*(2): 141–148.

Garside, J.R. and Nhemachena, J.Z. (2013) 'A concept analysis of competence and its transition in nursing'. *Nurse Education Today*, *33*(5): 541–545.

General Medical Council (2013) *Good Medical Practice*. Updated 2019. Available at: www.gmc-uk.org/-/media/documents/good-medical-practice---english-20200128_pdf-51527435.pdf. (accessed 23 April 2022).

Giacomino, K., Caliesch, R. and Sattelmayer, K.M. (2020) 'The effectiveness of the Peyton's 4-step teaching approach on skill acquisition of procedures in health professions education: A systematic review and meta-analysis with integrated meta-regression', *PeerJ*, *8*: e10129.

Gilmour, J.A., Kopeiki, A. and Douché, J. (2007) 'Student nurses as peer-mentors: Collegiality in practice', *Nurse Education in Practice*, *7*(1): 36–43.

Gingerich, A., Sebok-Syer, S.S., Larstone, R., Watling, C.J. and Lingard, L. (2020) 'Seeing but not believing: Insights into the intractability of failure to fail', *Medical Education*, *54* (2020): 1148–1158.

Gittinger, F.P., Lemos, M., Neumann, J.L., Förster, J., Dohmen, D., Berke, B., Olmeo, A., Lucas, G. and Jonas, S.M. (2022) 'Interrater reliability in the assessment of physiotherapy students', *BMC Medical Education*, *22*(2022): 1–10.

Goldsmith, J., Clarke, B. and Cross, S. (2009) 'The art of learning to teach inter-professionally', *Practice Nursing*, *20*(8): 414–416.

Gopee, N. (2001) 'The role of peer assessment and peer review in nursing', *British Journal of Nursing*, *10*(2): 115–121.

Gopee, N. (2002) 'Human and social capital as facilitators of lifelong learning in nursing', *Nurse Education Today*, *22*(8): 608–616.

Gopee, N. (2022) *Leading and Managing Healthcare*. London: Sage Publications.

Gopee, N. and Deane, M. (2013) 'Strategies for successful academic writing: Institutional and non-institutional support for students', *Nurse Education Today*, *33*(12): 1624–1631.

Gopee, N. and Galloway, J. (2017) *Leadership and Management in Healthcare*, 3rd edn. London: Sage Publications.

Gopee, N., Tyrell, A., Raven, S., Thomas, K. and Hari, T. (2004) 'Effective clinical learning in primary care settings', *Nursing Standard*, *18*(37): 33–37.

Gov.uk – Ofsted (2020) *Effective mentoring and a well-paced curriculum are key to high quality initial teacher education*. Available at: www.gov.uk/government/news/effective-mentoring-and-a-well-paced-curriculum-are-key-to-high-quality-initial-teacher-education (accessed 17 March 2022).

Gov.uk (2022) *Final report of the Ockenden review: Findings, conclusions and essential actions from the independent review of maternity services at the Shrewsbury and*

Telford Hospital NHS Trust. Available at: www.gov.uk/government/publications/final-report-of-the-ockenden-review (accessed 18 May 2022).

Gratrix, L. and Barrett, D. (2017) 'Desperately seeking consistency: Student nurses' experiences and expectations of academic supervision', *Nurse Education Today*, *48*(Jan.): 7–12.

Gray, M.A. and Smith, L.N. (2000) 'The qualities of an effective mentor from the student nurse's perspective: Findings from a longitudinal qualitative study', *Journal of Advanced Nursing*, *32*(6): 1542–1549.

Grealish, L. and Henderson, A. (2016) 'Investing in organisational culture: Nursing students' experience of organisational learning culture in aged care settings following a program of cultural development', *Contemporary Nurse*, *52*(5): 569–575.

Guba, E.G. and Lincoln, Y.S. (1989) *Fourth Generation Evaluation.* London: Sage.

Hall, K.M., Draper, R.J., Smith, L.K. and Bullough, R.V. (2008) 'More than a place to teach: Exploring the perceptions of the roles and responsibilities of mentor teachers', *Mentoring & Tutoring: Partnership in Learning*, *16*(3): 328–345.

Hallin, K. and Danielson, E. (2009) 'Being a personal preceptor for nursing students: Registered nurses' experiences before and after introduction of a preceptor model', *Journal of Advanced Nursing*, *65*(1): 161–174.

Hamilton, E.R., Rosenberg, J.M. and Akcaoglu, M. (2016) The substitution augmentation modification redefinition (SAMR) model: A critical review and suggestions for its use. *TechTrends*, *60*: 433–441.

Hamshire, C., Jack, K., Forsyth, R., Langan, A.M. and Harris, W.E. (2019) 'The wicked problem of healthcare student attrition', *Nursing Inquiry*, *26*: e12294, 1–8.

Handy, C. (1989) *Age of Unreason.* London: Business Books.

Handy, C. (2007) *Understanding Organizations* (4th edn; Kindle edition). Harmondsworth: Penguin.

Hauer, K.E., Oza, S.K., Kogan, J.R., Stankiewicz, C.A., Stenfors-Hayes, T., Cate, O.T., Batt, J. and O'Sullivan, P.S. (2015) 'How clinical supervisors develop trust in their trainees: A qualitative study'. *Medical Education*, *49*(8): 783–795.

Hauge, K.W., Bakken, H., Brask, O.D., Gutteberg, A., Malones, B.D. and Ulvund, I. (2019) 'Are Norwegian mentors failing to fail nursing students?', *Nurse Education in Practice*, *36*: 64–70.

Hawkins, P. and McMahon, A. (2020) *Supervision in the Helping Professions*, 5th edn. London: Open University Press.

Haycock-Stuart, E., Donaghy, E. and Darbyshire, C. (2016) 'Involving users and carers in the assessment of preregistration nursing students' clinical nursing practice: A strategy for patient empowerment and quality improvement?' *Journal of Clinical Nursing*, *25*(13–14): 2052–2065.

Health and Care Professions Council (HCPC) (2013) *Standards of Proficiency – Physiotherapists.* Available at: www.hcpc-uk.org/globalassets/resources/standards/standards-of-proficiency---physiotherapists.pdf (accessed 7 June 2022).

Health and Care Professions Council (2014a) *Standards of Proficiency – Paramedics.* Available at: www.hcpc-uk.org/globalassets/resources/standards/standards-of-proficiency---paramedics.pdf?v=637106257480000000 (accessed 7 June 2022).

Health and Care Professions Council (2014b) *Standards of Proficiency – Operating Department Practitioners*. Available at: www.hcpc-uk.org/globalassets/resources/standards/standards-of-proficiency---odp.pdf?v=637106257360000000. (accessed 13 April 2022).

Health and Care Professions Council (2016) *Standards of Conduct, Performance and Ethics*. Available at: www.hcpc-uk.org/standards/standards-of-conduct-performance-and-ethics (accessed 17 June 2022).

Health and Care Professions Council (2017) *Standards of Education and Training*. Available at: Standards of education and training (hcpc-uk.org) (accessed 13 April 2022).

Health and Care Professions Council (2018) *Standards for Continuing Professional Development*. Available at: www.hcpc-uk.org/standards/standards-of-continuing-professional-development (accessed 1 May 2022).

Health and Care Professions Council (2021) *What our Standards Say*. Available at: www.hcpc-uk.org/standards/meeting-our-standards/supervision-leadership-and-culture/supervision/what-our-standards-say/#:~:text='You%20must%20be%20open%20and,qualifications%20and%20skills'%20(9.2) (accessed 1 June 2022).

Health and Care Professions Council (2022) *Key Characteristics of Effective Supervision*. www.hcpc-uk.org/standards/meeting-our-standards/supervision-leadership-and-culture/supervision/approaching-supervision/key-characteristics-of-effective-supervision (accessed 30 May 2022).

Health Education England (HEE) (2014) *Values Based Recruitment Framework*. Available at: www.hee.nhs.uk/our-work/values-based-recruitment. (accessed 3 June 2022).

Health Education England (2017) *Nursing Associate Curriculum Framework*. Available at: www.hee.nhs.uk/sites/default/files/documents/Nursing%20Associate%20Curriculum%20Framework%20Feb2017_0.pdf (accessed 15 March 2022).

Health Education England (2018) *National Framework for Simulation-Based Education (SBE)*. Available at: www.hee.nhs.uk/sites/default/files/documents/National%20framework%20for%20simulation%20based%20education.pdf (accessed 7 May 2022).

Health Education England (2019) *Enhancing Supervision for Postgraduate Doctors in Training*. Available at: www.hee.nhs.uk/sites/default/files/documents/SupervisionReport_%20FINAL1.pdf. (accessed 4 September 2022).

Health Education England (2022a) *Clinical Supervisor*. Available at: www.nwpgmd.nhs.uk/educator-development/standards-guidance/clinical-supervisor (accessed 1 June 2022).

Health Education England (2022b) *Clinical/Educational Supervisors*. Available at: www.yorksandhumberdeanery.nhs.uk/faculty/elearning/clinicaleducational_supervisors (accessed 8 March 2022).

Health Education England (2022c) *Person-Centred Care*. Available at: www.hee.nhs.uk/our-work/person-centred-care (accessed 9 May 2022).

Health Education England (2022d) *PARE – Practice Assessment Record & Evaluation.* Available at: https://onlinepare.net (accessed 8 April 2022).

Health Education England (2022e) *NHS Education Funding Guide 2020 – 2021 Financial Year.* Available at: www.hee.nhs.uk/our-work/education-funding-reform/nhs-education-funding-guide (accessed 2 June 2021).

Hean, S., Clark, J.M., Adams, K., Humphris, D. and Lathlean, J. (2006) 'Being seen by others as we see ourselves: The congruence between the in-group and outgroup perceptions of health and social care students', *Learning in Health and Social Care*, 5(1): 10–22.

Heaslip, V. and Scammell, J.M.E. (2012) 'Failing underperforming students: The role of grading in practice assessment', *Nurse Education in Practice*, 12(2): 95–100.

Hegarty, J. (2017) 'Schema to demonstrate maintenance of professional competence for Nurses and Midwives: Results of a National Mixed Methods Study presented at NET2017 conference'. Available at: www.advance-he.ac.uk/knowledge-hub/schema-demonstrate-maintenance-professional-competence-nurses-and-midwives-results (accessed 1 May 2022).

Heirs, B. and Farrell, P. (1986) *The Professional Decision Thinker.* London: Sidgwick & Jackson.

Helminen, K., Johnson, M., Isoaho, H., Turunen, H. and Tossavainen, K. (2017) 'Final assessment of nursing students in clinical practice: Perspectives of nursing teachers, students and mentors', *Journal of Clinical Nursing*, 26(23–24): 4795–4803.

Henderson, A., Cooke, M., Creedy, D.K. and Walker, R. (2012) 'Nursing students' perceptions of learning in practice environments: A review', *Nurse Education Today*, 32(3): 299–302.

Heron, J. (2009) *Helping the Client: A Creative Practical Guide*, 5th edn. London: Sage Publications.

Heyns, T., Botma, Y. and Van Rensburg, G. (2017) 'A creative analysis of the role of practice development facilitators in a critical care environment', *Health SA Gesondheid*, 22(Dec.): 105–111.

Highe, L. (2020) 'The cultural change from mentor to practice assessor/supervisor', *Evidence-Based Nursing*. Blog posted 16 February. Available at: The cultural change from mentor to practice assessor/supervisor – Evidence-Based Nursing blog (bmj.com) (accessed 30 May 2020).

Hill, R., Woodward, M. and Arthur, A. (2020) 'Collaborative learning in practice (CLiP): Evaluation of a new approach to clinical learning', *Nurse Education Today*, 85: 1–6.

Holland, K. and Lauder, W. (2012) 'A review of evidence for the practice learning environment: Enhancing the context for nursing and midwifery care in Scotland', *Nurse Education in Practice*, 12(1): 60–64.

Holt, J., Coates, C., Cotterill, D., Eastburn, S., Laxton, J., Young, C. and Mistry, H. (2010) 'Identifying common competences in health and social care: An example of multi-institutional and inter-professional working', *Nurse Education Today*, 30(3): 264–270.

Houghton, T. (2016) 'Assessment and accountability: Part 2 – managing failing students', *Nursing Standard, 30*(41): 41–49.

Hughes, C. (1999) 'The dire in self-directed learning', *Adults Learning, 11*(2): 7–9.

Hughes, L.J., Mitchell, M. and Johnston, A.N.B (2016) '"Failure to fail" in nursing – A catch phrase or a real issue? A systematic integrative literature review', *Nurse Education in Practice, 20*(September): 54–63.

Hughes, L.J., Mitchell, M.L. and Johnston, A.N.B. (2021) 'Moving forward: Barriers and enablers to failure to fail – A mixed methods meta-integration', *Nurse Education Today, 98*: 1–7.

Hughes, S.J. and Quinn, F.M. (2013) *Quinn's Principles and Practice of Nurse Education*, 6th edn. Andover: Cengage Learning EMEA.

Hunt, L.A., McGee, P., Gutteridge, R. and Hughes, M. (2016) 'Manipulating mentors' assessment decisions: Do underperforming student nurses use coercive strategies to influence mentor's practical assessment decisions?' *Nurse Education in Practice, 20*(Sept.): 154–162.

Hutchison, T. and Cochrane, J. (2014) 'A phenomenological study into the impact of the sign-off mentor in the acute hospital setting', *Nurse Education Today, 34*(6): 1029–1033.

Institute for Apprenticeships & Technical Education (IATE) (2022a) *Registered Nurse Degree (NMC 2018)*. Available at: www.instituteforapprenticeships.org/apprentice ship-standards/registered-nurse-degree-nmc-2018 (accessed 2 April 2022).

Institute for Apprenticeships & Technical Education (2022b) *End-Point Assessment Plan for Registered Nurse Fully Integrated Degree Apprenticeship Standard*. Available at: www.instituteforapprenticeships.org/media/5919/st0781_v14_registered_ nurse_16_fullyintegrated-ap-for-publication_adjustment_15022022.pdf (accessed 2 April 2022).

Institute for Apprenticeships & Technical Education (2022c) *Developing an End-point Assessment Plan*. Available at: www.instituteforapprenticeships.org/developing- new-apprenticeships/developing-an-end-point-assessment-plan (accessed 5 April 2022).

Jack, K., Hamshire, C. and Chambers, A. (2017) 'The influence of role models in undergraduate nurse education', *Journal of Clinical Nursing, 26*(23–24): 4707–4715.

James Paget University Hospitals NHS Foundation Trust (2017) *The Journey of Collaborative Learning in Practice (CLiP) at JPUH*. Available at: PowerPoint presentation (hee.nhs.uk) (accessed 17 May 2022).

Jarvis, P. (2010) *Adult Education and Lifelong Learning Theory and Practice*, 4th edn. New York: Routledge.

Jayasekara, R., Smith, C., Hall, C., Rankin, E., Smith, M., Visvanathan, V. and Friebe, T. (2018) 'The effectiveness of clinical education models for undergraduate nursing programs: A systematic review', *Nurse Education in Practice, 29*(Mar.): 116–126.

Jeffs, T. (2003) 'Quest for knowledge begins with a recognition of shared ignorance', *Adults Learning, 14*(6): 28.

Jervis, A. and Tilki, M. (2011) 'Why are nurse mentors failing to fail student nurses who do not meet clinical performance standards?' *British Journal of Nursing, 20*(9): 582–587.

Johns, C. (2017) *Becoming a Reflective Practitioner*, 5th edn. Chichester: Wiley Blackwell.

Johnson, E.A. (2017) *Working Together in Clinical Supervision: A Guide for Supervisors and Supervisees*. New York: Momentum Press Health.

Joint Information Systems Committee (JISC) (2022) *Principles of Good Assessment and Feedback*. Available at: www.jisc.ac.uk/guides/principles-of-good-assessment-and-feedback# (accessed 10 May 2022).

Joint Royal Colleges Ambulance Liaison Committee (JRCALC) & the Association of Ambulance Chief Executives (2021) *UK Ambulance Services Clinical Practice Guidelines 2021*. Available at: https://aace.org.uk/clinical-practice-guidelines (accessed 21 June 2022).

Jokelainen, M., Turunen, H., Tossavainen, K., Jamookeeah, D. and Coco, K. (2011) 'A systematic review of mentoring nursing students in clinical placements', *Journal of Clinical Nursing, 20*(19–20): 2854–2867.

Jones, D.S. and Podolsky, S.H. (2015) 'Perspectives: The history and fate of the gold standard', *The Lancet, 385*(9977): 1502–1503.

Joyce, B., Calhoun, E. and Hopkins, D. (2009) *Models of Learning: Tools for Teaching*, 3rd edn. Maidenhead: Open University Press.

Kandola, D., Graham, R. and Wagner, U. (2022) 'Midwifery basics: Blood transfusions in the postnatal period – addressing the theory–practice gap', *The Practising Midwife, 25*(5): 14–17.

Kelton, M.F. (2014) 'Clinical coaching: An innovative role to improve marginal nursing students' clinical practice', *Nurse Education in Practice, 14*(6): 709–713.

Kendall-Raynor, P. (2007) 'Nurse cleared in supervision case is to face NMC', *Nursing Standard, 21*(17): 9.

Kerry, T. and Mayes, A.S. (eds) (1995) *Issues in Mentoring*. London: Routledge/Open University.

Kilminster, S.M., Jolly, B.C., Grant, J. and Cottrell, D. (2007) 'AMEE Guide No. 27: Effective educational and clinical supervision', *Medical Teacher, 29*(1): 2–19.

King's College London (2020) *Midwifery Ongoing Record of Achievement*. Available at: www.kcl.ac.uk/nmpc/assets/practice-learning/context-document-mora.pdf (accessed 22 May 2020).

Kirwan, C., Szafranska, M., Coveney, K., Horton, S. and Carroll, L. (2022) 'Midwifery students' experiences of objective structured clinical examinations: A qualitative evidence synthesis', *Nurse Education Today, 113*(2022): 1–11.

Knight, K.H., Leigh, J., Whaley, V., Rabie, G., Matthews, M. and Doyle, K. (2021) 'The supervisor conundrum', *British Journal of Nursing, 30*(20): 1156.

Knowles, M.S. (2020) *The Adult Learner: The Definitive Classic in Adult Education and Human Resource Development*, 9th edn. London: Routledge.

Koffka, K. (1935) *Principles of Gestalt Psychology*. Available at: https://psycnet.apa.org/record/1935-03991-000 (accessed 13 June 2022).

Kohler, W. (1925) 'The mentality of apes', in S. Nolen-Hoeksema, B. Fredrickson, G.R. Loftus and C. Lutz (eds) (2014) *Atkinson and Hilgard's Introduction to Psychology*, 16th edn. Andover, Hampshire: Cengage Learning.

Kolb, D.A. (2014) *Experiential Learning: Experience as the Source of Learning and Development*, 2nd edn. Hoboken, NJ: Pearson FT Press.

Kouzes, J.M. and Posner, B.Z. (2017) *The Leadership Challenge*, 6th edn. San Francisco, CA: Jossey-Bass.

Kramer, M. (1974) *Reality Shock: Why Nurses Leave Nursing*. St Louis, MO: Mosby.

Kulju, K., Stolt, M., Suhonen, R. and Leino-Kilpi, H. (2016) 'Ethical competence: A concept analysis', *Nursing Ethics*, 23(4): 401–412.

Lait, J., Suter, E. and Deutschlander, S. (2011) 'Inter-professional mentoring: Enhancing students' clinical learning', *Nurse Education in Practice*, 11(3): 211–215.

Lakasing, E. and Francis, H. (2005) 'The crisis in student mentorship', *Primary Health Care*, 15(4): 40–41.

Lancer, N., Megginson, D. and Clutterbuck, D. (2016) *Techniques for Coaching and Mentoring*, 2nd edn. London: Routledge.

Lane, M. (2014) 'Students' perceptions in relation to paramedic educator (ped) roles'. *Journal of Paramedic Practice*, 6(4): 194–199.

Lankshear, A. (1990) 'Failure to fail: The teacher's dilemma', *Nursing Standard*, 4(20): 35–37.

Lavender, R.J.B. (2017) 'What can dyslexic paramedic students teach us about mentoring? A case study', *Journal of Paramedic Practice*, 9(5): 202–206.

LearnPac Systems UK (2020) *What is the Difference between Statutory and Mandatory Training?* Available at: www.mandatorytraining.co.uk/blogs/statutory-and-mandatory-training-video-courses/what-is-the-difference-between-statutory-and-mandatory-training (accessed 1 May 2022).

Lee, N. (2011) 'An evaluation of CPD learning and impact upon positive practice change', *Nurse Education Today*, 31(4): 390–395.

Leggat, S.G., Balding, C. and Schiftan, D. (2014) 'Developing clinical leaders: The impact of an action learning mentoring programme for advanced practice nurses', *Journal of Clinical Nursing*, 24(11/12): 1576–1584.

Legislation.gov.uk (2020) *Directive 2013/55/EU of the European Parliament and of the Council*. Available at: www.legislation.gov.uk/eudr/2013/55/contents (accessed 14 June 2022).

Lester, S. and Costley, C. (2010) 'Work-based learning at higher education level: Value, practice and critique', *Studies in Higher Education*, 35(5): 561–575.

Lister, S., Hofland, J., Grafton, H. and Wilson, C. (eds) (2021) *The Royal Marsden Manual of Clinical Nursing Procedures* (Royal Marsden Manual Series), 10th edn. Oxford: Wiley-Blackwell.

Lockeman, K.S., Appelbaum, N.P., Dow, A.W., Orr, S., Huff, T.A., Hogan, C.J. and Queen, B.A. (2017) 'The effect of an inter-professional simulation-based education program on perceptions and stereotypes of nursing and medical students: A quasi-experimental study', *Nurse Education Today*, 58(Nov.): 32–37.

Manchester Metropolitan University & Health Education North West (2015) *Simulated Patient Common Framework*. Available at: www.ewin.nhs.uk/sites/default/files/SP%20Common%20Framework%20and%20Checklist_version%20for%20websites.pdf (accessed 29 June 2022).

Manley, K., Martin, A., Jackson, C. and Wright, T. (2018) 'A realist synthesis of effective continuing professional development (CPD): A case study of healthcare practitioners' CPD', *Nurse Education Today*, 69(Oct.): 134–141.

Manninen, K., Karlstedt, M., Sandelin, A., von Vogelsang, A. and Pettersson, S. (2022) 'First and second cycle nursing students' perceptions of the clinical learning environment in acute care settings: A comparative crosssectional study using the CLES+T scale', *Nurse Education Today*, 108(Jan.): 1–6.

Mannion, R. and Davies, H. (2018) 'Understanding organisational culture for healthcare quality improvement', BMJ, 363(Open Access): 1–4.

Marshall, J.E. (2012) 'Developing midwifery practice through work-based learning: An exploratory study', *Nurse Education in Practice*, 12(5): 273–278.

Maslow, A.H. (1987) *Motivation and Personality*, 3rd edn. London: Harper & Row.

Mathisen, C., Heyn, L.G., Jacobsen, T., Bjørk, I.T. and Hansen, E.H. (2022) 'The use of practice education facilitators to strengthen the clinical learning environment for nursing students: A realist review', *International Journal of Nursing Studies*. https://doi.org/10.1016/j.ijnurstu.2022.104258

Maxwell, R.J. (1984) 'Quality assurance in health care', *British Medical Journal*, 288(6428): 1470–1472.

Maynard, S.P., Mertz, L.K.P. and Fortune, A.E. (2015) 'Off-site supervision in social work education: What makes it work?', *Journal of Social Work Education*, 51(3): 519–534.

McCarthy, S., O'Raghallaigh, P., Woodworth, S., Lim, Y.L., Kenny, L.C. and Adam, F. (2016) 'An integrated patient journey mapping tool for embedding quality in healthcare service reform', *Journal of Decision Systems*, 25(suppl.): 354–368.

McCormack, B. and McCanse, T. (2017) *The Person-centred Practice Research Centre (CPcPR): Ageing Research*. Available at: www.nhsresearchscotland.org.uk/uploads/tinymce/Brendan%20McCormack%20presentation.pdf (accessed 9 May 2022).

McCormack, B., Manley, K. and Titchen, A. (2013) *Practice Development in Nursing and Healthcare*. Oxford: Wiley-Blackwell.

McGivney, V. (2003) *Adult Learning Pathways: Through Routes or Cul-de-Sacs?* Leicester: National Institute of Adult Continuing Education.

McGregor, D. (1987) *The Human Side of Enterprise*. London: Penguin.

McLeod, F., Jamison, C. and Treasure, K. (2018) 'Promoting interprofessional learning and enhancing the pre-registration student experience through reciprocal cross professional peer tutoring', *Nurse Education Today*, 64: 190–195.

Mead, D. (2011) 'Views of nurse mentors about their role', *Nursing Management*, 18(6): 18–23.

Megginson, D., Clutterbuck, D., Garvey, B., Stokes, P. and Garrett-Harris, R. (2006) *Mentoring in Action: A Practical Guide*. London: Kogan Page.

Merriam-Webster (2022) *Dictionary*. Available at: www.merriam-webster.com/ dictionary/theory (accessed 13 June 2022).

Middleton, L. and Llewellyn, D. (2016) 'How to record and evidence continuing professional development for revalidation', *Nursing Standard, 30*(44): 42–46.

Mikkonen, K., Elo, S., Miettunen, J., Saarikoski, M. and Kääriäinen, M. (2017) 'Development and testing of the CALDs and CLES+T scales for international nursing students' clinical learning environments', *Journal of Advanced Nursing, 73*(8): 1997–2011.

Millar, L., Conlon, M. and McGirr, D. (2017) 'Students' perspectives of using the hub and spoke model to support and develop learning in practice', *Nursing Standard, 32*(9): 41–49.

Milligan, F., Wareing, M., Preston-Shoot, M., Pappas, Y., Randhawa, G. and Bhandol, J. (2017) 'Supporting nursing, midwifery and allied health professional students to raise concerns with the quality of care: A review of the research literature', *Nurse Education Today, 57*(Oct.): 29–39.

Mint Human Resources (2022) *Honey and Mumford Learning Style Questionnaire*. Available at: Free Online Mumford and Honey Learning Styles Questionnaire (mint-hr.com) (accessed 12 February 2022).

Moniz, T., Arntfield, S., Miller, K., Lingard, L., Watling, C. and Regehr, G. (2015) 'Considerations in the use of reflective writing for student assessment: Issues of reliability and validity', *Medical Education, 49*(9): 901–908.

Moore, A. (2018) 'Preceptorship scheme aims to give new nurses a flying start', *Nursing Standard, 32*(22): 18–20.

Moore, L. (2010) 'Work-based learning and the role of managers', *Nursing Management, 17*(5): 26–29.

Moore, L., Lavoie, A., Bourgeois, G. and Lapointe, J. (2015) 'Donabedian's structure-process-outcome quality of care model: Validation in an integrated trauma system', *Journal of Trauma and Acute Care Surgery, 78*(6): 1168–1175.

Morley D. (2016) 'Applying Wenger's communities of practice theory to placement learning'. *Nurse Education Today, 39*(April 2016): 161–162.

Morley, D.A., Wilson, K. and McDermott, J. (2017) 'Changing the practice learning landscape', *Nurse Education in Practice, 27*(Nov.): 169–171.

Moroney, T., Gerdtz, M., Brockenshire, N., Maude, P., Weller-Newton, J., Hatcher, D., Molloy, L., Williamson, M., Woodward-Kron, R. and Molloy, E. (2022) 'Exploring the contribution of clinical placement to student learning: A sequential mixed methods study', *Nurse Education Today, 113*(June): 1–7.

Mullins, L. (2019) *Organisational Behaviour in the Workplace*, 12th edn. Harlow (UK): Pearson Education.

Nancarrow, S.A., Wade, R., Moran, A., Coyle, J., Young, J. and Boxall, D. (2014) 'Connecting practice: A practitioner centered model of supervision', *Clinical Governance: An Internation Journal, 19*(3): 235–252.

National Committee of Inquiry into Higher Education (NCIHE) (1997) *Higher Education in the Learning Society (The Dearing Report)*. Norwich: HMSO.

National Institute for Health and Care Excellence (NICE) (2014) *Safe Staffing for Nursing in Adult Inpatient Wards in Acute Hospitals*. Available at: www.nice.org.uk/guidance/sg1 (accessed 27 February 2022).

National Institute for Health and Care Excellence (NICE) (2022) *NICE Pathways – Everything NICE says on a topic in an interactive flowchart*. Available at: https://pathways.nice.org.uk (accessed 3 March 2022).

National Institute for Health and Care Research (NIHR) (2022) *Health Technology Assessment*. Available at: www.journalslibrary.nihr.ac.uk/HTA/# (accessed 23 April 2022).

Neary, M. (2000) 'Responsive assessment of clinical competence (Part 1)', *Nursing Standard*, 15(9): 34–36.

Nevalainen, M., Lunkka, N. and Suhonen, M. (2018) 'Work-based learning in health care organisations experienced by nursing staff: A systematic review of qualitative studies', *Nurse Education in Practice*, 29(Mar.): 21–29.

Ng, J.Y. (2014) 'Combining Peyton's four-step approach and Gagne's instructional model in teaching slit-lamp examination', *Perspectives on Medical Education*, 3(6): 480–485.

NHS Education for Scotland (2017) *Flying Start NHS: Definitive guide to the programme*. Available at: https://learn.nes.nhs.scot/1915/flying-start-nhs/flying-start-nhs-definitive-guide-to-the-programme (accessed 18 March 2022).

NHS Education for Scotland (2019) *Practice Learning Handbook: For practice supervisors and practice assessors*. Available at: www.nes.scot.nhs.uk/media/f3ajj03l/handbook_supervisor_and_assessor.pdf (accessed 23 May 2022).

NHS Education for Scotland (2021) *Practice Education Facilitator (PEF) and Care Home Education Facilitator (CHEF) National Priorities for July 2021 – March 2023*. Available at: www.nes.scot.nhs.uk/media/cjqhix33/national-pef-chef-priorities-2021_-2023.pdf (accessed 17 March 2022).

NHS Employers (2019) *Advanced Practice and Enhanced Practice*. Available at: www.nhsemployers.org/articles/advanced-practice-and-enhanced-practice (accessed 9 May 2022).

NHS England (2016) *Leading Change, Adding Value: A Framework for Nursing, Midwifery and Care Staff*. Available at: www.england.nhs.uk/wp-content/uploads/2016/05/nursing-framework.pdf (accessed 14 May 2022).

NHS England (2017a) *A-EQUIP: A model of clinical midwifery supervision*. Available at: www.england.nhs.uk/publication/a-equip-a-model-of-clinical-midwifery-supervision (accessed 31 March 2022).

NHS England (2017b) *Change Model*. Available at: www.england.nhs.uk/ourwork/qual-clin-lead/sustainableimprovement/change-model (accessed 17 September 2017).

NHS England (2022) *Improvement Capability Building and Delivery Team*. Available at: www.england.nhs.uk/sustainableimprovement (accessed 23 April 2022).

NHS England National Quality Board (NQB) (2014) *How to Ensure the Right People, with the Right Skills, are in the Right Place at the Right Time: A guide to establishing nursing, midwifery and care staffing capacity and capability*. Available at: www.

england.nhs.uk/wp-content/uploads/2013/11/nqb-how-to-guid.pdf   (accessed 14 June 2022).

NHS England and NHS Improvement (NHSEI) (2021) *Maternity and Neonatal Services Update*. Available at: www.england.nhs.uk/wp-content/uploads/2021/11/board-item-6-251121-maternity-and-neonatal-update.pdf (accessed 18 May 2022).

Noh, G.O. and Park, M.J. (2022) 'Effectiveness of Incorporating Situation-Background-Assessment-Recommendation (SBAR) methods into simulation-based education for nursing students: A quasi-experimental study', *Nurse Education Today*, 109(Feb.): 1–8.

Nolen-Hoeksema, S., Fredrickson, B., Loftus, G.R. and Lutz, C. (2014) *Atkinson and Hilgard's Introduction to Psychology*, 14th edn. Hampshire: Cengage Learning.

Notarnicola, I., Petrucci, C., De Jesus Barbosa, M.R., Giorgi, F., Stievano, A. and Lancia, L. (2016) 'Clinical competence in nursing: A concept analysis', *Professioni infermieristiche* (an Italian journal), 69(3): 174–181.

Nursing and Midwifery Council (NMC) (2008) *Standards to Support Learning and Assessment in Practice*. Available at: www.nmc.org.uk/standards-for-education-and-training/standards-to-support-learning-and-assessment-in-practice (accessed 9 May 2022).

Nursing and Midwifery Council (NMC) (2017) *Enabling Professionalism in Nursing and Midwifery Practice*. Available at: www.nmc.org.uk/globalassets/sitedocuments/other-publications/enabling-professionalism.pdf (accessed 1 July 2022).

Nursing and Midwifery Council (NMC) (2018a) *Standards for Student Supervision and Assessment*. London: NMC. Available at: www.nmc.org.uk/globalassets/sitedocuments/standards-of-proficiency/standards-for-student-supervision-and-assessment/student-supervision-assessment.pdf. (accessed 27 March 2022).

Nursing and Midwifery Council (2018b) *The Code: Professional standards of practice and behaviour for nurses, midwives and nursing associates*. Available at: www.nmc.org.uk/standards/code (accessed 13 March 2022).

Nursing and Midwifery Council (2018c) *Future Nurse: Standards of Proficiency for Registered Nurses*. Available at: www.nmc.org.uk/globalassets/sitedocuments/standards-of-proficiency/nurses/future-nurse-proficiencies.pdf (accessed 9 April 2022).

Nursing and Midwifery Council (2018d) *Standards Framework for Nursing and Midwifery Education*. London: NMC. Available at: www.nmc.org.uk/globalassets/sitedocuments/standards-of-proficiency/standards-framework-for-nursing-and-midwifery-education/education-framework.pdf (accessed 3 April 2022).

Nursing and Midwifery Council (2018e) *Standards for Pre-Registration Nursing Programmes*. Available at: www.nmc.org.uk/globalassets/sitedocuments/standards-of-proficiency/standards-for-pre-registration-nursing-programmes/programme-standards-nursing.pdf (accessed 24 May 2022).

Nursing and Midwifery Council (2018f) *Standards of Proficiency for Nursing Associates*. www.nmc.org.uk/globalassets/sitedocuments/standards-of-proficiency/nursing-associates/nursing-associates-proficiency-standards.pdf (accessed 7 June 2022).

Nursing and Midwifery Council (2019a) *Standards of Proficiency for Midwives.* Available at: www.nmc.org.uk/globalassets/sitedocuments/standards/standards-of-proficiency-for-midwives.pdf (accessed 23 April 2022).

Nursing and Midwifery Council (2019b) *Assessment for Progression.* Available at: www.nmc.org.uk/supporting-information-on-standards-for-student-supervision-and-assessment/academic-assessment/what-do-academic-assessors-do/assessment-for-progression (accessed 3 April 2022).

Nursing and Midwifery Council (2021a) *Council approves continued use of recovery standards to increase flexible use of simulation.* Available at: www.nmc.org.uk/news/news-and-updates/council-approves-continued-use-of-recovery-standards-to-increase-flexible-use-of-simulation (accessed 3 May 2021).

Nursing and Midwifery Council (2021b) *Keep Records of all Evidence and Decisions.* Available at: www.nmc.org.uk/employer-resource/local-investigation/guiding-principles/record-evidence-decisions. Accessed Date: 23 June 2022.

Nursing and Midwifery Council (2021c) *What is Revalidation?* Available at: www.nmc.org.uk/revalidation/overview/what-is-revalidation (accessed 2 May 2022).

Nursing and Midwifery Council (2022a) *Research into Pre-Registration Programme Requirements.* Available at: www.nmc.org.uk/education/programme-of-change-for-education/research-preregistration-programme-requirements (accessed 3 May 2022).

Nursing and Midwifery Council (2022b) *Quality Assurance Handbook – MAY 2022.* Available at: www.nmc.org.uk/search/?q=Quality+Assurance+Handbook+%E2%80%93+MAY+2022 (accessed 28 June 2022).

Nursing and Midwifery Council (2022c) *Raising Concerns: Guidance for nurses, midwives and nursing associates.* Available at: www.nmc.org.uk/standards/guidance/raising-concerns-guidance-for-nurses-and-midwives (accessed 3 May 2022).

Nursing and Midwifery Council (2022d) *Standards of Proficiency for Specialist Community Public Health Nurses.* Available at: www.nmc.org.uk/standards/standards-for-post-registration/standards-of-proficiency-for-specialist-community-public-health-nurses2/ (accessed 15 December 2022).

Nygren, F. and Carlson, E. (2017) 'Preceptors' conceptions of a peer learning model: A phenomenographic study', *Nurse Education Today, 49*(Feb.): 12–16.

O'Driscoll, M.F., Allan, H.T. and Smith, P.A. (2010) 'Still looking for leadership: Who is responsible for student nurses' learning in practice?', *Nurse Education Today, 30*(3): 212–217.

Olofsson, A., Taube, K. and Ahl, A. (2015) 'Academic achievement of university students with dyslexia', *Dyslexia, 21*(4): 338–349.

Orton, H.D., Prowse, J. and Millen, C. (1993) *Charting the Way to Excellence* (Ward Learning Climate Project). Sheffield: Sheffield Hallam University.

Panda, S., Dash, M., John, J., Rath, K., Debata, A., Swain, D., Mohanty, K. and Eustace-Cook, J. (2021) 'Challenges faced by student nurses and midwives in clinical learning environment: A systematic review and meta-synthesis', *Nurse Education Today, 101*(July): 1–12.

Papastavrou, E., Dimitriadou, M., Tsangari, H. and Andreou, C. (2016) 'Nursing students' satisfaction of the clinical learning environment: A research study', *BMC Nursing*, 15(44): 1–10.

Peters, R.S. (1966) *Ethics and Education*. London: Allen & Unwin.

Peters, R.S. (1973) *The Philosophy of Education* (Oxford Readings in Philosophy). Oxford: Oxford University Press.

Peyton, J.W.R (ed.) (1998) *Teaching and Learning in Medical Practice*. Rickmansworth, Herts: Manticore Europe.

Phillips, B.N., Turnbull, B.J. and He, F.X. (2015) 'Assessing readiness for self-directed learning within a non-traditional nursing cohort', *Nurse Education Today*, 35(3): e1–e7.

Phillips, T., Schostak, J. and Tyler, J. (2000) *Practice and Assessment in Nursing and Midwifery: Doing it for real*. Available at: https://eric.ed.gov/?id=ED463398 (accessed 30 May 2022).

Piaget, J. (1962) 'The stages of intellectual development of the child', in I. Roth (ed.), *Introduction to Psychology*. Milton Keynes: Lawrence Erlbaum Associates (LEA)/Open University.

Pienaar, M., Orton, A.M. and Botma, Y. (2022) A supportive clinical learning environment for undergraduate students in health sciences: An integrative review. *Nurse Education Today*, 119(3):105572. DOI:10.1016/j.nedt.2022.105572

Polit, D.F. and Beck, C.T. (2021) *Essentials of Nursing Research: Appraising Evidence for Nursing Practice*, 10th edn. London: Lippincott, Williams and Wilkins.

Power, A. and Farmer, R. (2017) 'Pre-registration midwifery education: Do learning styles limit or liberate students?' *British Journal of Midwifery*, 25(2): 123–126.

Proctor, B. (2011) 'Training for the supervision alliance: Attitude, skills and intention', in J.R. Cutcliffe, K. Hyrkas and J. Fowler (eds), *Routledge Handbook of Clinical Supervision: Fundamental International Themes*. London: Routledge. Chapter 3.

Public Health England (PHE) (2021) *Newborn and Infant Physical Examination (NIPE) Screening Programme Handbook*. Available at: Newborn and infant physical examination (NIPE) screening programme handbook – GOV.UK (www.gov.uk) (accessed 17 May 2022).

Quality Assurance Agency for Higher Education (QAA) (2009) *Personal Development Planning: Guidance for institutional policy and practice in higher education*. Available at: www.qaa.ac.uk/docs/qaas/enhancement-and-development/pdp-guidance-for-institutional-policy-and-practice.pdf?sfvrsn=4145f581_8 (accessed 9 May 2022).

Quality Assurance Agency for Higher Education (2010) *Code of Practice for the Assurance of Academic Quality and Standards in Higher Education, Section 3: Disabled students*. Available at: https://nadp-uk.org/wp-content/uploads/2015/02/2010-Code-of-practice-for-academic-qual-standards.pdf (accessed 13 June 2022).

Quality Assurance Agency for Higher Education (2014) *Setting and Maintaining Academic Standards: The frameworks for higher education qualifications of UK degree-awarding bodies (UK Quality Code for Higher Education Part A)*. Available at: www.qaa.ac.uk/docs/qaa/quality-code/qualifications-frameworks.pdf (accessed 5 April 2022).

Quality Assurance Agency for Higher Education (2018) *Assessment (UK Quality Code for Higher Education: Advice and Guidance)*. Available at: www.qaa.ac.uk/quality-code/advice-and-guidance/assessment (accessed 15 April 2022).

Quality Maternal and Newborn Care (2022) *Framework for Maternal and Newborn Care*. Available at: www.qmnc.org/about-qmnc/framework-for-quality-maternal-and-newborn-care/. Accessed date: 12 November 2022.

Race, P. (2014) *Making Learning Happen: A Guide for Post-Compulsory Education*, 3rd edn. London: Sage Publications.

Ramsden, P. (2003) *Learning to Teach in Higher Education*, 2nd edn. London: RoutledgeFalmer.

Renfrew, M.J., McFadden, A., Bastos, M.H., Campbell, J., Channon, A.A., Cheung, N.F., Silva, D.R.A.D., Downe, S., Kennedy, H.P., Malata, A., McCormick, F., Wick, L. and Declercq, E. (2014) 'Midwifery and quality care: findings from a new evidence-informed framework for maternal and newborn care'. *The Lancet*, *384*(9948): 1129–1145.

Rogers, A. and Horrocks, H. (2010) *Teaching Adults*, 4th edn. Maidenhead: Open University Press/McGraw-Hill Education.

Rogers, C. (1983) *Freedom to Learn in the 80s*. Columbus, OH: Charles Merrill.

Rogers, C. and Freiberg, H.J. (1994) *Freedom to Learn*, 3rd edn. Upper Saddle River, NJ: Pearson Education.

Rossler, K.L. and Tucker, C. (2022) 'Simulation helps equip nursing students to care for patients with dementia', *Teaching and Learning in Nursing*, *17*(1): 49–54.

Rowntree, D. (1987) *Assessing Students: How Shall We Know Them?* London: Kogan Page.

Roxburgh, M., Conlon, M. and Banks, D. (2012) 'Evaluating hub-and-spoke models of practice learning in Scotland, UK: A multiple case study approach', *Nurse Education Today*, *32*(7): 782–789.

Royal College of Nursing (RCN) (2012) *Quality with Compassion: The future of nursing education* (Willis Commission Report). Available at: https://cdn.ps.emap.com/wp-content/uploads/sites/3/2012/11/Willis-Commission-report-2012.pdf (accessed 23 May 2022).

Royal College of Nursing (2016) *RCN Mentorship Project 2015: From today's support in practice to tomorrow's vision for excellence*. Available at: www.rcn.org.uk/professional-development/publications/pub-005455 (accessed 24 March 2021).

Royal College of Nursing (2017) *Helping Students Get the Best from their Practice Placements* (A Royal College of Nursing Toolkit), 3rd edn. Available at: www.richmondtraininghub.net/wp-content/uploads/2017/10/PUB-006035.pdf (accessed 23 May 2022).

Royal College of Nursing (2018) *Advanced Level Nursing Practice*. Available at: www.rcn.org.uk/Professional-Development/publications/pub-006896 (accessed 22 June 2022).

Royal College of Nursing (2021) *NMC Introduces New Recovery Standard Offering Simulated Learning to Students*. Available at: www.rcn.org.uk/news-and-events/news/uk-nmc-introduces-new-recovery-standard-offering-simulated-learning-to-students-covid-19-180221 (accessed 6 May 2022).

Royal College of Nursing (2022a) *Using a Coaching Model in Practice Supervision.* Available at: Using a Coaching Model in Practice Supervision | Practice-based learning | Royal College of Nursing (rcn.org.uk) (accessed 25 May 2022).

Royal College of Nursing (2022b) *Neurodiversity Guidance: For employers, managers, staff and students.* Available at: www.rcn.org.uk/Professional-Development/publications/neurodiversity-guidance-uk-pub-010-156 (accessed 16 June 2022).

Saher, A., Alib, A.M.J., Amani, D. and Najwan, F. (2022) 'Traditional versus authentic assessments in higher education', *Pegem Journal of Education and Instruction, 12*(1): 283–291.

Saltiel, D. (2017) 'Supervision: A contested space for learning decision making', *Qualitative Social Work, 16*(4): 533–549.

Sanders, C.E. (2018) *Lawrence Kohlberg's Stages of Moral Development Psychology.* Available at: www.academia.edu/39038945/Lawrence_Kohlbergs_stages_of_moral_development_PSYCHOLOGY_WRITTEN_BY (accessed 1 July 2022).

Sawyer, T., Eppich, W., Brett-Fleegler, M., Grant, V. and Cheng, A. (2016) 'More than one way to debrief: A critical review of healthcare simulation debriefing methods', *Simulation in Healthcare, 11*(3): 209–217.

Scammell, B. (1990) *Communication Skills.* Basingstoke: Macmillan.

Schein, E.H. (2017) *Organizational Culture and Leadership,* 5th edn. Hoboken, NJ: John Wiley & Sons.

Schon, D. (1995) *The Reflective Practitioner: How Professionals Think in Action.* Aldershot: Arena.

Scott, B., Rapson, T., Allibone, L., Hamilton, R., Mambanje, C.S. and Pisaneschi, L. (2017) 'Practice education facilitator roles and their value to NHS organisations', *British Journal of Nursing, 26*(4): 222–227.

Scullion, P.A. (2010) 'Models of disability: Their influence in nursing and potential role in challenging discrimination', *Journal of Advanced Nursing, 66*(3): 697–707.

Shivers, E., Hasson, F. and Slater, P. (2017) 'Pre-registration nursing students' quality of practice learning: Clinical learning environment inventory (actual) questionnaire', *Nurse Education Today, 55*(Aug.): 58–64.

Skills for Health (2022) *The Care Certificate Standards.* Available at: www.skillsforhealth.org.uk/wp-content/uploads/2020/11/Care-Certificate-Standards.pdf (accessed 12 April 2022).

Skinner, B.F. (1971) *Beyond Freedom and Dignity.* New York: Alfred Knopf.

Smith, R. and Rennie, D. (2014) 'Evidence based medicine: An oral history (Editorial)', *BMJ, 348*(7942): g371.

Society for Simulation in Healthcare (SSH) (2022) Healthcare Simulation Dictionary, 2nd edn – 2.1. Available at: www.ssih.org/dictionary (accessed 7 May 2022).

Stacey, G., McGarry, J., Aubeeluck, A., Bull, H., Simpson, C., Sheppard, F. and Thompson, S. (2014) 'An integrated educational model for graduate entry nursing curriculum design', *Nurse Education Today, 34*(1): 145–149.

Steinaker, N.W. and Bell, M.R. (1979) *The Experiential Learning: A New Approach to Teaching and Learning.* New York: Academic Press.

Stewart, K.R. and Hand, K.I. (2017) 'SBAR, communication, and patient safety: An integrated literature review', *MEDSURG Nursing, 26*(5): 297–305.

Stickley, T. (2011) 'From SOLER to SURETY for effective non-verbal communication', *Nurse Education in Practice, 11*(6): 395–398.

Strauss, S.E., Glasziou, P., Richardson, W.S. and Haynes, R.B. (2019) *Evidence-Based Medicine: How to Practice and Teach EBM*, 5th edn. Edinburgh: Elsevier.

Suliman, M. and Warshawski, S. (2022) 'Nursing students' satisfaction with clinical placements: The contribution of role modelling, epistemic authority, and resilience – a cross- sectional study', *Nurse Education Today, 115*: 1–6.

Tanner, K. (2014) 'Increasing objectivity in the assessment of interpersonal skills and attitude', *Journal of Paramedic Practice, 6*(11): 566–571.

Taylor, N., Wyres, M., Green, A., Hennessy-Priest, K., Phillips, C., Daymond, E., Love, R., Johnson, R. and Wright, J. (2021) 'Developing and piloting a simulated placement experience for students', *British Journal of Nursing, 30*(13): S19–S24.

Tee, S.R., Owens, K., Plowright, S., Ramnath, P., Rourke, S., James, C. and Bayliss, J. (2010) 'Being reasonable: Supporting disabled nursing students in practice', *Nurse Education in Practice, 10*(4): 216–221.

Thiroux, J. and Krasemann, K. (2014) *Ethics, Theory and Practice*, 11th edn. Harlow: Pearson Education.

Thomas, M. and Westwood, N. (2016) 'Student experience of hub and spoke model of placement allocation: An evaluative study', *Nurse Education Today, 46*(Nov.): 24–28.

Thorne, S. (2020) 'Rethinking Carper's personal knowing for 21st century nursing', *Nursing Philosophy, 21*(4): 1–7.

Tickle, N., Creedy, D.K., Carter, A.G. and Gamble, J. (2022) 'The use of eportfolios in pre-registration health professional clinical education: An integrative review', *Nurse Education Today, 117*(Oct.): 1–16.

Tremayne, P. and Hunt, L. (2019) 'Has anyone seen the student? Creating a welcoming practice environment for students', *British Journal of Nursing, 28*(6): 369–373.

Tweed, A., Graber, R. and Wang, M. (2010) 'Assessing trainee clinical psychologists' clinical competence', *Psychology Learning and Teaching, 9*(2): 50–60.

University of St Andrews (2022) *Learning Agreement*. Available at: www.st-andrews. ac.uk/students/study-abroad/academic/agreement (accessed 13 June 2022).

van Wijngaarden, J.D.H., Dirks, M., Dippel, D.W.J., Minkman, M. and Niessen, L.W. (2006) 'Towards effective and efficient care pathways: Thrombolysis in acute ischaemic stroke', *Qjm, 99*(4): 267–272.

VARK Learning Limited (2022) *The VARK Questionnaire (version 8.01)*. Available at: The VARK Questionnaire | VARK (vark-learn.com) (accessed 12 February 2022).

Velásquez, S.T., Ferguson, D., Lemke, K.C., Bland, L., Ajtai, R., Amezaga, B., Cleveland, J., Ford, L.A., Lopez, E., Richardson, W. and Saenz, D. (2022) Interprofessional communication in medical simulation: Findings from a scoping review and implications for academic medicine. *BMC Medical Education, 22*(1): 1–12.

Viney, R. and McKimm, J. (2010) Mentoring. *British Journal of Hospital Medicine, 71*(2): 106–109.

Wace, C. (2022) 'University payout over student's death', *The Times*, 21 May, p. 27.

Walia, S. and Marks-Maran, D. (2014) 'Leadership development through action learning sets: An evaluation study', *Nurse Education in Practice, 14*(6): 612–619.

Wang, Y., Literature, X., Liu, Y. and Shi, B. (2022) 'Mapping the research hotspots and theme trends of simulation in nursing education: A bibliometric analysis from 2005 to 2019', *Nurse Education Today*. https://doi.org/10.1016/j.nedt.2022.105426.

Warne, T., Johansson, U., Papastavrou, E., Tichelaar, E., Tomietto, M., Van den Bossche, K., Moreno, M.F.V. and Saarikoski, V.M. (2010) 'An exploration of the clinical learning experience of nursing students in nine European countries', *Nurse Education Today*, *30*(8): 809–815.

Waskett, C. (2010) 'Clinical supervision using the 4S model 1: Considering the structure and setting it up', *Nursing Times*, *106*(16): 12–14.

Watts, P.I., McDermott, D.S., Alinier, G., Charnetski, M., Ludlow, J., Horsley, E., Meakim, C. and Nawathe, P.A. (2021) 'Healthcare simulation standards of best practice™ simulation design', *Clinical Simulation in Nursing*, *58*: 14–21.

Way, S., Fisher, M. and Chenery-Morris, S. (2019) 'An evidence-based toolkit to support grading of pre-registration midwifery practice', *British Journal of Midwifery*, *27*(4): 251–257.

Webb, C. and Shakespeare, P. (2008) 'Judgements about mentoring relationships in nurse education', *Nurse Education Today*, *28*(5): 563–571.

Webber, E. (2017) *Building Successful Communities of Practice*. London: Blurb.

Welsh Assembly Government (2009) *Post Registration Career Framework for Nurses in Wales*. Available at: https://gov.wales/sites/default/files/publications/2019-03/post-registration-career-framework-for-nurses-in-wales.pdf (accessed 8 May 2022).

Wenger, E. (2000) *Communities of Practice: Learning, Meaning and Identity*. Cambridge: Cambridge University Press.

Wilkinson, J.E., Rushmer, R.K. and Davies, H.T.O. (2004) 'Clinical governance and the learning organization', *Journal of Nursing Management*, *12*(2): 105–113.

Williams, B., Perillo, S. and Brown, T. (2015) 'What are the factors of organisational culture in health care settings that act as barriers to the implementation of evidence-based practice? A scoping review', *Nurse Education Today*, *35*(2): e34–e41.

Williamson, G. (2009) 'Student support on placement: The student experience and staff perceptions of the implementation of placement development team', *The 2009 RCN International Nursing Research Conference: Book of Abstracts* (Section 9.1.3): 107.

Wong, B.S.H. and Shorey, S. (2022) 'Nursing students' experiences and perception of peer feedback: A qualitative systematic review', *Nurse Education Today*, *116*: 1–8.

Yang, K., Nisbet, G. and McAllister, L. (2017) 'Students' experiences and perceptions of inter-professional supervision on placement', *International Journal of Practice-based Learning in Health and Social Care*, *5*(2): 1–18.

Young, P., Moore, E., Griffiths, G., Raine, R., Stewart, R., Cownie, M. and Frutos-Perez, M. (2010) 'Help is just a text away: The use of short message service texting to provide an additional means of support for health care students during practice placements', *Nurse Education Today*, *30*(2): 118–123.

INDEX